Geriatric
Physical Diagnosis

Geriatric Physical Diagnosis

A Guide to Observation and Assessment

MARK E. WILLIAMS, M.D.

McFarland & Company, Inc., Publishers
Jefferson, North Carolina, and London

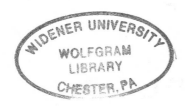

LIBRARY OF CONGRESS CATALOGUING-IN-PUBLICATION DATA

Williams, Mark E.
Geriatric physical diagnosis : a guide to observation and
assessment / Mark E. Williams.
p.   cm.
Includes bibliographical references and index.

ISBN-13: 978-0-7864-3009-3

library binding : 50# alkaline paper ∞

1. Geriatrics — Diagnosis.   2. Older people — Diseases — Diagnosis.
3. Physical diagnosis.   I. Title.
[DNLM: 1. Physical Examination — methods.   2. Aged.   WT 141 W725g 2008]
RC953.W55   2008
618.97'075 — dc22   2007017507

British Library cataloguing data are available

Manufactured in the United States of America

*McFarland & Company, Inc., Publishers
Box 611, Jefferson, North Carolina 28640
www.mcfarlandpub.com*

To my wife,
JANE CLARK WILLIAMS,
the most loving and perceptive person I know,

and to my sons,
JOHN and JAMES

Acknowledgments

"At times our own light goes out and is rekindled by a spark from another person. Each of us has cause to think with deep gratitude of those who have lighted the flame within us."

— **Albert Schweitzer**

"Piglet realized that while he had a very small heart, it could hold a considerable amount of gratitude."

— **A. A. Milne**

Although this book is attributed to a single author, it is really a gift from a number of individuals. My thanks to them is hardly adequate. Most of the material I have learned by interacting with elderly people, teaching physical diagnosis to medical students and medical residents, reading and rereading books and articles, regretting my own mistakes, and occasionally recognizing the mistakes of others. Because of this, I am deeply indebted to the authors, role models, students, residents and patients I have encountered over the past twenty-five years. Special mention must go to Dr. Joseph Sapira whose textbook *The Art and Science of Bedside Diagnosis* appeared in 1990. This book validated my commitment to physical diagnosis and taught me many valuable lessons. Its profound influence is reflected throughout this book.

I especially wish to acknowledge Nortin Hadler, M.D., my brilliant mentor and my first internal medicine attending physician when I was an inexperienced third-year clinical clerk. He introduced me to the depth of physical diagnosis and I am grateful for his enduring impressions, provocative insights, and eternal patience. It was a rare privilege for me to work with him at the patient's bedside through my early medical career and later as attending physicians on parallel inpatient services. Without his guidance my life course would have been profoundly different. A large portion of Chapter 2 is taken from an article in *The New England Journal of Medicine* we co-authored over 20 years ago.

I also thank T. Franklin Williams, M.D., my geriatric fellowship director and friend, who devoted time and attention to show me firsthand the ways of the skilled and experienced geriatrician. His values and insights

have had a considerable influence on my geriatric practice and my approach to elderly patients.

Doctors Sara Bass and Jason Higey deserve
special mention for their cheerful receptive-
ness to read and critique early versions of this
book's outline and for their help in suggesting possible charts and illustrations. A word
of special thanks goes to Doctors Phil Smith,
Serge Joffy, and Michael Gorjanc for their help
in researching the historical vignettes. I also
express my gratitude to Ole Daniel Enersen
of Whonamedit.com for his willingness to
share biographical material from his excellent

website. Inspiration for the illustrations came
from a variety of sources.

I owe a special debt of gratitude to Dr.
Ian Stevenson who read early versions of the
manuscript.

My former secretary, Ann Bossems, proof-
read the entire first draft and offered considerable technical assistance. Tina Jones also provided technical help.

Finally, this book would not be possible
without the encouragement and patience of
my wife, Jane, and sons, John and James. Their
love and support form the core of my personal
and professional life.

Table of Contents

Preface

The goal of this book is to assist the curious, motivated clinician in becoming a more perceptive observer of elderly patients and in improving his or her skills in geriatric bedside diagnostic examination. Achieving this goal will depend on the clarity of presentation in this book and on the learner's patience, self-discipline, and honesty in studying and practicing the appropriate skills. As a martial arts instructor once taught me, practice does not make perfect; only perfect practice makes perfect.

The physical examination is an essential part of the geriatric assessment. Exemplary technique coupled with a caring manner immediately reflects the clinician's competence to the patient and family members. This approach is especially satisfying when it promptly leads to a patient's relief of suffering and distress. And it shows the maturity and grounding of the clinician. Information of significant diagnostic and therapeutic value flows between the patient and perceptive clinician during the conscientious physical examination.

Medical observation is an active, creative process, part of what we already do in the midst of our daily activities. It is highly portable and efficient and is useful in other areas of our personal growth and conscious evolution. For example, we can learn that precise observation requires our undivided attention. The greatest block to full observation is having things sink into a familiar context. Ultimately we may come to realize that virtually everything we do is based on habit. Work and concentrated effort are required to address habits, and the first step is to appreciate their power and impact on our clinical data gathering and our reactions to events. Our habits are subtle, and recognizing them can be a challenge, but without our appreciation of their presence overcoming them is impossible. With effort, over time we can slowly develop the capacity to anticipate our habitual action and open up the possibility of conscious action. We must be alert to our habits and be able to change our state of consciousness from our normal waking state to a state of high concentration when the task requires it.

The intention of medical observation is to appreciate the truth in the light of the moment, the reality behind the appearance. Medical observation allows us to appreciate the connections between a patient's appearance, dress, language, and behaviors. These connections reflect a person's unified sense of self with specific clues of occupations, illnesses, and past events. In addition, these observations allow us to determine a person's state of mental function by examining the congruity of this self-revelation. Medical observations also facilitate explanation and verification by providing the substantiating evidence that underlies a clinical impression. These observations can provide a basis of clinical taxonomy for various states such as dementing illness. Chapter 3 will cover an approach to observations of appearance, dress, language, and behaviors. How they can be used to help determine a person's mental function is the subject of Chapter 22.

Do we really need another textbook of physical diagnosis? Surprisingly, no other textbook concentrates on geriatric physical examination. Physical diagnosis skills, a core aspect of geriatric care, are declining, perhaps on the mistaken notion that advanced technology can replace skillful bedside diagnostic examination. Increasingly, answers to clinical questions are given in clinical laboratory and imaging terms rather than in physical findings. Recently I asked an attentive medical resident about one of my patients who had an exacerbation of congestive heart failure. In response,

the resident offered me the serum level of brain naturetic peptide, the degree of pulmonary congestion on chest x-ray and the ejection fraction on cardiac echo. The resident did not feel the need to examine the patient for an S3 gallop, distended neck veins, pulmonary rales, an enlarged liver and pedal edema.

Every day, numerous elderly people undergo technological procedures for human predicaments that could have been identified by a careful history and thoughtful physical examination — more rapidly and efficiently and at less expense and inconvenience. In addition, health workers often care for elderly people in settings such as the home, assisted living facility, or nursing home that are distant from diagnostic technology. While the core of the book is physical diagnosis in elderly people, the skills herein can be applied to younger individuals.

The text also includes historical vignettes and anecdotes of great physical diagnosticians to stimulate interest in the evolution of clinical skills and to challenge learners to add to the growing chrestomathy of helpful techniques. These historical diversions also recreate the ambiance of bedside teaching rounds where the excitement of unexpected findings and circumstances typify the learning environment. Moreover, the vignettes acknowledge the great debt we owe to the giants on whose shoulders we stand. This debt should give us gratitude for the past, a sense of service for the present, and an understanding of our responsibility for the future.

There is a fundamental tension between geographic-and-organ-system teaching approaches. This book is organized geographically, generally following the order of the basic exam. In addition, there is a problem-based section within each chapter that shows approaches to specific regional complaints.

This book is not meant to be an exhaustive, evidence-based review of bedside clinical medicine. Diagnostic utility and useful observations have been favored over interesting but useless minutiae. The approach is unapologetically personal and shows one individual's way to systematically examine an elderly person. This approach is what I use in my daily clinical practice. I do not perform all elements of the examination on each patient. For example, the Rinne and Weber hearing evaluations are not always a part of my basic examination. However, they have a place in my clinical repertoire, and they can be constructive in the appropriate clinical setting.

Useful observations and techniques refined through over thirty years of active, hands-on, clinical practice form the basis of the work. I have been privileged to teach physical diagnosis at the bedside for over twenty-five years at the University of Rochester, the University of North Carolina, and the University of Virginia. My style of writing reflects a perceptual approach to education that attempts to communicate the nature of the experience of performing the examination, rather than to simply list the repertoire. This approach is challenging because it is difficult to communicate the nature of the psychology of the examiner and the *conscious experience* of performing the examination.

I agree with Alice in the epigraph that illustrations embellish a text. Drawings are generally superior to photographs and sometimes even to videos, since they can often show what cannot be seen otherwise. There is a reason that this ancient form of visual aid to education has stood the test of time. Financial constraints did not allow me the luxury of working with a professional medical illustrator, so my own line drawings, inspired by a number of sources, complement the text. My hope is that my lack of artistic ability will be overlooked in favor of the illustrations' utility in communicating key concepts.

Clinicians are already seeing increasing numbers of elderly people, and the demographic changes in our society grow more compelling with each census. The leading edge of the baby boom generation is just turning 65, and the number of elderly people will have doubled from 35 million in 2000 to over 70 million in 2030. With exacerbating factors of a birth dearth and increased life spans, many social observers predict that concern for elderly people will skyrocket in less than a decade. Clinicians must be well prepared for this demographic imperative. The need for exemplary geriatric physical diagnosis skills can only increase, and each of us will benefit if this need is fulfilled.

A Personal Note

If I were to pick up a book on the more subtle aspects of the geriatric physical examination written by someone in his mid-fifties I would want to know something about the credentials and qualifications of that author.

I grew up in the rural South and never considered old people any different from anyone else. My hometown community was one where people spoke to each other on the street, took long walks after supper, and knew each other's joys and sorrows.

From early childhood I was intrigued with perceptive puzzles (such as finding the hidden objects in a picture; finding 10 differences between pictures A and B; identifying which 2 of the 8 butterflies are exactly alike, and so on)—usually in my favorite childhood "journal," *Highlights for Children*.

In elementary school I learned about magic tricks and developed an interest in magical performance. In its essence, magic teaches the psychology of deception for purposes of entertainment. An unintended consequence was that I learned to appreciate the critical distinction between appearance and reality. In junior high school I discovered Sir Arthur Conan Doyle and omnivorously read the entire canon of Sherlock Holmes stories, attracted by the interplay between meticulous observations and sophisticated reasoning.

My family was not affluent, but fortunately I was able to attend college on a full scholarship. In medical school my attention was drawn to physical diagnosis, and I read several classic textbooks as well as numerous original descriptions of physical signs and conditions. My very first internal medicine ward attending as a fresh third-year student was Dr. Nortin Hadler, an absolutely stellar diagnostician and one of the most intelligent persons I know. His brilliant role modeling at the bedside showed me what was possible and formed the core of my bedside diagnostic skills. I am still striving to approach his level of clinical acumen.

As a clinical clerk I began to feel uneasy. I felt that something was not quite right. Major scientific advances were elegant and held great promise to relieve suffering, but the application of this knowledge was often ineffective. I also saw far too many instances where old people were not being treated like people.

When I was an internal medicine resident in the mid 1970s, leading medical journals were publishing articles on the "geriatric imperative," and Robert Butler had won a Pulitzer Prize for his book *Why Survive? Being Old in America*. I completed my residency and was chosen to be a Robert Wood Johnson Clinical Scholar. This two-year program confirmed and strengthened my sense of social responsibility to the aging. In the late 1970s, with the full support of my wife, I decided on geriatric medicine as a career and became one of the first group of physicians to receive formal fellowship training in the area. The problem was how to pursue instruction in this relatively new discipline. Fellowship programs were limited and none had a convincing track record. I set two strict criteria to guide my search: the program must have a director with substantial hands-on experience in caring for elderly people, and there must be a large facility to serve as a training site. In retrospect, the decision was easier than it seemed at the time, and in 1980 my wife and I moved to Rochester, New York, for me to work with Dr. T. Franklin Williams at the Monroe Community Hospital. There I spent almost five years immersed in learning the essential features of effective care to older people.

In the mid–1980s I was offered the best job in the country: developing geriatric programs and activities at my alma mater, the University of North Carolina. Another extraordinary stroke of good fortune placed my new office adjacent to Dr. Mack Lipkin, Sr., one of the giants of clinical medicine in the 20th century, who had retired to North Carolina to continue his teaching and writing. We established a close friendship, sharing clinical pearls, numerous conversations, and tuna fish sandwiches. I was stunned when one day Dr. Lipkin asked me to be his personal physician. Our relationship deepened and I was honored to share the most personal insights and perceptions of a wise, sensible, and articulate physician. I felt the aging process from the inside out, witnessing it in Dr. Lipkin, my other geriatric patients, and myself.

Again, however, I have begun to sense that things are not quite right. I have seen the technical (impersonal) aspects of medicine advancing at a rate unparalleled in human history. Meanwhile, the closer interpersonal qualities of the doctor-patient relationship have not seemed to keep pace. Of course, there are many reasons for this, and this book is not an attempt to rectify the current situation. Nonetheless, the quality of that relationship may be improved if clinicians have a more complete knowledge of the geriatric physical examination. And so I have focused my attention on providing useful information on geriatric physical diagnosis to clinicians. This interest — and a little goading by students and residents requesting additional clinical education — eventually led to the book you now hold.

Three strict principles guide my writing:

1. The emphasis is on clinical observation and connecting the observations into a useful, practical, perceptive framework.

2. The writing style should convey my conviction that elderly people should receive the best possible care.

3. The inner state of the clinician should be shared to help show the conscious evolution, that purification of experience, which parallels the acquisition of new clinical and perceptive skills.

Because I am primarily a clinician, most of the material comes from my own reading, clinical experience and personal philosophy. However, I claim no originality for the material, as my experience is the product of a vast variety of sources: instructors and mentors, current and past textbooks, journal articles and periodicals, discussions with students and colleagues, and interactions with my patients and their families. It will not surprise me if my opinions are not uniformly shared by others. After all, there are many ways to accomplish our objectives and professionals should be expected to disagree. But the more complete our understanding of geriatric physical diagnosis, the better prepared we will be to work with our elderly patients to develop an effective plan of care. Ultimately we will all be the beneficiaries of the health care system of the future and so we will get the healthcare in our old age that we plan for and deserve. Who amongst us does not deserve the very best?

CHAPTER 1

General Principles

"Begin at the beginning and go on till you come to the end; then stop."
— **Lewis Carroll**

"The most essential part of a student's instruction is obtained ... not in the lecture-room, but at the bedside. Nothing seen there is lost; the rhythms of disease are learned by frequent repetition; its unforeseen occurrences stamp themselves indelibly in the memory."

— **Oliver Wendell Holmes, M.D.**

"Mediocrity knows nothing higher than itself, but talent instantly recognizes genius."
— **Sir Arthur Conan Doyle**

The fact that you are reading this says a lot about your interest and commitment to improve your care of elderly people. It is important that you commit yourself to excellence. Mediocrity has no place in the care of older adults. If you have not already done so, you will need to develop the self-discipline, patience and restraint necessary to maintain focus and avoid distractions.

EXAMINER PSYCHOLOGY

The psychology of the examiner is the first consideration. Careful clinicians must be able to focus their attention and awareness. Their inner state is one of complete attention to the patient's concerns and appreciation of the special quality of the present moment. The examiner's overall intention is to help, to be of assistance to a person explicitly asking for relief of distress and implicitly seeking guidance or support. In addition, the technique of the clinician reflects the grounding and maturity of the examiner. You must be totally focused on the patient with no thoughts or inner dialogue on any other matter. You are giving the other person your most priceless possession: your undivided attention.

PERCEPTIVE CAPACITY

The second consideration is to work hard to increase your perceptive capacity. This is not as easy as it sounds. There are three types of knowledge: general, specialized, and perceptive. General knowledge is what is in the textbook or encyclopedia. Take basketball as an example. If we look up "basketball" in an encyclopedia we get a particular type of information: the history of the game, number of players on a team, basic rules, referees' signals and a listing of past championship teams. Specialized knowledge is what an informed fan would know: which teams had a good recruiting year, which team plays well against a particular opponent, whose star player has a nagging injury. This body of knowledge is not found in the encyclopedia. The third type of knowledge is perceptive knowledge: what is it like to be out on the basketball court with the ball in a game situation? This framework helps us appreciate that most healthcare education is either general or specialized knowledge: lists, tables, flow charts, algorithms, decision trees or clinical pathways. While this important information has its place in clinical care, very little time is spent teaching what it is like *to do*.

Perceptive knowledge is challenging to share. Consider the following example. My favorite childhood magazine, *Highlights for Children*, always had a page filled with hidden pictures. Underneath the drawing there were items to find: ball, spoon, scissors, etc. The perceptive educational challenge is this: How would you teach someone how to become expert at finding the hidden pictures? Just pointing them out would initially help a beginning learner but at some stage the person would say, "Yes, I see it now that you point it out, but how did you do it?" Think about how you would approach this educational challenge (assuming for a moment you are a skillful hidden-picture finder).

One difficulty in sharing perceptive knowledge is that we have a limited perceptive vocabulary. It is cumbersome to communicate perceptive insights without a descriptive vocabulary. Another factor limiting the sharing of perceptive knowledge is that there are few role models with the requisite experience who also are willing and able to communicate their techniques. To do so also requires a willingness to expose one's vulnerabilities to others. While this lack of suitable instructors is unfortunate, a greater problem is that there are even fewer committed students. Some students seem to crave excitement, stimulation or entertainment, rather than gaining additional perceptive knowledge. They do not seem to be willing to invest the required effort in learning and refining advanced techniques of physical diagnosis. Many times I have heard, "Those clinical signs are wonderful. Is there a quick reference I can have that summarizes them?" It is the exceptional student who asks, "What skills do I need to learn in order to be able to do that?" Your interest in this book suggests that you are the latter type of student.

REVERENCE FOR THE PATIENT

Francis Ward Peabody said in a classic 1927 monograph in *JAMA* (*The Journal of the American Medical Association*) that the art of caring for the patient is to care for the patient. He also wrote, "The treatment of a disease may be entirely impersonal; the care of a patient must be completely personal." This succinct advice epitomizes the need for the craftsmanship of caring.

My sons used to collect sports cards. While I cannot tell the valuable cards from the common cards, I can sort them fairly accurately by watching how my sons handle them. The rare rookie card of a star athlete is handled with a sense of reverence. In fact, we can observe how people handle objects they perceive to be valuable by how they manipulate them. There is a precious delicacy of the touch, with attention to each nuance in movement. The pottery bowl or rare book commands total concentration with an obvious appreciation for the material or artistic value. In the same way it is easy to identify the caring student (or clinical practitioner) by how he or she takes the patient's hand to begin the physical examination. Again, there is a sense of conscious appreciation, respect and reverence.

A HEALING ATMOSPHERE

Conscientious information gathering requires awareness of the premise and dynamics of the clinical encounter and structuring the environment to facilitate communication. The attitudes of physicians and other healthcare personnel strongly influence the quality of information available from the history. The premise of the clinical relationship is the expectation of reducing morbidity and improving function and quality of life by whatever means possible. The premise, not to eliminate the cause of the distress (which may be impossible in many circumstances) but to relieve the distress itself, is important to emphasize because the presence of disease and the development of symptoms are not always closely related (see Chapter 2). This key insight leads to palliative care and frees healthcare providers from the frustration, anxiety, and sense of vulnerability that results from cure-oriented expectations.

Attention to a few specific environmental considerations can improve communication with an older person and put them at ease. Because some older people have visual impairments, techniques to improve nonverbal cues are useful. For example, to improve visual information physicians should avoid having a

Goal	Possible Strategies
Put the person at ease	• Introduce yourself and shake hands
	• Sit reasonably close
	• Smile
	• Maintain comfortable eye contact
	• Give the person your undivided attention
	• Ask about the person's level of comfort
Overcome potential sensory impairments	• Sit at eye level directly facing the person to allow lip reading
	• Do not sit with your back to a window or bright light source since this puts your face in silhouette
	• Speak slowly and clearly without over-articulation
	• Do not shout
	• Use an amplifier or stethoscope if patient has significant hearing difficulty
Reduce distractions	• Do not take excessive notes or continually type on a laptop computer
	• Decrease ambient noise
	• Minimize interruptions
	• Keep the room temperature appropriate
	• Use comfortable furniture

Table 1.1. Ways to improve communication during the interview

strong light behind them (such as a window) because it puts the face in silhouette. Another useful technique is to reduce the distance between participants. As a rule of thumb, the optimal distance is that at which the interviewer begins to feel uncomfortably close. For individuals with hearing impairment, the volume of the voice must be raised without raising the pitch or by lowering the pitch. Shouting, which raises the pitch, defeats the purpose because high-frequency sounds are characteristically affected more profoundly than lower-frequency sounds in the aging ear. Shouting can also produce significant discomfort because the failing ear may become more sensitive to loud sounds through the process of acoustic recruitment. If no hearing amplifier is available, sometimes you can place a stethoscope in the patient's ears and talk slowly and clearly into the bell to improve communication.

Adjusting environmental conditions can improve communication with an older person. Office equipment should be practical and comfortable. Plush furniture may be stylish and handsome, but dysfunctional for persons with arthritic conditions. Older persons often prefer a simple straight-backed chair with armrests (for assistance in standing). Another important way to improve communication is to sit. The importance of sitting is inversely proportional to the time available for the encounter: the less time available, the greater the importance of sitting. Besides providing a

common level for eye contact, sitting helps to neutralize the appearance of impatience and haste. The appearance of impatience inhibits communication by magnifying a hierarchical relationship (physician over patient), rather than establishing a partnership to solve problems. The professional may nonverbally communicate that he or she is more interested in the problem or disease than in the person who is experiencing the distress.

RECOGNIZE UNIQUENESS

As we age, we become more unique and differentiated and less like one another. There is more biologic variability among octogenarians than neonates. Anyone who has attended a high school or college reunion can attest to the fact that some individuals age very slowly over a ten-year period while others seem to have aged several decades. Because of this increasing biologic variability with aging, our approach must be individualized. A "one size fits all" strategy will not fit an older person. Algorithmic approaches, decision trees, clinical pathways, and management guidelines are likely to be less than optimal if uncritically applied to elderly people. Tailoring our approach involves appreciating the older person as a person.

CHAPTER 2

The Approach to the Elderly Patient

"He who loves practice without theory is like the sailor who boards ship without a rudder and compass and never knows where he may cast."

— **Leonardo da Vinci**

"You ought not attempt to cure the eyes without the head, or the head without the body, so neither ought you to attempt to cure the body without the soul; and this is the reason why the cure of many diseases is unknown to the physicians of Hellas, because they disregard the whole which ought to be studied also; for the part can never be well unless the whole is well."

— **Plato**

The approach to the elderly person requires a perspective different from that needed for medical evaluation of younger persons. The spectrum of symptoms is different; the manifestations of distress are more subtle; and the implications for maintaining independence are more compelling. Improvement is sometimes less dramatic and slower to appear. Diagnosis is often different in older patients compared to younger ones. Chronic illnesses are more common and the presentation of disease is frequently nonspecific in elderly people. The most common presenting complaints are mental status changes, behavioral changes, pain, urinary incontinence, gait disturbance or a fall, and weight loss. As a result of this nonspecific presentation, symptoms are difficult to interpret.

The value of most medical interventions in old age can be measured by their influence on independence. An older person's ability to manage daily activities cannot be determined confidently from the length of the problem list. The crucial issue is the elderly person's ability to function, because the discomfort and disability produced by even incurable conditions generally can be modified. A conventional disease-specific perspective may not lend itself to developing strategies that best serve the older patient. The benefits of rehabilitation need to be emphasized in developing an effective, comprehensive plan of care for functionally impaired older persons.

PERCEPTIONS OF AGING

The striking increase in average life expectancy during the twentieth century rates as one of the major events of our time. We are in the midst of a social revolution, not in new ideology, but in our changing population patterns. For the first time in human history, infants in fortunate nations like ours can expect to live well into their seventies and beyond. This demographic revolution increases pressure on resources, as it also creates further social change and new opportunities for older persons. Such rapid changes have left most of us living in the past with our generally negative attitudes about aging and elderly people. Most of us still view old people as physically decrepit or in rapid, inevitable decline. Mentally, they are viewed as forgetful or childish, with little ability to learn and adapt; socially and economically, they are often considered a burden. The same outmoded beliefs are embedded in many of our healthcare and social programs. With such stereotypes, where is the expectation and encouragement for their continuing capacity to enrich their own lives and to enrich society?

These deep-seated cultural stereotypes do not accurately describe the new wave of elderly persons or their potential contributions to society. Today's aging individuals are typically far from decrepit. Fewer than 25 percent experience any significant disability and fewer than 5 percent are in nursing homes. Intellectually they thrive when given new opportunities to learn and grow. Given suitable occupation, they work with zest and competence well beyond the traditional age of retirement. Many have an emotional maturity and the kind of wisdom that comes only with age. In short, chronological age has virtually lost its meaning as a useful index of individual capacity.

To be sure, many old people have special needs for health care and other supports. But these cannot be provided knowledgeably without abandoning the old stereotypes, creating a broader public understanding of today's elderly population and its potential relationship to the rest of society. Such understanding will bring recognition of the many ways our later years can be more a culmination of life than prelude to death.

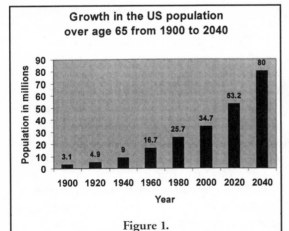

Figure 1.

Growth in the U.S. population over age 65 from 1900 to 2040. Source: U.S. Census Bureau using median series estimates for projections from 2020–2040.

DIFFERENCES BETWEEN AGES

What is aging? Aging is a nearly ubiquitous biologic process characterized by progressive, predictable, inevitable evolution and maturation until death. Aging is not the accumulation of disease, although aging and disease are related in subtle and complex ways. A fundamental principle is that biologic and chronological age are not the same. Different individuals age at different rates and within our bodies aging occurs in different organ systems at different rates influenced primarily by our socioeconomic status and our lifestyle choices. For example, smoking cigarettes seems to accelerate the aging in the pulmonary and cardiovascular systems.

Normal aging in the absence of disease is a remarkably benign process. In physiological terms, normal aging involves the steady erosion of organ system reserves and homeostatic controls. This erosion is evident only during periods of maximal exertion or stress. Mark Twain reportedly said there is no difference between an old man and a young man, as long as they are both sitting. The limits of homeostatic maintenance eventually reach a critical point (usually in advanced age), such that relatively minimal insults cannot be overcome, resulting in the person's death over a relatively short time. Consequently, any morbidity apparent to the person is compressed into the last period of life. Deviations from this ideal represent the effects of superimposed disease.

Aging also causes important changes in body composition and in the structural elements of tissues. Between the ages of 25 and 75, the lipid compartment expands from 14 to 30 percent of the total body weight, while total body water (mainly extracellular water) and lean muscle mass decline. This change in body composition has important implications for nutritional planning, metabolic activity and the use of drugs by older persons. For example, the lipid soluble drugs such as diazepam remain in the bodies of older persons for a much longer time than they remain in younger persons. Aging changes have also been documented in connective tissue and the isomeric forms of structural proteins.

PRESENTATION OF ILLNESS

Three factors influence the presentation of disease in an older person: the underreporting of illness, changes in the patterns of illness, and altered responses to illness. A common myth is that older persons are hypochondriacal and frequently burden the healthcare system with trivial complaints. In fact, older people may underreport significant symptoms of illness. The reasons for underutilization of healthcare services by older persons may result from personal attitudes and social isolation. One prevalent attitude is ageism: the belief that old age is inextricably linked with disability and morbidity. In other words, all old people are the same and they are falling apart. This belief reduces the demand for health care, since the manifestations of disease may be dismissed as age-related changes, leading people to say, "What do you expect at my age?"

A second factor contributing to the underreporting of illness by older persons is the perception of an unresponsive system of care. This apparent unresponsiveness may take several forms, such as inconvenient office locations, inadequate parking facilities, abbreviated encounters with physicians, and apparently uninterested or discourteous health personnel. Depression is another factor limiting the desire in some older persons for interaction with the healthcare system. This condition reduces the desire for improvement — "What do I have to gain?" Depression is a significant geriatric illness because it is both prevalent and treatable. Denial, another reason suggested for the underreporting of illness by older persons, may result from fear of economic, social, or functional consequences. Economic fears may be justified because of the high cost of clinical encounters, especially to persons who saved their resources without planning for unstable economic trends. A final relevant psychological factor is the isolation often experienced by many older persons through the loss of a spouse, migration of children and death of friends. Isolation reduces opportunities for receiving reactions to personal appearance, state of health, ideas, or attitudes.

The second factor influencing the presentation of illness in some older persons is an altered pattern or distribution of illness. Some conditions such as hip fracture, Parkinson's disease, or polymyalgia rheumatica are relatively restricted to later life. In addition, some diseases become more prevalent with advanced age. Examples of conditions with an increased prevalence in older persons include vascular disorders, cardiopulmonary disease, malignancy, malnutrition, myxedema, neurodegenerative disorders, and tuberculosis. Because of these altered patterns of illness, the physician must understand the epidemiological implications to interpret various signs and symptoms. For example, jaundice, a sign often suggesting viral hepatitis in young people, usually results from gallbladder disease or malignancy in an older person. Another example is psychotic symptoms such as delusions or hallucinations which suggest possible schizophrenia or bipolar illness in young people and dementia or medication side effects in elderly people.

The accumulation of multiple chronic disorders is another special feature of illness presentation in older persons. Four of every five persons over age 65 have at least one chronic illness. Symptoms of one condition may either exacerbate or mask symptoms of another, frequently complicating clinical evaluation. For example, symptomatic arthritis may mask the expression of severe cardiovascular disease if a person, by limiting physical activity, does not stress the heart.

Altered response of older persons to illness is yet another dimension of geriatric health behaviors. A person's perception of illness may be modified by attitudinal factors, social factors, and changes in the sensory organs. Manifestations of clinically important disease may be attenuated in older persons, particularly those who are frail and disabled. For example, angina pectoris may be absent or less dramatic in older persons (especially elderly women) with ischemic cardiac disease.

A final factor relevant to geriatric physical diagnosis is that symptoms in one organ system may reflect abnormalities in another. An acutely ill older person frequently presents with confusion, anorexia, involutary weight loss, urinary incontinence, unsteady gait (or the effects of a fall), or combinations of these and other symptoms. For example, an older person with a urinary tract infection may present with confusion and disorientation. As a result of this nonspecific presentation of illness, the effective clinician must exercise meticulous attention to expeditiously evaluate acute changes in an older person's health status.

THE CLINICIAN'S PERSPECTIVE

How critical is it for the physician to determine the precise nature of the underlying disease when helping an elderly person cope with illness? Certainly, the quest to define the disease causing a person's distress is important when the disease is reversible, remediable, or both. Almost by definition, this search is not a dominant issue in the management of many chronic conditions, such as heart failure or chronic arthritides. Nonetheless, the clinical algorithm that mandates the initial "ruling out" of the remediable disease permeates clinical teaching and practice. Since the seventeenth century, a first principle of medical practice has been the mandate to define the one disease that underlies a patient's distress. Treatment directed at this underlying disease represents the most direct and effective way to alleviate symptoms. Despite the overwhelming success of this disease-illness paradigm, its limitations cannot be disregarded: some features of illness (the manifestations or symptoms of distress) are independent of disease (the anatomic or physiological derangement). Many diseases do not necessarily produce illness or symptoms that lead to clinical presentation, and the quality of the illness may not be predictable from knowledge of the disease. For example, knowing the extent of disease in a patient with rheumatoid arthritis does not allow one to predict confidently that patient's capacity to work. The search for reversible disease, although important, is a secondary issue in the management of chronic illness and may even be detrimental if the physician-patient relationship is predicated on uncovering reversible disease.

Three arguments that favor precise determination of the underlying disease are particularly compelling: (1) identifying reversible or remediable disease is obviously rewarding, (2) clinical uncertainty is thereby reduced, and (3) accurate prognosis through an understanding of the condition's natural history should be useful. But do these arguments pertain to chronic illness in an elderly person?

The discovery of reversible disease in chronically ill elderly patients remains an important medical responsibility. However, this search for remediable disease should not be the focus of the clinical encounter. If it is the focus, what is the basis of the doctor-patient relationship when all reversible diseases have been excluded? Contrary to the situation in acute illness in which the expeditious discovery of remediable disease is an imperative, the search for reversible disease in chronically ill people can be pursued in a more leisurely manner. Most experienced physicians readily define and treat remediable conditions in their elderly patients. Often, iatrogenic problems (especially drug toxicities, unnecessary screening tests, and abuse of physical and chemical restraints) are the reversible processes identified.

A disease-specific focus, however, deemphasizes the dominant issue in the management of chronic illness, which is the maximization of the patient's productivity, creativity, well-being, and happiness. This goal of improving patient quality of life, function and satisfaction to the utmost is usually achieved without curing the underlying disease.

The need to reduce clinical uncertainty, to leave no stone unturned, is another rationale for defining disease in the setting of chronic illness. A common argument is that a patient may be spared unnecessary diagnostic procedures once the underlying condition is totally defined. The decision about how far to proceed with diagnostic evaluation is ultimately a joint contract between the patient and the physician. The benefit of a diagnostic procedure derives from the likelihood that it will yield meaningful information. In chronic illness in elderly people, information meaningful in the definition of disease is elusive. Diagnostic tests are an exercise reflecting more the need to allay clinicians' anxiety than to resolve clinical uncertainty, and they are often counterproductive. If it is justifiable to make illness the primary concern of both participants, many diagnostic tests become irrelevant.

The third argument for defining disease in chronically ill people is to allow accurate prognosis. Because prognosis generally involves estimating the remaining life span, its value is maximal in diseases that markedly influence longevity. For such diseases, prognostic estimates facilitate therapeutic decisions. For example, treatment regimens that are especially toxic or risky are usually reserved for circumstances in which longevity is immediately threatened. Small reductions in life expectancy are a less important concern in the management of chronic disease and become nearly irrelevant for many elderly people. Even for some less chronic problems, many patients seem to prefer improved quality of life to extended life span.

Another factor that limits the utility and accuracy of prognostic estimates in geriatric patients relates to the constancy of the human life span. If the age at which patients have their first infirmity continues to increase, then the overall period of infirmity must decrease, assuming that life span remains constant. In view of this compressed morbidity, delaying the onset of progression of chronic illness becomes as important as curing the underlying chronic disease. Furthermore, most of the disability experienced by elderly people results from diseases (such as atherosclerosis, diabetes

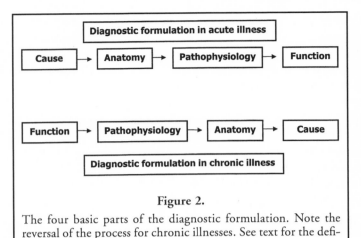

Figure 2.

The four basic parts of the diagnostic formulation. Note the reversal of the process for chronic illnesses. See text for the definition of the parts of the formulation.

mellitus, osteoarthritis, or chronic obstructive pulmonary disease) that represent exaggerations of normal age-related physiological decline, thus raising them above a clinical threshold. Because the problem is one of the rate, not the fact of decline, a "cure" would require defining the determinants of the threshold. For example, what specific factors determine the clinical threshold above which a physician should prescribe medications for elderly patients with glucose intolerance? Does the maintenance of a euglycemic state (or having a glycated hemoglobin in the normal range) with medications constitute a cure? Defining these threshold determinants and their relation to the quality of illness is a matter of some urgency. Otherwise, "prognosis" will continue to predict the number of chronic diseases at death — hardly an overriding patient concern. Even such a limited prognostic inference is confounded because elderly people manifest such wide biologic variability.

Understanding the difference between illness and disease is part of the treatment of elderly people, with function rather than disease as the focus. The effective physician appreciates that an increase in diagnostic capability does not substitute for care. And diagnostic efficiency does not necessarily improve the patient's quality of life or life expectancy. In fact, functioning can often be im-

proved without knowledge of what disease the patient has, but knowledge of the illness can provide the necessary information. For example, treatment of urinary incontinence due to detrusor instability focuses on reduction of bladder contractions, increasing of bladder capacity, and improvement of confidence and self-esteem (see Chapter 24). Treatment does not depend on knowing whether the bladder instability is due to brain trauma, cerebrovascular accidents, dementia caused by Alzheimer's disease, or any other irreversible process. Knowledge of the illness, rather than the underlying disease, allows the physician to help the patient to a greater degree. When the patient is treated in this way, both physician and patient avoid the disappointment and frustration of not being able to define or cure the primary disease that underlies the illness of urinary incontinence.

When a diagnosis does need to be made, it can usually be made more effectively in the elderly patient by reversing the usual order of the diagnostic thought process. In younger patients, there are four basic parts to the diagnostic formulation: The first is etiology, which may range from bacteria to poverty; the second is anatomy, i.e., what would be seen if the body were dissected today; the third is pathophysiology; and the fourth is the functioning of the patient. In elderly people, the key points remain the same, but the order of importance — the order in which these factors need to be considered — tends to be reversed. Functioning is the first step to consider.

THE IMPORTANCE OF FUNCTION

The ability to continue living independently is a critical issue for all elderly persons.

Loss of this ability is a serious illness which, in this country, often leads to institutionalization. In some instances, the loss of independence is a manifestation of overt organ-system dysfunction (such as severe heart failure), but that is the exception. Why should an elderly person with reasonably well-preserved visceral, mental, and musculoskeletal function be afflicted with the illness of loss of independence?

Manual dexterity, extensively validated in numerous studies, appears to be intimately and principally associated with the ability to live independently. Manual function is quantified by timing the performance of simple tasks (such as writing a sentence, opening a door, or stacking checkers). In one of my early research studies, the least sensitive of the manual tasks surpassed in sensitivity any other traditional measure studied, including a battery of standard assessments and findings on physical examination in predicting disability. The quantification of manual inefficiency in elderly patients provides important information for making clinical decisions that relate to the probability that the patient will lose independence. This reference holds in spite of the enormous differences in other characteristics seen in groups of elderly people.

An important implication of these observations is that measurements of illness, when they are properly quantitated, are superior to strictly disease-oriented indices in defining certain health needs. Because of the ubiquity of chronic disease and the lack of objective physiological markers of aging, most geriatric assessments use measurements of disability (or illness). Even in the studies just described, no difference in pathoanatomic state (disease) could be discerned in the functioning of the rheumatologic, neurological, ophthalmologic, or other organ systems. We do not know how to account for the difference in manual ability; yet, as a vital sign of functioning, the measurement reflects the risk of the loss of independence, and the impairment in hand function may even be responsible for this loss.

THE GERIATRIC ASSESSMENT

Geriatric assessment means getting to know the older person. The basic principles of the assessment are shown in Table 2.1.

The rest of this book is devoted to helping you improve your skills to perform this assessment in an effective manner.

In overview, the assessment process begins when the physician first sees the patient. The clinician's overall impression of the older person's health is an important aspect of the preliminary examination. The way a person walks into the room and sits down, the nature of the handshake, the manner of dress, the type of language, and the many other specific observations all combine to produce a general impression of the elderly person's health. Chapter 3 will address these initial impressions in detail. Important inferences regarding functional cardiovascular and respiratory

---

Table 2.1. Basic principles of clinical geriatric assessment

PRINCIPLE

- Pay attention
- Avoid causing discomfort or indignity
- Use meticulous observations and proper technique
- Search for signs of dysfunction, disease, and disability
- Evaluate physical, mental, and social functions and eliminate iatrogenic factors

capacity and basic nutritional status can be made from observations of exposed skin at the hands, arms, face, and head. Skin and nails often reveal signs of systemic disease, vitamin deficiency, and occupational trauma or hypertrophy. Recent loss of weight can be judged from clothing that is too large, especially at the collar and the waist.

While taking the history, the physician can make important observations regarding visual acuity, hearing, articulation, vocabulary, manner of delivery, and mental status. If carefully structured and attentively pursued, the interview can serve as the physical examination of the intellect. The physician uses the patient's language and behavior during the history taking to assess his or her degree of mental resiliency, flexibility, attentiveness, and general attitude. Any change from expected behavior or from previous patient behavior should be noted and usually prompt additional inquiry.

SUMMARY

The approach to the elderly person requires a perspective different from that needed for the medical evaluation of younger persons. The spectrum of complaints is different; the manifestations of distress are more subtle; the implications for function are more important; and improvements are sometimes less dramatic and slower to appear. The differential diagnosis of various problems is often different. Presentations are frequently nonspecific (mental status changes, behavioral changes, urinary incontinence, gait disturbance, or weight loss). The crucial issue is the elderly person's ability to function. Understanding the difference between illness and disease is a prerequisite to the care of patients affected by incurable disorders. Educated palliation in the absence of substantive information regarding this discrepancy is the art of medicine. Because elderly patients often present with several chronic diseases, many of which are irreversible, cure-oriented physicians are especially vulnerable to frequent disappointments. More important, even though many chronic conditions are incurable, the discomfort or disability they produce may be substantially modified. If this concept is not realized and addressed, elderly patients with irreversible chronic diseases may receive less than optimal care from physicians seeking cures. The degree to which we as physicians can assist chronically ill people reflects our understanding of human discomfort and our sensitivity to personal distress. If we maintain a purely disease-specific focus, we may have difficulty thinking about strategies to best serve our patient. Defining pathological entities may be less complicated than intervening in the illness of the patient, but the latter constitutes healing.

CHAPTER 3

Initial Impressions

"How can I be orderly with this? It's like counting the leaves in a garden, along with the song notes of partridges, and crows. Sometimes organization and computation become absurd."

— **Rumi**

"Let him, on meeting a fellow-mortal, learn at a glance to distinguish the history of the man, and the trade or profession to which he belongs.... [I]t sharpens the faculties of observation, and teaches one where to look and what to look for. By a man's fingernails, by his coat-sleeve, by his boots, by his trouser-knees, by the callosities of his forefinger and thumb, by his expression, by his shirt cuffs — by each of these things a man's calling is plainly revealed. That all united should fail to enlighten the competent inquirer in any case is almost inconceivable."

— **Sir Arthur Conan Doyle**

The physical examination of the elderly person begins at the moment the clinician sees the patient and continues until the clinical encounter is complete. My basic premise is that each of us makes a statement of who we are (or perhaps more accurately who we think we are) and that this self-revelation is reflected to others through the choices that we make in our appearance, dress, language, and behaviors. Human choices are not random, so appreciating the nature of this self-expression can be very useful. Each of us is cultivating a "look," and it is not a random event in the way we wear our hair, the fit of our clothing, what we choose to show off about our selves and those things we wish to hide. Normally this self-expression is congruent and in everyday life we subliminally make a value judgment about the person (pleasant, eccentric, attention-seeking, sincere, self-centered, etc.) and continue our personal or professional interaction. Incongruities in this self-presentation are important diagnostic clues and require further inquiry. The appreciation and identification of these incongruities is crucial to diagnosing dementing illnesses. In this regard, the clinical interview becomes the "physical examination of the intellect." This concept is expanded in Chapter 22. This chapter will review a basic framework of the fundamental observations within each of the categories of appearance, dress, language and behavior.

Table 3.1. Description of classic facies

Condition	Facial Findings	Other Visible Clues
Acromegaly	Jaw prominence; enlarged nose, lips, brow	Large hands with enveloping pillow-like feel to the handshake
Amyloidosis	Periorbital purpura (raccoon eyes) after abrupt increase in venous pressure such as a cough	Note: raccoon eyes also suggest basilar skull fracture
Cushing's Syndrome	Moon face where buccal fat pads obscure the ears from the front	Red cheeks, easy bruising
Depression	Worn, weary look; poor eye contact; forced smile	Stooped posture
Klippel-Feil Syndrome	Exaggerated forward head position	Congenital abnormality of cervical spine
Mitral Stenosis	Flushed cheeks, drawn look to face making the nose seem prominent	Atrial fibrillation, exertional dyspnea
Myotonic Dystrophy	Dull, sad eyes; bilateral ptosis atrophy of facial muscles; male pattern baldness	Sternocleidomastoid atrophy, difficulty releasing the handshake
Myxedema	Coarse features, coarse dry hair, periorbital edema, facial puffiness, loss of lateral eyebrows (Queen Anne's sign)	Large tongue; dirty appearing hyperkeratotic elbows
Nephrotic Syndrome	Periorbital puffiness, lassitude, dullness	Grayish sallow complexion in renal failure
Paget's Disease	Frontal bossing producing a large "Mr. Magoo" head	Possible hearing aids from deafness
Parkinson's Disease	Expressionless mask face; dull eyes; slow facial movements	Several days' beard on neck from inability to see it due to stooped posture
Polycythemia Rubra Vera	"Man in the moon face" with concave facial profile resembling a nutcracker	Ruddy complexion
Scleroderma	Small, tight mouth, small oral opening, minimal wrinkles with shiny skin; narrow pinched nose	Tightening of fingers with loss of transverse creases and finger pad
Seborrhea	Waxy flaking on eyebrows and nasolabial crease	Possible signs of Parkinsonism, HIV if appearance is abrupt
Smoker (Chronic)	Excessive facial wrinkles, hollow cheeks, thin vertical cracks along lips	Sunken yet bright-appearing eyes
Stroke	Facial asymmetry; facial droop with loss of nasolabial fold	Upper extremity hemiparesis

APPEARANCE

The initial appreciation of the patient derives from an impression of their body in overview as well as specific features of the individual's uniqueness. These identifying characteristics form the observational basis of our individuality and provide essential clues of the person's inner and outer states. The patient's gender is an obvious initial observation. A fundamental clinical question is whether the patient looks acutely ill, chronically ill or generally well. Does the apparent age (how old the patient looks) match the chronological age (how many birthdays the patient has celebrated)? Perhaps the apparent age reflects biologic age, overall health and well-being better than the chronological age. Some nonagenarians look decades younger than their years and their life expectancy seems to correlate with their apparent age rather than their chronological age. One caveat is that surgery or severe illness can appear to age them many years over days or weeks.

Body Size, Shape and Proportion

The observant clinician notes the patient's body size, shape and proportions. For example, is the patient overweight or are there signs of weight loss such as temporal wasting or, if more severe, loss of the buccal fat pad? Increases in abdominal fat may suggest increased risk of diabetes mellitus and premature vascular disease. Skin findings may be obvious over the face, arms, legs or other areas of exposed skin. Is there the pallor of anemia, the bronze tone of jaundice, the lemon yellow tint of pernicious anemia, the hyperpigmentation of Addison's disease, the ruddy complexion of hypertension or alcoholism, the ecchymosed arm of a recent fall or possible abuse?

Look carefully at the patient's overall habitus and posture. The hunched forward position of kyphosis may reflect previous anterior vertebral compression fractures from osteopenia. The presence of assistive devices such as wheelchairs, canes, or walkers provides obvious clues of ambulation difficulty. Musculoskeletal deformities such as amputations, the arthritic changes of rheumatoid arthritis, the unilateral contractures of cerebrovascular disease or the frontal bossing of Paget's disease may be immediately visible.

Specific Appearances

Some diseases create specific appearances that in some circumstances allow the likely diagnosis to be made on sight (see Table 3.1). Reviewing artwork of conditions such as Park-

Table 3.2. Common causes of delirium in elderly people	
Cause	*Examples*
• Drugs	Intoxication, medication adverse effect, substance abuse, poisoning, withdrawal
• Endocrine disorders	Thyroid, adrenal, pituitary, pancreas
• Low oxygen, low glucose	
• Infection (fever)	
• Renal failure	
• Infarction	Heart, brain, other organs
• Underlying acute illness	Malignancy, fracture, brain condition, gastrointestinal illness, pain
• Metabolic disorders	Electrolyte abnormalities, calcium abnormality

insonism, myxedema, depression, acromegaly, and chronic lung disease can refresh your memory and sharpen your skills. Do not be in a rush to make a spot diagnosis.

Adventitious Movements

Notice the presence of any adventitious movements. Restlessness is a worrisome sign in a bedfast or nursing home patient and suggests delirium until proven otherwise (see Table 3.2).

Virtually any medical condition is a potential cause of delirium but the common things to consider are drug toxicity, infection, metabolic disorder, or an acute cardiac, pulmonary, or neurological event. Alcohol or drug withdrawal is an underappreciated cause. Often individuals in withdrawal will have damp feet (see Table 3.3 for adventitious movements).

Type of Movement	Location	Nature of Movement	Clinical Name	Condition
Tremor (rhythmic oscillation)	Hands at rest (usually asymmetric)	Pill rolling of thumb and hand at rest	Resting tremor	Parkinsonism
	Hands	Fine, worse with anxiety	Physiological tremor	Anxiety, drugs, hyperthyroidism
	Hands (with movement)	Coarse, flapping, worse when approaching target	Intention tremor	Cerebellar disease
	Hands and head	Smooth and rapid	Essential tremor	Basal ganglia
Twitching (movement fragment)	Eye, face, shoulder, hand	Repetitive wink, shoulder shrug, throat clearing	Tic	Habit, behavioral disorders
Brief shake	Upper extremity	Brief, meaningless	Chorea	Basal ganglia, dopamine excess
Jerking (very fast)	Extremity	Sudden kick or arm flinch	Myoclonus	Broad differential but consider Creutzfeldt-Jakob Disease in rapidly progressive dementia
Writhing	Face, extremity	Slow, sinuous	Athetosis	Damage to corpus striatum
Flailing	One upper extremity	Violent and rapid	Hemiballismus	Subthalamic stroke
Chewing	Mouth and tongue	Repetitive, strange, peculiar	Tardive dyskinesia	Medication side effect

Table 3.3. Adventitious movements

In addition to restlessness, any stereo-typic limb movements, such as tremor, chorea, or athetosis, provide clues to the person's neu-rological or behavioral status. Rhythmic head bobbing from side to side suggests tricuspid insufficiency while forward and backward bob-bing (de Musset's sign) reflects a wide pulse pressure usually from aortic insufficiency. A wide pulse pressure can also cause a crossed leg to bob up and down with the pulse. An essential tremor can produce irregular head nodding. Occasionally elderly people with se-vere behavioral problems or psychiatric illness will quietly rock back and forth in their chair.

Self-Care and Makeup

A person's attention to self-care is a use-ful reflection of his or her physical, cognitive and affective state since personal maintenance is one of the first areas to be neglected if a sys-tem is stressed. The presence of makeup in an older woman generally implies well-being (or recent improvement if the patient has been ill). Care in the application reflects the extent of functionally adequate vision and upper ex-tremity motor coordination. Over-application may reflect vanity and a strong desire to look much younger. Heavy eyebrow coloration may be an attempt to hide eyebrow hair loss, per-haps due to hypothyroidism, SLE, or syphilis. The timing of the last hairdo provides a clue to when an older woman last felt reasonably well. Check the hair length to see how far hair has grown (approximately one-half inch every six weeks). Aggressive nutrient replacement in an undernourished person may accelerate hair growth. Perfume suggests well-being or use as camouflage. If the patient is wearing nail pol-ish, the distance from the cuticle to the line of polish gives the approximate date of applica-tion since nails grow about 0.1mm/day. Picked-at nail polish reflects nervousness and agitation. Toenail polish suggests unusual flex-ibility, a friendly helper, or perhaps pampered affluence.

DRESS (DIAGNOSTIC CLUES FROM CLOTHING)

Observing the older person's choice of clothing helps in appreciating their socioeco-nomic status, personality, culture, interests, and state of health. However, the interpreta-tion must be circumspect: the clothing may have come from a second-hand store. None-theless, the disciplined observer can identify when a person who is well off financially is trying to look less conspicuous by dressing down with the garments of a less economically advantaged elderly person. In addition, fash-ion speaks to certain self-awareness as to what "age" or style feels most comfortable to the in-dividual. Incongruities are especially reveal-ing and should be noted: an expensive but frayed suit could signify change in fortune.

Clothing Style and Fit

Pay attention to the style and fit of cloth-ing. Check the belt for the amount and rate of weight gain or loss. A rule of thumb is ap-proximately 15 pounds per belt loop. The thickest dark black mark reflects the usual belt placement and fainter marks suggest recent changes. Cerebral dominance can sometimes be inferred from the differential wear on the shirt cuffs with the more worn, shiny texture indi-cating the dominant side. (You could infer that I am in academic medicine from observing my shiny pants knees, since I am on them a lot.)

The person who shows up in the clinic wearing pajamas or a nightgown probably has a major chronic illness. If they also have a suit-case with them, they have been hospitalized in the past and are expecting to be hospitalized today. Bulges in shirt or pants pockets may give clues to personal mythology. (What specific items do you keep with you? What is the personal significance of each item?) While it is not usually practical or appropriate to ask, it is fascinating and quite revealing to observe what people choose to keep with them in their pockets, wallets or purses. One approach shared by Dr. Stefan Gravenstein is to ask to see the photograph on the person's driver's license. This allows an unobtrusive look at items in the wallet or purse including changes in physical appearance, the birth date, cards from organizations, amount of cash, clutter, wear and other flotsam and jetsam of daily life.

Clothing Material and Color

Notice the patient's choice of clothing material and color. What basic statement are they making? Are they drawing attention to themselves or trying to blend in? Is the clothing trendy, flashy, tasteful, conservative, or practical? What economic status does the clothing reflect? What is being hidden and what is being revealed? The person who is totally covered may have photosensitivity. Neck coverings such as a scarf or turtleneck could be hiding a thyroidectomy or tracheotomy scar. What does the person feel comfortable showing off about him or herself?

An elderly woman wearing a sweater on a hot summer day might have the cold intolerance of hypothyroidism, while the elderly man feeling comfortable wearing only a short-sleeve cotton shirt in the winter suggests an increased risk of accidental hypothermia. Fa-

Table 3.4. Urine colors

Urine Color	Possible Causes	Comments
Red	Hematuria, porphyria, Serratia marcescens, or ingestion of blackberries, aniline dyes (food coloring), beets (beeturia), phenytoin, phenolphthaleine	Beeturia is a sign of iron deficiency anemia. The red beet pigment is transported across the gut wall by the iron transport system and is filtered by the kidneys. The red urine disappears with iron replacement.
Brown	Hemaglobinuria, myoglobinuria, methemoglobinuria, bilirubin or ingestion of phenol, cresol, phenhydrazine, metronidazole, nitrofurantoin, phenothiazines	
Orange	Dehydration, urate crystals, or ingestion of rifampin, senna, pyridium, rhubarb, Vitamin B supplements	
Bright yellow	Bilirubin, or ingestion of Beta-carotene supplements, Vitamin B supplements, aniline dyes	
Blue or Green	Pseudomonas aeruginosa infection, or ingestion of asparagus, carotenoids, methylene blue, aniline dyes, urised, risanpin	
Black	Alkaptonuria, alphamethyldopa, or sorbitol ingestion	In alkaptonuria the urine turns black on standing; older patients will have slate gray ears

cial tissue tucked in a sleeve may reflect raw emotions or seasonal rhinitis. Uniforms provide immediate inferences to the person's occupation and its value to the individual. Hobbies or special interests, such as fishing flies or Masonic membership, may be reflected on a necktie or tie tack. The elderly man wearing his Phi Beta Kappa tie is trying to tell you something.

Fastidiousness and Clothing Stains

The degree of fastidiousness is also important since people pay less attention to self-care when they are ill. The collar of a well-worn shirt can provide evidence of skin dryness or oiliness, makeup, and general hygiene. A collar size over 17 reveals an increased risk of obstructive sleep apnea. Stains on clothing can be a clue to hobbies or occupation (paint, plaster), or poor hygiene (dirt, food, body fluids). The absence of sweat in the presence of fever suggests anhidrosis. A fishy odor to sweat can be a sign of schizophrenia, uremia, zinc oxide or excess fish oil supplementation. Sweat (or urine) that smells like violets raises the question of possible turpentine ingestion.

Burns on clothing can reflect impaired mental status, inattention or drug effect. A rosette of small round burns under the neck on the anterior chest (rosette sign) produced from cigarette ash falling onto the chest suggests a smoker with coexistent drug or alcohol abuse who nods off while smoking. Some occupations and hobbies requiring welding or soldering can increase the risk of burns on clothing.

Stains on Underwear

Stains on underclothing reflect general self-awareness of hygiene and state of health. Orange or red staining of undergarments suggests rifampin. (Could the person have tuberculosis?) The color of stool stains may be a clue to ingestion or illness, such as the light tan (acholic) color in liver disease. Darker than normal stool color suggests gastrointestinal bleeding (maroon, purplish black or tarry), or the ingestion of iron (greenish black), charcoal (coal black) or bismuth (dark gray black). Mineral oil ingestion produces an oily stain on undergarments because the anal sphincter cannot completely contain oil (although it can exquisitely differentiate and contain solid, liquid and gas). Urine stains come in a variety of colors, each with its own differential (see Table 3.4).

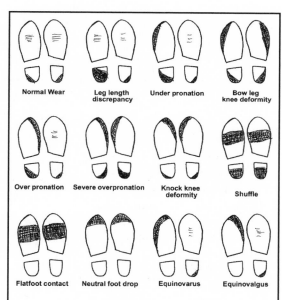

Figure 3. Patterns of Shoe Wear.

Normal walking produces slight wear on the outer portions of the heels. Leg length discrepancy causes excess heel wear on the longer limb. Underpronation of the foot increases the wear on the lateral sole and heel. The bowleg deformity tends to produce bilateral wear on the lateral aspect of the soles and heels. Overpronation causes wear on the medial sole, while severe overpronation affects both the sole and the heel. The knock-knee deformity tends to cause wear on the medial aspects of the soles, with relatively normal heel wear. Shuffling causes wear across the heel and sole, while flatfoot contact mainly affects the sole. Neutral foot drop (bilateral in this drawing) increases the wear to the toe. Equiovarus foot drop wears the lateral sole (but not the heel) because of underpronation. Equinovalgus foot drop produces excess wear to the medial portion of the toe of the sole.

Shoes

Shoes tell the story of their owner. Notice the coordination of shoes with the rest of the clothing. The type of shoe is informative, too. Are they casual, dressy, athletic, or made for work or walking? Are the shoes well cared for or is there a pattern of neglect? If the patient is only wearing one shoe or one shoe has an open toe, consider gout, trauma, arthritis, or bunions. Shoes with no laces or laces that are undone imply significant edema, inflamed feet, or limited dexterity. The patterns of shoe wear also provide important information. Excess wear on the toe relative to the heel suggests foot drop. Differential wear on one side is seen in hemiparesis, leg length discrepancy, and scoliosis.

Jewelry and Ornaments

Ornaments are interesting reflections of personality and interests. The amount and quality of jewelry reflects the taste and economic status of the owner. Rings can provide clues to education, age (estimate from class ring graduation year), clubs, organizations, and marital status (obviously not infallible). The absence of a ring heralded by a light-toned shiny band of skin at the base of the left ring finger may suggest depression or suicide risk. A tight-fitting ring implies edema while a loose,

Table 3.5. State assignment of the first three digits of Social Security Numbers

Number	State	Number	State	Number	State
001–003	New Hampshire	400–407	Kentucky	530	Nevada
004–007	Maine	408–415	Tennessee	531-539	Washington
008–009	Vermont	416–424	Alabama	540–544	Oregon
010–034	Massachusetts	425–428	Mississippi	545–573	California
035–039	Rhode Island	429–432	Arkansas	574	Alaska
040–049	Connecticut	433–439	Louisiana	575–576	Hawaii
050-134	New York	440–448	Oklahoma	577–579	Dist. of Columbia
135-158	New Jersey	449–467	Texas	580	Virgin Islands
159–211	Pennsylvania	468–477	Minnesota	581-584	Puerto Rico
212–220	Maryland	478–485	Iowa	585	New Mexico
221-222	Delaware	486–500	Missouri	586	Pacific Islands*
223–231	Virginia	501–502	North Dakota	587–588	Mississippi
232–236	West Virginia	503–504	South Dakota	589–595	Florida
237–246	North Carolina	505–508	Nebraska	596–599	Puerto Rico
247–251	South Carolina	509–515	Kansas	600–601	Arizona
252–260	Georgia	516–517	Montana	602–626	California
261-267	Florida	518–519	Idaho	627–645	Texas
268–302	Ohio	520	Wyoming	646–647	Utah
303–317	Indiana	521-524	Colorado	648–649	New Mexico
318–361	Illinois	525	New Mexico	700–728	Railroad workers
362–386	Michigan	526–527	Arizona		
387–399	Wisconsin	528–529	Utah		

*Guam, American Samoa, Philippine Islands, Northern Mariana Islands

Note: This table is no longer technically accurate as the Social Security Administration has added numbers for some states. However, when your elderly patient received his or her number, this was the formula.

wrapped ring reflects weight loss. A black stain under a gold-colored ring or necklace is a soft sign of diabetes mellitus. Tie tacks, necklaces, earrings, pins, medallions, and key chains may tell of hobbies, clubs, education, profession, and religious beliefs. A person wearing a copper bracelet has arthritis and believes in talisman. Some people wear their Social Security Number on their jewelry. The first digit of the Social Security Number tells the region of the U.S. from which the card was applied, while the first 3 digits tell the state (see Table 3.5).

LANGUAGE

Appearance and dress form the basis of our initial impressions of patients, and their general state of health. On this stage of static observations a dynamic communication occurs between the physician and patient. Language is a major part of this interaction.

The Rate and Delivery of Speech

The first part of the language assessment is called paralanguage, which deals with the rate and delivery of speech. In essence, para-language addresses the manner of speech. How do patients say what they say? The aphasia classification of fluency is based on paralanguage (see Table 3.6).

The strength of the person's voice is a useful marker of overall "vitality." This concept can be especially helpful in assessing a familiar patient over the telephone. Illness seems to compromise the patient's voice projection providing a clue to a change in their status. Paralanguage also addresses the speech rate, pitch, volume, degree of articulation, and quality of the delivery. For example, anxious individuals may speak at a rapid rate at a higher than normal pitch. New onset of soft speech may be a clue to Parkinsonism.

Another aspect of paralanguage concerns pauses and pause intervals. The pause interval is the time from the end of your utterance to the beginning of the person's response. Normally this interval varies based on the content. Strong, emotionally charged content tends to shorten the pause interval and subliminally we may think, "I struck a nerve." Unfamiliar content lengthens the interval. If you were asked, "Give me a one-sentence summary of the second law of thermodynamics," there might be a pause. But if the pauses are always short we might consider hyperthyroidism, autonomic

Table 3.6. Classification of the Primary Aphasia Syndromes				
Aphasia Type	*Fluency*	*Comprehension*	*Repetition*	*Comments*
Broca's	non-fluent	intact	impaired	Paresis of right arm
Transcortical motor	non-fluent	intact	intact	
Mixed transcortical	non-fluent	impaired	intact	
Global	non-fluent	impaired	impaired	
Anomic	fluent	intact	intact	
Conduction	fluent	intact	impaired	
Isolation	fluent	impaired	intact	Very rare
Wernicke's	fluent	impaired	impaired	Also right superior quadrantanopsia
Thalamic	fluent	variable	intact	Fluent dysarthria after mutism

overactivity or anxiety. Excessively long pause intervals might signify depression, Parkinsonism, medication effect or myxedema.

The Content of Speech

The next component of language assessment is a general linguistic analysis. This is an analysis of the content of the communication. In other words, does the language make sense? The key question is, "Are the thoughts complete?" Can the person communicate a coherent flow of concepts or ideas? Some individuals show digressions from the main theme of the conversation, digressing from the digressions and never returning to the main point. We all know people who communicate this way, so a deviation from their normal communication pattern is more revealing than a stable communication pattern. Incomplete thoughts reflect more significant communication difficulty. Does the patient show awareness of the implications of answers (insight), anticipation of an answer, or evidence of abstract thinking? These would tend to show higher cortical function. Humor does not always indicate higher function unless it is spontaneous to the moment. Some very demented elderly people can relate extremely humorous stories from a well-practiced repertoire.

More Subtle Linguistic Analysis

The linguistic analysis can become even more specialized. The person's choice of words may be a marker of intellectual vitality. The descriptive richness is revealed in colorful verbs and adjectives. The use of personal pronouns may mirror the emotional distance. For example, the use of the word "my" often indicates emotional closeness. ("My doctor asked me to see you today.") The complexity of syntax also reflects overall education and mental capacity.

Specific Content Issues

Specific content issues include evidence or examples of dysfunction, rate of progression, and the nature of adaptations. In evaluating mental status (see Chapter 22) it is useful to see if the person can take a "mental walk" and use his or her imagination to provide spatial information. For example, "Mrs. Smith, if you met me at the front door of your house and you invited me inside, tell me what we would see." People with dementia have difficulty using their imagination and have extreme difficulty with this task. Context specificity refers to the concept that the boundaries of the answer are contained in the question. People with dementia may easily answer a question but not within the appropriate boundary. For example, in response to "What specific plants did you plant in your garden?," "I planted annuals and perennials" is a few categories of abstraction removed from the question's intent.

BEHAVIORS

Observing behaviors is easy but interpreting behaviors is difficult. It is extremely easy to extrapolate too much from behavioral observations. Nonetheless, some emotions are clearly revealed in gestures. Cultural context is critical in interpreting behaviors. The overall harmony and congruence of the observations are the keys to understanding the meaning of a behavior. Contradictions (apparent incongruities) are very revealing. For example, a nervous laugh could reflect either amusement or extreme discomfort or both.

Facial Expression

The core of our emotional life is conveyed on the twenty-five square inches of the human face. Nothing is as well known as the subtle nuances of facial expression that ripple across the countenance like waves on the ocean. In fact, the actual change in expression reflecting an altered mood is very slight. Most details of facial expression are comprised primarily of eye and mouth movements.

The Use of the Eyes

According to mythologist Joseph Campbell, the twelfth century troubadours of Europe said, "The eyes are the messengers of the heart — they search for what the heart seeks to possess." Eye movement sends a variety of emotion. For example, eyes that are downcast, with the face turned away, may show low self-esteem. Gaze aversion occurs if a topic makes one feel uncomfortable or guilty. If students are asked questions they think they should be able to answer but cannot, their eyes immediately look toward their feet. In grief, the brow is furrowed and the eyes are clenched. The eyes of depression sometimes view the world through partially closed lids: the brows are always involved, often slightly raised and bent into an inverted "V." Raised eyebrows suggest disbelief and the jaw muscles may tighten. A sideways glance reflects suspicion, uncertainty, or rejection. Frowns are easily recognized as signs of displeasure or confusion.

If the lower eyelid rises, it shows plainly that the person is not sure they believe what you are telling them. If the lower lid, in addition to being raised, is brought in towards the nose, it indicates frank disbelief. If your message is not registering, the upper lid will be lowered and the eyeball will be slightly raised to meet it. If the upper lid completely covers the iris to the pupil, the patient's mind is sluggish. If the upper lid covers the top half of the pupil, this indicates the patient is indifferent. When the upper lid comes down only to the top edge of the pupil, the patient is interested and attentive. If the upper lid covers half the width of the top arc of the iris, the patient's mind is very attentive. If the upper lid touches the edge of the iris, it is a positive indication that the mind is attentive, but feelings have been aroused. Proptosis suggests hyperthyroidism. More specific eye observations are covered in Chapter 8.

Eye Contact

Eye contact is normally evident during 30–60% of a conversation. Limited eye contact implies the person is hiding something, perhaps a sense of low self-esteem. Eye contact increases if one feels defensive, aggressive or hostile. Excessive eye contact (over 60%) implies the person is interested in the other person more than the subject of the conversation. (The extremes are lovers and fighters.)

Abstract thinkers seem to have more eye contact than concrete thinkers. Perhaps they have a better ability to integrate information and are less distracted by eye contact. Eye contact with a slight one-sided smile means that the person is weighing your actions.

The Mouth

The mouth also clearly transmits the inner state of the person. In sadness or depression the mouth is often stretched and the lip margins may be thinned. The mouth tends to show anger by being tightly compressed. An open mouth with clenched teeth and tightly drawn eyes suggests significant pain.

Smiles

Interpreting smiles is a useful skill to cultivate. The simple smile is open and relaxed, with the mouth pulled up toward the ear and the eyes are slightly closed with a tight lower lid. False smiles tend to be less relaxed with eyes that are open and the corners of the mouth moved laterally rather than up toward the ear. This smile is polite but has no depth or sense of sincerity.

Hand and Arm Gestures

Hand and arm movements are another core element of behavior. Gestures are hand signals that send visual signs of openness, doubt, frustration, inner conflict, and self-esteem. For example, a clenched fist shows determination or aggression. A broad scissors movement (resembling a basketball referee's call of "no basket") suggests "no way." Finger pointing is assertive. Palm movements also convey useful information. A hard karate chop onto an open palm suggests a desire to cut through a problem. Holding both palms up is often a sign that implores for agreement, while having both palms down is a restraining gesture for people to remain cool-headed. Palms facing directly ahead as if stopping traffic are front-repelling and signify protest. Palms with the backs facing ahead are embracing, and reflect a comfort seeker. Sidewise palms (like a hand shake) while talking suggest a desire for nego-tiation.

Open hands signal sincerity, openness, and pride as does unbuttoning the coat. Arms crossed on chest can be a sign of defensiveness or simply a posture of comfort. One useful clue is to check the hands to see if they are re-laxed or fist-like. Standing with hands on hips implies readiness or dedication.

Placing the hand to the cheek with the forefinger pointing reflects the patient's criti-cal evaluation. Chin stroking is a sign of con-sideration or that the patient is making a judg-ment and considering your remarks. Pinching the bridge of the nose (usually with closed eyes) indicates great concern and thought over the decision. Nose twitching is a sign of doubt or negation. (Beware — sometimes a nose itches, but with practice you can tell the difference.) A hand covering the mouth suggests astonish-ment, self-doubt, or deceit.

Signs of Frustration

Several gestures reflect frustration. For example, arms spread while hands grip edge of table is a posture demanding attention. Sit-ting with the hand on the occiput with the head bowed is another reflection of inner frus-tration. A fist is a clue to determination, ex-treme emphasis, or anger. Tugging at the ear reflects a desire to interrupt.

Signs of Inner Conflict

Signs of inner conflict include perspira-tion that may indicate nervousness, infection or a withdrawal syndrome, or hands pinching and fidgeting. These fidgeting gestures imply a need for reassurance. Finger gestures, such as thumb sucking, nail biting, or picking at the cuticle or nail polish, convey anxieties, inner conflicts, and apprehensions. Tightly clenched hands show an intense inner tension, as does hand-wringing. A pointed finger says, "Look there," and is often used to reprimand, ad-monish, discipline, or drive home a point. Gripping the wrists suggests needing self-control; this reflects putting on the brakes.

Signs of Self-Esteem

Signs of self-esteem include placing the palm to the back of the neck. This is a defen-sive, bending posture. On the other hand, steepling the fingers as if in prayer reflects con-fidence, and self-control. The hand height when steepling, if high enough, can show a proud, smug demeanor.

Sitting on the edge of the chair implies readiness and a person who is action-oriented. The patient who sits leaning back with crossed legs and making a kicking movement reflects boredom and impatience. A person sitting with a leg over the arm of the chair signals indiffer-ence and an uncooperative attitude. Sitting with the chair back to one's chest is a sign of dominance or aggression. Leaning back with hands supporting one's head signals a sense of superiority, while fidgeting implies nervous-ness. Tugging at pants suggests that decision-making is in process. Sitting with locked an-kles signals inner tension and significant stress. On the other hand, sitting with the hands at back of the neck, leaning back, with straight posture, and the shins out, suggests authority and self-confidence.

Postures

Standing postures are also very revealing to the observant physician. The specific approach to gait analysis is covered in Chapter 23. The pace, stride length and posture signal the emotions and overall vitality. Frail individuals tend to walk slower and without the usual rhythmic cadence of a normal gait. A rapid walk with free-hand swing means the person is goal-oriented and used to pursuing objectives. Walking with one's hands always in pockets suggests secretiveness, a critical nature, and often enjoyment of playing a devil's advocate role. The elderly person who scuffles with their head down signals dejection.

The individual who walks with hands on hips denotes sudden bursts of energy. These individuals are sprinters rather than long-distance runners. Walking with one's hands behind the back with head bowed and at a slow pace shows that one is preoccupied. The person who walks with chin raised, arm swing exaggerated, and legs stiff, reflects self-satisfaction and pomposity.

Miscellaneous Behaviors

There are some other behaviors that can be seen frequently in the clinical setting. The head tilted to the side is often an attempt at persuasion.

Moving close to speak confidentially can be an aggressive gesture that is used to dominate or direct. Short breaths can signify respiratory distress or general frustration. "Tsk, tsk" implies frustration or disgust, while rapid jerky movements reflect nervousness. "Whew" suggests relief, and frequent throat clearing reflects nervousness. Jingling money in pockets may show preoccupations.

CHAPTER 4

The Vital Signs

The pragmatic rule is that the meaning of a concept may always be found, if not in some sensible particular which it directly designates, then in some particular difference in the course of human experience which its being true will make. Test every concept by the question, "What sensible difference to anybody will its truth make?" and you are in the best possible position for understanding what it means and for discussing its importance.

— **William James**

To know that you do not know is the best.
To pretend to know when you do not know is a disease.

— **Lao-tzu**

Vital signs are literally signs of life. Obtain them with care and precision. They are performed so routinely that it is easy for us to get sloppy and to cut corners, taking the pulse for only fifteen seconds and multiplying by 4, for example, or estimating the respiratory rate rather than directly measuring it. Always collect the vital signs attentively, accurately, carefully and completely.

TEMPERATURE

Normal aging can impair thermoregulation predisposing elderly, people to hypothermia and heat stroke. The oral temperature used to be taken by a mercury-filled thermometer held by the patient under the tongue for three minutes. Modern devices estimate temperature digitally using probes resembling Popsicle sticks. (Am I dating myself?) The rectal temperature averages one degree Fahrenheit higher than the simultaneously obtained oral temperature. The axillary temperature averages about one degree lower than the oral temperature. Other areas used to measure temperature have included the tympanic membrane. Although the "normal" temperature of 98.6° was originally determined from axillary temperatures, the accepted "normal" oral temperature is 98.6° Fahrenheit. A higher axillary temperature than oral temperature suggests hyperthyroidism (Lucatello's sign).

Potential Artifacts

Potential artifacts in temperature measurement include cerumen impaction in the otic thermometers, improper placement of the oral thermometer in the mouth (not really under the tongue), mouth breathing (over 20 breaths per minute) while using an oral thermometer, and factitious fever. A simultaneous oral and immediately voided urine temperature measurement while observing the patient can sometimes uncover factitious fevers since the urine temperature and oral temperatures should be comparable. Fortunately, factitious fever in elderly people is uncommon. There is diurnal temperature variation of between one-half and two degrees (lower in the morning and higher in the afternoon).

FEVER

Because of impaired thermoregulation with aging, some older persons will not mount an appropriate febrile response to serious illness. As a result, the lack of fever does not rule out infection or inflammation in an ill elderly person. Fever is defined as an oral temperature greater than 100°F, although some authorities do not consider a fever significant until the temperature exceeds 38.5°C (101.3°F). For some elderly persons with consistently low basal temperatures such as 97°F, an increase of two degrees may represent a fever. Fever generally implies inflammation or infection. Fever is usually associated with an increase in the pulse of eight to ten beats per minute for each Centigrade degree of fever (Liebermeister's rule). Infection with intracellular organisms can cause a bradycardia with fever, the "pulse-temperature dissociation" (Jean Faget's exception to Liebermeister's rule originally described for Yellow Fever). Organisms that can produce pulse-temperature dissociation are shown in Table 4.1. Failure of the rectal temperature to drop after sitting in a cool bath for fifteen minutes suggests typhoid fever (Baruch's sign).

Fever Patterns

Fever patterns, seldom documented in the medical chart anymore, are sometimes helpful in figuring out the underlying cause. Sustained fevers that show little change throughout the day raise the possibility of Gram-negative infections. A persistent low-grade

---

Table 4.1. Organisms that can produce temperature-pulse dissociation

Type of Organism	*Examples*
Gram-negative bacteria	Salmonella typhi (typhoid fever), Brucella species
	Leptospira interrogans
	Francisella tularensis
	Chlamydia species (pneumonia)
	Legionella pneumophila (Legionnaire's disease)
Tick-borne species	Rickettsia species
	Orientia tsutsugamushi (scrub typhus)
	Coxiella burnetii (Q fever) (inhaled infection, not from a tick bite)
	Babesia (babesiosis)
Viruses	Dengue fever virus
	Yellow fever virus
Others	Corynebacterium diphtheriae (diphtheria)
	Plasmodium species (Malaria)

fever with two peaks each week suggests viral illnesses such as Dengue fever or West Nile virus. Relapsing fevers have some afebrile days in between febrile days. Hodgkin's disease occasionally produces Pel-Ebstein's relapsing fever with intervals from days to weeks.

Pieter Klaases Pel (1852–1919) was a popular Dutch physician who described Pel's ocular crisis in neurosyphilis. **Wilhelm Ebstein** *(1836–1912) was a German internist who described Ebstein's anomaly of the tricuspid valve, as well as a characteristic lesion in the terminal convoluted tubule in diabetic nephropathy. They each independently described the relapsing fever of a patient with splenomegaly.*

Examples of infectious agents causing relapsing fevers are Brucellosis (fever with activity and no fever with rest), and tuberculosis (also extrapulmonary TB). Fever twice a day (double quotidian fever) suggests gonococcal endocarditis.

Malaria has a characteristic pattern that indicates the organism. Fever every third day (tertian fever) suggests *P. vivax* or *P. ovale*. Fever on the fourth day (quartan fever) suggests *P. malariae*. Double quartan fevers occur every other day with mild and severe occurrences. Intermittent fevers that return to normal each day or remittent fevers that drop during the day but not to normal provide less help as diagnostic clues.

Fever over 41°C (106°F) in an elderly person suggests heat stroke. An elevated temperature can also indicate a central nervous system process such as hypothalamic dysregulation, malignant neuroleptic syndrome, sleep disorders, sedative withdrawal, or stroke.

Hypothermia

Hypothermia is defined as an oral temperature that is less than 95°F. Suspect hypothermia if the patient's temperature is less than 96°F. Normal thermometers do not read very low and even digital thermometers lose accuracy outside a narrow range. Hypothermia can occur during the summer. Conditions commonly producing hypothermia include hypothyroidism, hypoglycemia, Addison's disease, medication effect, severe acute illness, and exposure. In addition to low body temperature, some hypothermic individuals show a delayed *contraction* phase of deep tendon reflexes (as opposed to the delayed relaxation phase of myxedema) and Osborn "J" waves on the electrocardiogram (see Figure 4).

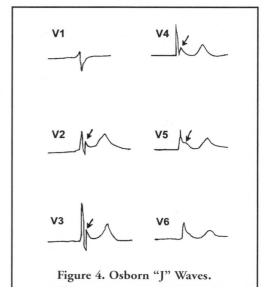

Figure 4. Osborn "J" Waves.
Osborn "J" waves are electrocardiographic evidence of a body temperature less than 95°F (hypothermia). The arrows on the figure point to the "J" waves in precordial leads V2–V5.

PULSE

When feeling the pulse, make a special point to appreciate the elastic quality of the vessel wall in addition to the pulse rate and the nature of the pulse wave. If you can still palpate the arterial wall distal to a point of occlusion, Osler's sign, you may have diagnosed atherosclerosis. In addition, check for peripheral vascular disease by simultaneously feeling the pulses on each side of the radials, femorals, dorsalis pedis, and posterior tibial. Appreciating a diminished pulse on one side implies a vascular process on that side.

The pulse beat following a premature contraction should feel perceptibly stronger due to the increased filling time produced by the compensatory pause. If the beat following the premature contraction is not stronger, think aortic outflow obstruction, such as hypertrophic obstructive cardiomyopathy. Feeling a diminished pulse after a premature contraction is Brockenbrough's sign of subaortic stenosis. When the pulse is irregular, compare the apical pulse rate with the peripheral pulse rate to see if there is a pulse deficit (a difference in the pulse rates) suggesting atrial fibrillation.

Subclavian Steal Syndrome

A diminished left radial pulse in an older person (usually a man) raises the possibility of subclavian steal syndrome (see Figure 5). The patient may present with vertigo, headache, left arm claudication or left eye visual disturbance

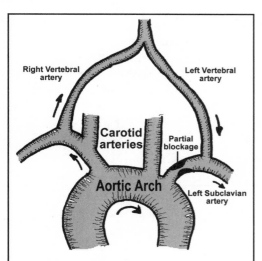

Figure 5. Subclavian Steal Syndrome.
The subclavian steal syndrome is caused by obstruction of the subclavian artery proximal to the take-off of the left vertebral artery. The blood travels from the right side, then retrograde down the left vertebral artery to bypass the blockage and supply the left arm. The common symptoms of the syndrome — headache, vertigo, or left eye visual disturbance with use of the left arm — are due to relative ischemia of the symptomatic structures.

when using his or her left arm. The syndrome is caused by obstruction of the subclavian artery proximal to the take off of the vertebral artery. The blood travels retrograde down the vertebral artery on the left to bypass the blockage and supply the arm. The symptoms are due to the relative ischemia of the symptomatic structures. Occasionally this syndrome can occur in vascular access lines (such as for hemodialysis) attached to an external jugular catheter.

Pulse Rate

The pulse is considered slow (bradycardia) if it is less than 60 beats per minute. In this situation consider third-degree heart block or medication effect as possible causes. A normal pulse rate ranges from 60 to 100 beats per minute. A rapid pulse rate or tachycardia is greater than 100 beats per minute. Palpating over a sensitive site should increase the pulse rate (Mannkopf's sign).

A pulse rate between 100 and 125 beats per minute suggests sinus tachycardia. Sinus tachycardia, an important sign of underlying illness, should not be dismissed as an incidental finding. If the patient has a peripheral AV fistula, sinus tachycardia slowed by compressing the artery proximal to the fistula is Branham's sign. Chronic sinus tachycardia caused by right heart hypertension stretching the atrial receptors is the Bainbridge reflex.

Francis Arthur Bainbridge (1874–1921) was an English physiologist who described the formation of lymph and contributed to the classification of parathyphoid bacteria. He also made important contributions to exercise physiology.

Causes of sinus tachycardia include congestive heart failure, myocardial infarction, fever, dehydration, anemia and hyperthyroidism. Pulse rates between 125 and 170 suggest atrial flutter with 2 to 1 block, while rates between 170 and 200 suggest paroxysmal atrial tachycardia. A pulse rate over 200 is a cause for serious concern because the etiology of the

Table 4.2. Heart rates, arrhythmias and possible causes

Pulse Rate (beats per minutes)	Type of arrhythmia	Possible Causes (not an exhaustive list)
Less than 60 (Symptoms are often not present until the heart rate drops below 50)	Bradycardia	• Medication effect • Third degree heart block (sick sinus syndrome) • Inferior myocardial infarction • Increased intracranial pressure • Infection • Hypothermia • Hypogycemia • Hypothyroidism
60 to 100	Normal	
75		• Possible atrial flutter with 4:1 block
100 to 150 Regular rhythm	Sinus tachycardia	• Pain • Fever • Hyperthyroidism • Infection • Hypoglycemia • Dehydration • Anemia • Medications • Myocardial infarction • Congestive heart failure • Right heart hypertension (Bainbridge reflex)
	Ventricular tachycardia	• Coronary artery disease • Cardiomyopathy • Medications
Greater than 100 Irregularly irregular rhythm	Atrial fibrillation with rapid ventricular response	• Myocardial infarction • Pulmonary embolism • Thyrotoxicosis • Electrolyte disorder
	Multifocal atrial tachycardia	
Greater than 150 Regular rhythm	Supraventricular tachycardia	

tachycardia is usually significant and it is likely that the tachycardia will progress to ventricular tachycardia.

How can you tell paroxysmal atrial tachycardia from sinus tachycardia? Paroxysmal atrial tachycardia begins abruptly and ends abruptly, while sinus tachycardia slowly accelerates and decelerates.

Pulse Rhythm

• *A regular rhythm* allows you to detect a rhythmic pattern and predict when every beat will occur.

• *A regularly irregular pulse occurs in a predictably irregular pattern.* When you feel this rhythm, strongly consider second-degree AV block. Look at the neck veins and consider obtaining an electrocardiogram. It is possible to appreciate whether or not the PR interval is increasing, based on watching the "a" wave and "c" wave of the jugular venous pulse (see Chapter 15). In second-degree AV block some

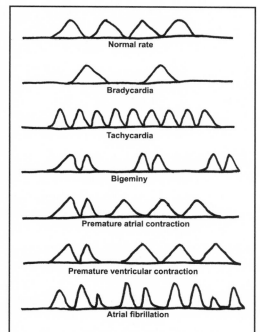

Figure 6. Pulse Rates and Rhythms.

A normal pulse rate with regular rhythm allows you to predict when the next beat will occur. A bradycardia is a pulse rate below 60 while a tachycardia is a rate greater than 100 beats per minute. Bigeminy is when beats are paired with a premature contraction occurring after each normal beat. Premature atrial contractures reset the timing of the atrial contraction, while premature ventricular contractions have a compensatory pause that allows the next normal beat to occur without resetting the timing. Atrial fibrillation is irregularly irregular: you cannot predict when the next beat will occur.

atrial impulses are blocked in the AV node while most are transmitted. A beat is regularly missed, such as three beats and then a missed beat. The AV block takes its name from the ratio of atrial contractions to ventricular contractions (typically a very constant ratio for each patient) such as 4:3 AV block (three beats, then a dropped beat). Mobitz type I, second-degree AV block is called Wenckebach where the PR interval lengthens with each beat until a beat is dropped.

> *Karel Frederik Wenckebach (1864–1940) was a Dutch internist who described the cardiac rhythm that bears his name. He also studied the effect of quinine on arrhythmias and authored an important paper on beriberi. Quinine pills used to be called Wenckebach's pills.*

> *Woldemar Mobitz (1889–1951) was a Russian surgeon who moved to Germany and became an extraordinary professor. His main interest was in cardiac rhythm disturbances, and he first reported the two types of second-degree AV block that bear his name.*

Mobitz type II AV block has no change in the PR interval, so the beats are simply dropped. Bigeminy, trigeminy, or quadrigeminy refer to paired atrial and ventricular contractions. Sometimes the ectopic beats are every third beat or every fourth beat.

• *Pulsus alternans,* where every other beat feels weak, suggests severe myocardial failure. If the electrocardiogram also shows electrical alternans with every other QRS amplitude being high and low, then the prognosis is poor. The key point is that this is not a bigeminal pulse. You can tell them apart because pulsus alternans beats are equally spaced while bigeminal beats are coupled. A more sophisticated method is to check the blood pressure and note that the pulse rate near the systolic blood pressure level in pulsus alternans seems to be one-half of the peripheral pulse rate. As the cuff pressure drops, the alternate beats appear similar to the pulsus parodoxus but their appearance is independent of the patient's respirations.

• *An irregularly irregular rhythm* suggests

atrial fibrillation. This rhythm should always catch you off guard, as it is unpredictable. If you find yourself getting into a predictable pattern, then consider paroxysmal atrial fibrillation or digitalis toxicity (especially in chronic atrial fibrillation). In any irregularly irregular rhythm, measure the pulse deficit by subtracting the radial pulse rate from the apical rate determined by auscultating the heart. Any pulse deficit suggests atrial fibrillation. Loss of the pulse deficit in atrial fibrillation suggests digitalis toxicity. Atrial fibrillation plus any sudden decline in function raises the possibility of embolic disease. Atrial fibrillation in the setting of dementia suggests multi-infarct disease rather than Alzheimer's disease. The causes of atrial fibrillation include ischemic cardiac disease, chronic hypertension, or hyperthyroidism.

How can you tell multifocal atrial tachycardia from atrial fibrillation? In multifocal atrial tachycardia there is no pulse deficit and it is easy to determine the blood pressure.

Premature Ventricular Contractions

Premature ventricular contractions (PVCs) should also be noted. The beat following the premature contraction should feel slightly stronger because the PVC is followed by a compensatory pause. The compensatory pause allows for increased ventricular filling and stroke volume of the following beat. If the beat following a PVC is not stronger but diminished, consider the possibility of idiopathic hypertrophic subaortic stenosis (Brockenbrough's sign) or severe left ventricular failure. Sometimes having the patient perform a stressful mental task (such as mentally reciting the months of the year backwards) can bring out a PVC, giving you the chance to assess the beat following the compensatory pause.

Premature Atrial Contractions

In contrast to the premature ventricular contractions, premature atrial contractions (PACs) do not produce a compensatory pause. In order to distinguish the PAC from the PVC, try tapping out the rhythm with your foot like a metronome. Have your foot tap down in synchrony with each beat of the pulse. PACs will change the timing so that the beat will occur on the up-count of your foot and will continue to occur on the up-beat. A PVC will occur on the up-beat, but the pulse will resume on the down-beat after the compensatory pause.

Factors Affecting the Pulse Wave

Stroke volume, peripheral resistance, degree of stenosis and the elasticity of the vessels affect the nature of the pulse wave. Pulse waves will not be as evident in a rigid artery. A bounding pulse, best appreciated by holding the patient's hand over their head, is generally produced by a higher peak and more rapid decline.

Estimating the Pulse Pressure

Try to develop a sense of the pulse pressure, the difference between the systolic and diastolic blood pressures (vide infra). For example, feeling bounding foot pulses in an octogenarian suggest a wide pulse pressure (greater than 60 millimeters of mercury). A wide pulse pressure can also be observed in visibly pulsing (and often tortuous) arteries. In elderly people a wide pulse pressure suggests aortic insufficiency, systolic hypertension, thyrotoxicosis, complete heart block, and fever.

Narrow pulse pressures (less than 30 millimeters of mercury) suggest acute hypotension, severe congestive heart failure, cardiac tamponade, pericardial constriction, or severe stenotic valvular heart disease, such as mitral or aortic stenosis.

Reviewing the Pulse Patterns

Pulse patterns include the weak thready pulse, the pulse with a delayed upstroke, the

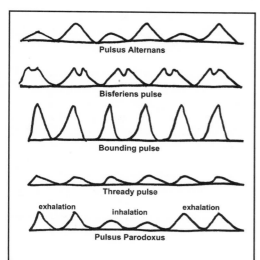

Figure 7. Pulse Patterns.

Pulsus alternans, when every other beat of the pulse feels weak, implies severe myocardial failure. Bisferiens pulse is feeling a double impulse with each beat. It usually suggests subaortic stenosis or valvular aortic stenosis. A bounding pulse implies a wide pulse pressure (greater than 60mmHg) such as with aortic insufficiency. A thready pulse implies a narrow pulse pressure (less than 30mmHg) often caused by acute hypotension, severe congestive heart failure, cardiac tamponade, pericardial constriction, or severe stenotic valvular heart disease, such as mitral or aortic stenosis. Reduction of the intensity of the pulse with inspiration suggests pulsus parodoxus. In extreme cases the pulse may completely disappear in inspiration.

pulse where every other beat is weak, or two pulses for each cardiac cycle. A weak and rapid pulse suggests severe congestive heart failure or shock. The delayed pulse is called "pulsus parvus et tardus" (small and slow-rising) and suggests aortic stenosis, severe arterial stenosis or aortic aneurysm. Pulsus alternans (vide supra), where every other beat feels weak, suggests severe myocardial failure. Bisferiens pulse is sometimes appreciated as a double pulse or a "fuzzy" feeling to your palpating fingers. If you suspect this, listen over brachial artery and gently push down on the proximal portion until you hear a soft compression bruit which is normal with vascular compression. In bisferiens pulse you will hear two soft bruits for

each cardiac cycle. The bisferiens pulse may be heard in IHSS, aortic stenosis or low peripheral resistance state. Bradycardia when palpating over an AV fistula is the Nicoladoni-Israel-Branham sign, with the claim that Nicoladoni independently described it in 1875, Israel in 1877, and Branham in 1890. A pulse that does not decrease when going from standing to lying suggests hypertension (Huchard's sign).

Pulse Variations with Respiration

Pulse variations can sometimes be noted with respiration. Changes in rate, with decreases in inspiration and increases in expiration, suggest sinus arrhythmia. In fact, this is a normal sign of adequate function of the autonomic nervous system. On the other hand (pun intended), reduction of the intensity of the pulse with inspiration suggests pulsus parodoxus (vide infra). In extreme cases the pulse may completely disappear in inspiration. This was the historical paradox: Where did the pulse go with inspiration since cardiac auscultation confirmed the presence of the heartbeat?

BLOOD PRESSURE

The gold standard of blood pressure measurement is a mercury manometer, although these are now being replaced due the biohazard of mercury. Some aneroid (gauge and needle) blood pressure cuffs are not accurate. Digital systems are accurate but have to be calibrated and monitored. If a blood pressure does not seem realistic (for example, finding a narrow pulse pressure in a patient with bounding pulses) then recheck the blood pressure manually.

Taking the Blood Pressure

Taking a blood pressure is like playing the piano; it is easy to do poorly and more difficult to do well. Make sure the blood pressure cuff is high enough on the biceps to provide access to the brachial artery. Check to assure the correct size cuff by configuring the lines on the cuff to match the correct range. A mid-arm circumference greater than 27cm is too large for the standard blood pressure cuff. The larger the arm the greater the *apparent* blood pressure, so the blood pressure obtained with a cuff that is too small will be artificially high. Using too large a cuff will not artificially lower the blood pressure and, in fact, it might elevate the apparent blood pressure.

Do not place the cuff over clothing. It is also important to make sure that the point of the brachial artery where you are listening is at the level of the heart. Listening above the heart level will reduce the blood pressure (as you might predict) while listening with your stethoscope placed below the heart level will increase the apparent blood pressure.

Begin the blood pressure determination by palpating the systolic and diastolic blood pressure. To accomplish this, palpate the brachial artery and pump up the blood pressure cuff until you feel the brachial pulse disappear. Slowly release the blood pressure cuff pressure by about 2mmHg per second until you feel the pulse return. That point where you first feel the pulse is the palpable systolic pressure. With very light palpation you can appreciate the vibratory thrill of the Korotkov sound. Continue to slowly lower the cuff pressure until the thrill disappears; that point is the palpable diastolic blood pressure. Now lower the cuff pressure to zero.

Nikolai Sergeievich Korotkov (1874–1920) was a Russian surgeon and an important pioneer of early 20th century vascular surgery. He studied the development of collateral circulation and spent his latter career performing surgery on disabled soldiers. His method of blood pressure measurement was reported in 281 words in a presentation in 1905. Here is the original description: "The cuff of Riva-Rocci is placed on the middle third of the upper arm; the pressure within the cuff is quickly raised up to complete cessation of circulation below the cuff. Then,

letting the mercury of the manometer fall, one listens to the artery just below the cuff with a children's stethoscope. At first no sounds are heard. With the falling of the mercury in the manometer down to a certain height, the first short tones appear; their appearance indicates the passage of part of the pulse wave under the cuff. It follows that the manometric figure at which the first tone appears corresponds to the maximal pressure. With the further fall of the mercury in the manometer one hears the systolic compression murmurs, which pass again into tones (second). Finally, all sounds disappear. The time of the cessation of sounds indicates the free passage of the pulse wave; in other words at the moment of the disappearance of the sounds the minimal blood pressure within the artery predominates over the pressure in the cuff. It follows that the manometric figures at this time correspond to the minimal blood pressure."

The next step is to perform the auscultatory blood pressure. To determine the systolic pressure, place the bell of your stethoscope (if your stethoscope has a bell) over the brachial artery as determined by your previous palpation. Pump up the blood pressure cuff to 10mmHg above the palpable blood pressure. Now lower the cuff pressure by 2mmHg per beat until you hear the first Korotkov sound; that point is the systolic blood pressure. Determine the diastolic pressure by continuing to slowly lower the pressure (2mmHg per heart beat) until you notice a muffling of the sound (some people will not have a muffling point) and note that value. Continue lowering the cuff pressure until the Korotkov sounds disappear; that is the diastolic blood pressure. In cases of high stroke volume such as aortic insufficiency, thyrotoxicosis, fever, anemia, or beriberi, or when the diastolic pressure seems to be zero, use the muffling point as the diastolic blood pressure instead of zero. Systolic hypertension in hyperthyroidism is Pende's sign. Fresh petechia below a tourniquet or blood pressure cuff suggests a platelet abnormality (Rumpel-Leede sign). (Theodor Rumpel [1862–1923] was a German surgeon from Hamburg. Stockbridge Carl Leede was an American physician, born in 1882.) Seeing several splinter-like petechiae at the elbow below the blood pressure cuff is a variant of the Rumpel-Leede sign called the Grocco-Frugoni sign.

Potential Artifacts

Unless you are careful, a number of potential errors can creep into your determination of the blood pressure (see Table 4.3). In rounding off errors, the blood pressure readings are often "rounded to eights and zeros." Values ending in one, three, or seven are rare. While these are technically errors, being off by one or two millimeters of mercury is usually not clinically significant. Nonetheless, making small, careless errors does not inspire confidence that other observations will be made and recorded more accurately. Another problem in blood pressure measurement is to release the cuff pressure too rapidly. Doing this can produce an abnormally high diastolic blood pressure or an abnormally low systolic blood pressure. Obviously, the slower the heart rate the more pronounced the magnitude of this artifact because the pressure gauge can travel quite a distance between beats.

Having the patient's arm too tense can increase the systolic blood pressure by more than 10mmHg. In fact, the ability to increase the systolic blood pressure by more than

Table 4.3. Potential errors in blood pressure measurement

Source of Error

- Placing the cuff over clothing
- Having a tight sleeve above the cuff
- Using the wrong sized cuff
- Placing the cuff incorrectly on the arm
- Not having the cuff placed at heart level
- Having the patient's arm too tense
- Lowering the pressure too rapidly
- Using aneroid or digital equipment that is not calibrated
- Pausing midway and re-inflating the cuff

10mmHg with isometric handgrip is a test of normal autonomic tone. White coat hypertension may be a variant of the tense arm noted above. Some people have an intense autonomic reaction when visiting a physician (even one not wearing a white coat). This autonomic drive can accentuate the blood pressure response. Home monitoring of the blood pressure usually shows lower blood pressure readings.

Lack of vascular compliance due to arteriosclerosis can increase the apparent systolic blood pressure. Extreme vascular stiffness generally increases the extrinsic pressure needed to compress the vessel, making both the systolic and diastolic blood pressures artificially high. To screen for this phenomenon check Osler's maneuver. First, feel the brachial pulse distal to the blood pressure cuff and inflate the cuff above the systolic pressure. If you can still feel the artery then it is too stiff (sometimes calcified) and the apparent blood pressure may be artificially high.

Sir William Osler (1849–1919) was a Canadian physician who transformed medical education by emphasizing the value of clinical experience. His studies led him to London, Berlin, Vienna, Leipzig, and back to his alma mater in Montreal, McGill. In 1884, he was offered the chair of clinical medicine at the University of Pennsylvania — he accepted based on the flip of a coin. When he later became the first professor of medicine at the new Johns Hopkins University School of Medicine, there were initially no students. He used this time to write The Principles and Practice of Medicine, published in 1892. In this same year, he married Grace Gross, the great-granddaughter of Paul Revere. His textbook was the most popular medical text of its time. When John D. Rockefeller was seeking guidance for his philanthropic endeavors, he turned to Frederick Gates, a fellow businessman and philanthropist. Gates had recently read Osler's text in its entirety and subsequently inspired Rockefeller to direct his foundation toward medical research. This led to the establishment of the Rockefeller Institute of Medical Research in New York.

Osler was known to be a man of immense personal charm who epitomized Peabody's saying that "the secret of patient care is caring for patients." He insisted on patients being treated as people, not as "interesting cases."

In his farewell speech at Johns Hopkins, Osler suggested that academics retire at age 60, and then be allowed one year of contemplation before being peacefully dispatched by chloroform. He did admit to being a little dubious of the plan, "as my own time is getting so short." "To study medicine without reading textbooks is like going to sea without charts," he said, "but to study medicine without dealing with patients is not going to sea at all."

A potentially serious error in blood pressure measurement is to miss an auscultatory gap. The gap is an apparent loss of the Korotkov sounds with their reappearance before reaching the diastolic blood pressure. The gap can make the diastolic blood pressure appear to be much higher than it really is. This can occur in situations where an excess amount of blood is pooled in the patient's arm. Most commonly it happens when the person taking the blood pressure lowers the cuff pressure to below systolic blood pressure and then re-inflates the cuff "just to be sure" of the systolic value. The significance of the auscultatory gap is to appreciate that it can occur and that the diastolic blood pressure is not the value at the gap.

Measuring the Blood Pressure in the Patient with Atrial Fibrillation

It is challenging to accurately measure the blood pressure in the setting of atrial fibrillation (AF) since the stroke volume changes from beat to beat and so the blood pressure also varies from beat to beat. How do you determine the blood pressure in the setting of AF? Joseph Sapira suggests averaging three blood pressures. Lower the cuff pressure very slowly until three beats can easily be heard; the first beat is the systolic blood pressure. Continue slowly lowering the pressure until you hear the last three beats; the last one represents the diastolic blood pressure.

Ventricular tachycardia changes the first Korotkov sound so that it varies with every beat. Supraventricular tachycardia does not change the Korotkov sound with each beat.

The Pulse Pressure

The pulse pressure is the difference between the systolic and diastolic blood pressure. Normally the pulse pressure is 25–50% of the systolic blood pressure. Noting an abnormally low (narrow) pulse pressure suggests

Table 4.4. Common causes of wide and narrow pulse pressures	
Pulse Pressure	*Possible Causes*
Wide pulse pressures (greater than 60mmHg)	• Aortic insufficiency • Systolic hypertension • Thyrotoxicosis • Fever • Complete heart block • Paget's disease of bone • Anemia • Thiamine deficiency
Narrow pulse pressures (less than 30mmHg)	• Severe aortic stenosis • Hypotension • Severe congestive heart failure • Cardiac tamponade • Pericardial constriction

decreased stroke volume from aortic stenosis, tachycardia, pericardial constriction or tamponade.

Abnormally wide pulse pressure suggests large stroke volumes. A clue is feeling bounding pulses in an old person's feet. Wide pulse pressures are seen in aortic insufficiency, fever, anemia, hyperthyroidism, and sometimes Paget's disease. An abnormally wide pulse pressure in just one limb suggests an AV fistula distal to the site of blood pressure cuff placement. (Note the pulse slow down when the artery is occluded for the systolic blood pressure, Branham's sign.)

Measuring Systolic Gradients in the Extremities

Sometimes it is important to measure the blood pressure in both arms, for example when you suspect an ascending aortic aneurysm. The *lower* blood pressure is the abnormal one. (There is no way for an arm to increase its blood pressure.) Differences greater than 10mmHg are abnormal.

To measure systolic gradients in the arms and legs, first measure the systolic blood pressure in the legs with the patient supine. Either place the blood pressure cuff around the calf and use the dorsalis pedis pulse or use a thigh cuff and use the popliteal artery. Next, measure the blood pressure in the arm, also with the patient supine. Arm blood pressures greater than legs suggest significant atherosclerosis. Leg blood pressures are normally no more than 15mmHg greater than arm blood pressures. If the pressure difference is more than 15mmHg, then consider Hill's sign of aortic insufficiency, aortic dissection, or vascular occlusion of the upper extremities. (Could this old person have Buerger's disease or Takayasu's disease?)

Checking for Orthostatic Hypotension

Measure the supine blood pressure, then have the patient stand, and immediately recheck the blood pressure. Normally the systolic blood pressure will drop slightly and the diastolic blood pressure will rise a little to maintain mean arterial pressure. Classically orthostatic hypotension is a drop between supine and standing blood pressure of 20mmHg systolic or 10mmHg diastolic. If you know the patient is in shock (hypotensive) then orthostatic measures will not add useful information. The basic causes of orthostatic hypotension are volume depletion (the pulse will increase with the orthostatic change), neurological or autonomic dysfunction (pulse often will not increase with the orthostatic drop), cardiac failure or pheochromocytoma. Sitting blood pressure can be used when patient weakness prevents standing, but the legs should be dependent. Just sitting the person in bed is not sufficient.

Pulsus Paradoxus

• *What is the paradox in the title?* The paradox is that you can hear the heart sound at the apex but cannot feel the pulse in the periphery. Where did the pulse go? That was the historical paradox. The pulsus paradoxus is caused by increased right ventricular pressure that crowds the left ventricular outflow and reduces the left ventricular stroke volume. In addition, increased negative thoracic pressure can reduce left atrial filling. Pericardial fluid dynamics may accentuate these mechanisms. Idiopathic hypertrophic subaortic stenosis can give a "paradoxical" paradoxical pulse, with an increase in the systolic blood pressure with inspiration and a decrease with expiration.

• *How to check for a pulsus paradoxus.* After determining the blood pressure, repeat the blood pressure reading, carefully noting the systolic pressure with expiration. (Do not have the patient take a deep breath or otherwise change the respiratory pattern.) Very slowly continue lowering the blood pressure reading at no more than 2mmHg per beat until there is no loss of the Korotkov sounds with inspiration. (The beat frequency will seem to double at this point.) Note that reading. The difference between the systolic blood pressure in expiration and not hearing a loss of beats with inspiration is the paradoxical pulse (pulsus paradoxus). A pulsus of more than 10mmHg is abnormal.

• *Measurement of the pulsus paradoxus in atrial fibrillation.* Atrial fibrillation can make the determination of pulsus challenging. First, sense the basic underlying brachial arterial rate. Measure the blood pressure as described above. Let the cuff pressure go to zero and inflate the cuff to 10mmHg above the previously measured systolic pressure. Very slowly lower the cuff pressure when the patient passively expires, until you hear the first beats of the systolic pressure. (Note this value.) Sense the loss of beats (apparent slowing of the rate) during inspiration. Continue to very slowly lower the cuff pressure until no change in the rate seems to occur during inspiration. (Note that value.) The difference between the systolic pressure and the pressure where no change in rate occurs with inspiration is the pulsus paradoxus.

Most patients with significant pericardial tamponade physiology will have a pulsus paradoxus. Asthma will produce a pulsus when the FEV1 is less than 0.7 liters. Approximately 30% of cases of pulmonary embolism will have a pulsus. Any condition that creates significantly different ventricular filling pressures such as aortic insufficiency, end-stage left ventricular failure, or atrial septal defect can reduce the pulsus paradoxus.

Valsalva's Maneuver

Valsalva's maneuver is forced continuous expiration *for about 25 seconds* against a closed glottis (not puffing out the cheeks or holding your nose). The goal is to produce about 40mmHg of airway pressure. If the patient has difficulty simply bearing down, place a straw in the tubing of a blood pressure cuff and ask the patient to try to blow the pressure to 100mmHg (no one can but almost everyone will Valsalva trying to accomplish the task). Another approach is to place your hand on the patient's abdomen and have them push against it while holding their breath.

Antonio Mario Valsalva (1666–1723) was an Italian anatomist who learned microscopic anatomy from Malpighi (1628–1694). His remarkable book on the human ear, published in 1704, became the gold standard on the subject for over a century. In it he described and drew even the minute muscles and nerves of the ear, subdividing the ear into its internal, middle, and external parts, and he showed an original method of inflating the middle ear (Valsalva's maneuver). Valsalva coined the term Eustachian tube, one of the earliest known eponyms, named for Eustachio Manfredi (1674–1739). Valsalva also noted that motor paralysis occurs on the opposite side to the cerebral lesion, both in stroke and in cases of cranial injury. He made important contributions to surgery (inventing a number of useful surgical instruments), public health (he served as Inspector of Public Health in Bologna and investigated human and veterinary epidemics), and psychiatry (calling for humane treatment of insane persons).

There are four phases to the Valsalva. Phase I is onset and produces an increase in the blood pressure with no increase in pulse. It is due to aortic compression.

Phase II is the mid-strain and produces a decrease in blood pressure and an increase in the pulse due to decreased venous return and increased sympathetic tone.

Phase III is the release of the Valsalva that produces decrease in blood pressure and no change in the pulse due to blood staying in the lungs.

Phase IV is the recovery producing a blood pressure increase and pulse decrease due to increased venous return and increase in sympathetic activity.

Abnormalities in the Valsalva response suggest autonomic dysfunction. Look for loss of the reflex bradycardia that should occur on the release phase. Any cause of autonomic dysfunction can affect the Valsalva including diabetic autonomic neuropathy, chronic renal failure, and drugs.

RESPIRATIONS

The respiratory rate is straightforward to determine. Count the respirations for a minute and observe the pattern and degree of respiratory effort. Moving the diaphragm without moving any air does not count as a breath.

Respiratory Rate

The normal respiratory rate for elderly people living independently is 12 to 18 breaths per minute. The normal rate in long-term care patients is 16 to 25. No normal person has a respiratory rate of 20 or more.

An increased respiratory rate (tachypnea) is more than 20 breaths per minute (or more than 25 breaths per minute for a long-term care patient). Tachypnea suggests infection (especially sepsis), reactive airways disease (in COPD exacerbation the patient has air trapping and cannot empty the lungs), congestive heart failure (patient pants in mid-respiration), pulmonary embolus (very few patients with pulmonary embolus have respiratory rates less than 16), and metabolic acidosis. A respiratory rate over 30 in a patient with suspected abdominal disease suggests primary chest disease with referred symptoms to the abdomen. A decreased respiratory rate (less than 10 breaths per minute) is a form of hypoventilation called bradypnea. Bradypnea is seen in severe myxedema, ingestion of CNS depressants (narcotics and benzodiazepines), and CNS disease (pontine hemorrhage, hypoglycemia, meningitis).

Respiratory Patterns

Stridor, a medical emergency, is a harsh musical sound that suggests partial airway obstruction. Stridor on inspiration and expiration implies airway obstruction at the glottis. Inspiratory stridor implies upper airway obstruction while stridor mainly during expiration suggests tracheal or bronchial obstruction.

Note whether the breathing is labored or not. Pursed lips breathing is seen in end-stage emphysema as the patient tries to increase the end expiratory pressure to maintain the small airways. Wheezing suggests small reactive air-

---

Table 4.5. Causes of abnormal resting respiratory rates

Respiratory Rate	*Possible Causes*
Bradypnea (Less than 10 breaths per minute)	• Hypothyroidism • Hypoglycemia • Hypothermia • Uremia • Medication effect (especially CNS depressants) • Pontine hemorrhage • Meningitis • Increased intracranial pressure
Tachypnea (24 or more breaths per minute)	• Infection (especially pneumonia) • Chronic obstructive pulmonary disease • Congestive heart failure • Metabolic acidosis • Pulmonary embolism • Pneumothorax • Pain

way obstruction. Labored breathing prevents airway closure and suggests pneumonia or acute abdomen.

Deep rapid respiration (an exaggeration of normal) in metabolic acidosis is Kussmaul's respiration. Kussmaul's respiration is classically associated with diabetic ketoacidosis. These patients may have an increase in tidal volume. Patients have difficulty with conversation, having to breathe in between phrases.

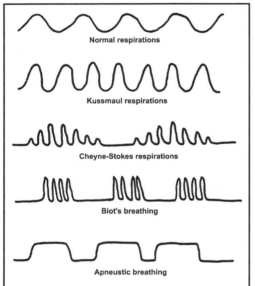

Figure 8. Respiratory Patterns.
Normal breathing is quiet and regular. Kussmaul's respirations are deep and rapid, and are generally seen metabolic acidosis (classically in diabetic ketoacidosis). The pattern of Cheyne-Stokes respiration is one of increasingly deep respirations followed by a steady diminution of breathing until an apneic episode occurs. The significance of Cheyne-Stokes respiration is prolonged circulatory time or primary neurological disease. Biot's breathing is characterized by irregularly irregular breathing with sudden apneas. It suggests CNS disease, such as increased intracranial pressure or meningitis. Apneustic breathing is seen in severely ill patients with coma. The patient holds his or her breath at the end of inspiration until the Herring-Breuer (carotid body) reflex initiates exhalation. This breathing pattern suggests pontine disease.

Adolf Kussmaul, (1822–1902) a German internist, wrote with great authority on many subjects including psychology, pathology, and neurology. He was the first to attempt esophagoscopy and gastroscopy, and introduced gastric lavage. He is also credited with the introduction of pleural tapping. Kussmaul first described the voluntary mutism seen in psychosis (Kussmaul's aphasia), and considered his book on aphasia as one of his greatest accomplishments. He was also the first to diagnose mesenteric embolism, and to describe periarteritis nodosa. Kussmaul's sign is the increase in jugular venous pressure on inspiration reflecting limited expansion of the right ventricle.

The pattern of Cheyne-Stokes respiration is one of increasingly deep respirations followed by a steady diminution of breathing until an apneic episode occurs. The significance of Cheyne-Stokes respiration is prolonged circulatory time or primary neurological disease. Some patients will show pupillary dilation with rapid breathing and pupillary contraction with apnea. The differential diagnosis of Cheyne-Stokes respiration is primary CNS disease, CHF, meningitis, pneumonia, reaction to medications, and obesity.

John Cheyne (1777–1836) was the son of a Scottish surgeon. He studied medicine and pathology at Edinburgh University and wrote his first book — Essays of Diseases of Children — in 1801. He wrote Pathology of the Membrane of the Larynx and Bronchia, in 1809. He first described acute hydrocephalus in 1808. In 1809 he went to Dublin, where he became a physician at the Meath Hospital, and soon thereafter professor of medicine. In 1820 he became Physician General in Ireland. John Cheyne is considered by some to be the founder of Irish medicine.

William Stokes' (1804–1878) father, Whitley Stokes (1763–1845), succeeded John Cheyne as professor of medicine at Meath Hospital. William Stokes was a pioneer of physical diagnosis and introduced the stethoscope to Irish physicians. His monograph was the first paper on the stethoscope written in English. Stokes is also known for Stokes-Adams syndrome of syncope caused by ventricular fibrillation and for Stokes' law that states that the muscles overlying an inflamed organ may be paralyzed.

Biot's breathing is a sign of increased intracranial pressure (Biot's sign). It is characterized by irregularly irregular breathing (the "atrial fibrillation" of respiration) with sudden apneas. It suggests CNS disease, such as increased intracranial pressure or meningitis.

Apneustic breathing is seen in severely ill patients with coma. The patient holds each breath at the end of inspiration until the Herring-Breuer (carotid body) reflex initiates exhalation. This breathing pattern suggests pontine disease.

CHAPTER 5

The Hands and Wrists

"All we have to decide is what to do with the time that is given to us."
— **J.R.R. Tolkien**

"It is a capital mistake to theorize before one has data."
— **Sir Arthur Conan Doyle**

The hands are an excellent place to begin the geriatric assessment. In social terms, hands are the least threatening part of the body to touch. By beginning the examination with a careful look at the hands, the process immediately reflects the physician's attentive, meticulous, conscientious manner — competence — to the patient.

As discussed in Chapter 1, the reverent way that a physician approaches a patient reflects a critical part of the physician's inner state. Thoughtful observation also reveals that hands have a high density of useful information. For example, information is routinely gained about overall vitality, inner emotional state, cerebral dominance, occupations and hobbies, past medical history, neuromuscular function, cardiovascular function, rheumatic conditions, dermatological problems and risk of future functional decline. The general sequence of the examination is shown in Table 5.1.

Table 5.1. The sequence of the hand examination

- Shake hands
- Check nails
- Inspect fingers
- Examine joints
- Survey palms
- Evaluate neuromuscular function
- Compare hands
- Note skin conditions

SHAKE HANDS

Occasionally a diagnosis will become evident from the handshake. Inability to let go of the hand suggests myotonia. In hyperthyroidism the palms will be moist, a fine tremor may be evident, and palmar erythema will be visible. The handshake of an anxious patient may be similar but without the red palms. A very soft velvety feeling of the skin, reminiscent of feeling a baby's foot, suggests contralateral cerebrovascular disease. If the manual softness is bilateral, consider bilateral cortical disease such as Alzheimer's disease. The handshake of a patient with acromegaly is characteristic. The hand envelops your fingers like a soft pillow and has a full, smooth appearance. Parkinsonism can sometimes be evident by the underlying tremor and cogwheel rigidity.

Variations in the Size and Shape of the Hands

Gross irregularity of shape and size suggests rheumatoid arthritis, Paget's disease of bone or, rarely, neurofibromatosis. Unilateral enlargement of a hand can be seen in significant manual labor or arteriovenous aneurysm. Square dry hands should raise the consideration of myxedema.

EXAMINE THE NAILS

Elderly people carry the last six months of their medical record on the approximately ten square centimeters of keratin comprising the fingernails. The patient's manicure can reveal state of health, nutritional status, past events, personality, occupation and one's inner state (see Table 5.2). Systemic illness should show the nail changes in each of the nails on one hand. The thumb may reveal more extensive changes, given its increased size.

Nail growth

Nail growth is continuous. It takes about six months for a fingernail in an elderly person to completely grow out. Cold temperature can slow growth rates but not to any clinically significant degree (pun intended). The middle

---

Table 5.2. Potential information available from examining the fingernails

- Overall vitality
- Inner emotional state
- Cerebral dominance
- Past medical history
- Nutritional status
- Cardiovascular function
- Occupations and hobbies
- Rheumatic conditions
- Dermatological problems

finger nail grows the fastest followed by those of the forefinger and ring finger. Aging slows the growth rate from approximately three months in childhood to six months in 70-year-olds. Nails in elderly people are also thicker than in younger people. Thin nails in a postmenopausal woman raise the possibility of metabolic bone disease. The nails of the dominant hand grow slightly quicker than the nondominant nails, probably because minor trauma accelerates nail growth. Conversely, immobility slows the growth rate of fingernails. Understanding the growth rate is important because the time interval from a critical event can be es-

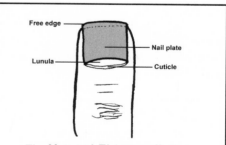

Figure 9. Normal Fingernail.

The visible portion of the nail plate extends from the cuticle to the free edge. The proximal white crescent is called the lunula. It takes approximately six months for the nail to grow from the cuticle to the free edge, so lesions seen on the nail can sometimes be dated by the location. For example, a white line halfway up the nail suggests acute illness three months earlier.

timated from the location of a nail lesion. For example, a white line appearing transversely halfway up the nail suggests an acute illness three months earlier. Regular observation will demonstrate its progression to the nail edge.

It is critical to examine the nails in adequate light. Gently rotate the nail in the light so that the reflection highlights all aspects of the nail (see Figure 9). Notice the lunula, the pale crescent-moon-like coloration at the base of the nail. Leukonychia stria and a pointed tent-like lunula suggests an excessive manicure and pushing on the cuticle (see Figure 10).

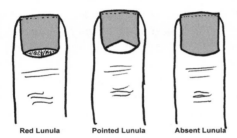

Red Lunula   Pointed Lunula   Absent Lunula

Figure 10. Abnormalities of the Lunula.
A red lunula is nonspecific but is often seen in cardiovascular illness such as congestive heart failure. A pointed lunula suggests repeated trauma, such as from excessive manicures or psychiatric illness. The absence of the lunula may reflect anemia or undernutrition.

Paronychias suggest stress and poor attention to hygiene. This can reflect depression, dementia, or psychiatric illness (see Table 5.3).

Table 5.3. Reflections of the person's inner state from the manicure

- Leukonychia stria and pointed lunula reveal cuticular trauma
- Picking off nail polish reflects nervousness and agitation
- Paronychias suggest stress
- Poor attention to hygiene raises the possibility of depression, dementia, or psychiatric illness

Nail Polish

Distance from base and line of polish gives approximate date of application. (Nails grow 0.1mm/day.) Picking at the polish reflects nervousness and agitation. Toenail polish suggests unusual flexibility or a friendly helper.

Beau's Growth Arrest Lines

In 1946, Beau described transverse lines in the substance of the nail as signs of previous acute illness. The lines look as if a little furrow had been plowed across the nail (see Figure 11). By noting its location on the nail, the approximate date of the illness can be determined. Moreover the depth of the line provides a clue to the severity of the illness. Illnesses producing Beau's lines include severe infection, myocardial infarction, hypotension, shock, or surgery. Intermittent doses of immunosuppressive therapy or chemotherapy can also produce Beau's growth arrest lines. Severe zinc deficiency has also been proposed as a cause of Beau's lines.

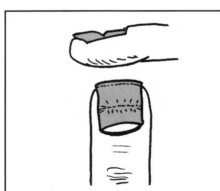

Figure 11. Beau's Growth Arrest Line.
Beau's line is a palpable transverse depression in the nail that indicates severe illness, such as severe infection, myocardial infarction, hypotension, shock, or surgery. Intermittent doses of immunosuppressive therapy or chemotherapy can also produce Beau's lines. The mechanism is growth arrest in the nail caused by the illness. The date of the insult can be timed from the location of Beau's line on the nail. Seeing the line about halfway up the nail in the illustration suggests an illness approximately three months ago.

Koilonychia (Spoon Nails)

Koilonychia gets its name from "koilos" which is the Greek word for spoon. The nail shape changes from mildly convex to frankly concave (see Figure 12). Spoon nails suggest iron deficiency, diabetes mellitus, or deficiency in sulfur-containing amino acids (especially cysteine or methionine). The thickness of the nail plate can help you to infer the underlying disorder. Soft, thin spoon nails are seen in iron deficiency and deficiency of amino acids. Since small amounts of insulin and growth hormone are necessary for amino acid transport, uncontrolled diabetes (hemoglobin A1C over 10) can produce koilonychias with thick nails (see

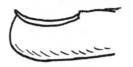

Figure 12. Spoon Nail.

In spoon nails the nail shape is concave. Ask yourself if a drop of water would stay on the nail without rolling off. If the answer is "yes, it would stay on the nail," then the nails are spoon nails. Spoon nails suggest iron deficiency, diabetes mellitus, or deficiency in sulfur-containing amino acids (especially cysteine or methionine).

Table 5.4). Rarely, spoon nails can be seen in Raynaud's phenomenon.

Table 5.4. Hand findings in diabetes mellitus		
Finding	*Differential diagnosis*	*Distinguishing features*
Spoon nails	Iron deficiency; deficiency in sulfur-containing amino acids; Raynaud's phenomenon	Thickness of nail plate: uncontrolled diabetes (hemoglobin A1C over 10) can produce thick spooned nails. Soft, thin spoon nails are seen in iron deficiency and deficiency of amino acids.
Beading of the nails	Thyroid disorder; vitamin B12 deficiency	Beading can be seen in any endocrine condition.
Dupuytren's contracture	Postmyocardial infarction; cirrhosis; Raynaud's phenomenon; syringomyelia	
Palmar xanthomas	Myxedema; renal failure; biliary cirrhosis; chronic pancreatitis; cobalt chloride toxicity	
Palmar erythema	Cirrhosis; alcoholism; hyperthyroidism; vitamin B deficiency; beriberi; rheumatoid arthritis; polycythemia rubra vera; tuberculosis; normal finding in 5% of the general population	Palms will also be sweaty with hyperthyroidism.
Atrophy of the interosseous muscles	Peripheral neuropathy; vascular disease	Fingers do not show atrophy.
Burning sensation of hands	Alcoholic neuritis; polyneuritis; lung cancer; lymphoma; gastric cancer; toxic neuritis; ischemic neuropathy; compartment syndromes	

To determine if a nail is spooned, perform the water drop test. Place a drop of water on the nail. If the drop does not slide off then the nail is flattened from early spooning. With practice you should be able to look at the nail and perform a mental water drop test.

Nail Deformities

Nail deformities may result from nutritional deficiency, infection, trauma and a variety of diseases (see Table 5.5). Test the soft-ness and flexibility of free edge by bending the nail gently downward. A firm, easy bending is normal. Next, examine the nail thickness by peering down on the fingertip. Thin, brittle nails suggest metabolic bone disease, thyroid disorder, or nutrient deficiency.

A central thin ridge can be seen in iron, folic acid, or protein deficiency (see Figure 13). Distal changes appear first and then move proximally. A central canal with a fir tree appearance is Heller's deformity, and is seen in peripheral arterial disease. Beading of the nails

Table 5.5. Useful observations of nail shapes	
Abnormal shape	*Possible associated illness*
Clubbing	• Lung cancer, pulmonic abscess, interstitial pulmonary fibrosis, sarcoidosis, beryllium poisoning, pulmonary arteriovenous fistula, subacute bacterial endocarditis, infected arterial grafts, aortic aneurysm, inflammatory bowel disease, sprue, neoplasms (esophagus, liver, bowel), hyperthyroidism
Spooned nails	• Iron deficiency, diabetes mellitus, deficiency in sulfur-containing amino acids (especially cysteine or methionine)
Transverse depression (Beau's growth arrest line)	• Significant acute illness (location of the line provides a clue to the timing of the illness)
Thin brittle nails	• Metabolic bone disease, thyroid disorder, systemic amyloidosis, severe malnutrition
Central nail ridge	• Nutritional deficiency (iron, folic acid, or protein)
Central canal	• Peripheral arterial disease, malnutrition, repetitive trauma
Nail pitting	• Psoriasis (random pits), alopecia areata (geometric rippled grid), eczema, lichen planus
Nail beading	• Endocrine disorders
Rough, sandpapered surface	• Autoimmune disease, psoriasis, chemical exposure, lichen planus
Thick coarse nails	• Onychomycosis, chronic eczema, peripheral vascular disease, Yellow nail syndrome, psoriasis
Separation of free edge	• Thyrotoxicosis, psoriasis, trauma, contact dermatitis, toxic exposures (solvents)
Curved or beaked nail of distal digit)	• Renal failure, hyperparathyroidism, psoriasis, systemic sclerosis
Nail destruction	• Trauma, paronychia, toxic epidermal necrolysis, chemotherapy, bullous diseases

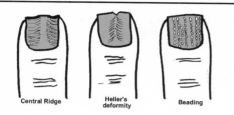

Figure 13. Abnormalities of Nail Shape.
These changes in nail shape can be useful clues to underlying illness. A central thin ridge can be seen in iron, folic acid, or protein deficiency. A central canal with a fir tree appearance is called Heller's deformity and implies peripheral arterial disease. Small longitudinal beads that resemble miniature candle wax dripping down the nail characterize beading. Beading of the nails suggests endocrine abnormalities, such as diabetes, thyroid disorder, and vitamin B12 deficiency.

suggests endocrine abnormalities such as diabetes, thyroid disorder, and vitamin B12 deficiency. Small longitudinal beads that resemble miniature candle wax dripping down the nail characterize beading.

Paronychias

Paronychias are common and result from infection along the edge of the nail. Water exposure is a risk factor. Paronychias suggest stress, trauma, bacterial infection, or herpetic whitlow. Healing can produce deformity along the side of the nail. Pseudomonas paronychia can turn the nail green.

Fungal infections frequently affect the nails. Candida species most commonly affect the fingernails while dermatophytes involve the toenails. Classically the entire nail is involved but some nails will be completely spared. There is usually heaped-up debris under the nail edge and the nail is dystrophic.

Onycholysis

The pulling away of the distal end of the nail is called onycholysis. Most commonly, onycholysis reflects thyrotoxicosis, trauma,

psoriasis, drug effect (especially tetracyclines), and chemical exposures. Sometimes anemia can produce onycholysis. In psoriasis there are pits in the nails in addition to the onycholysis. Lichen planus can also produce irregular, white, raised lesions on the distal nails.

Nail Discolorations

Minor trauma to the nail plate can injure the capillaries below the nail base. The result is a chalky white spot that appears on the nail. Multiple white patches can be seen, usually on single nails. More significant trauma produces a hematoma under the nail. Repetitive trauma from occupations such as farming can produce characteristic nail changes. Lilac discoloration along the free edge of the fingernail suggests syphilis (Millian's sign).

Vascular disease causes nail opacity. Raynaud's can cause brittle nails with longitudinal ridges and pterygia. Scleroderma produces dusky curved nails with characteristic soft tissue changes.

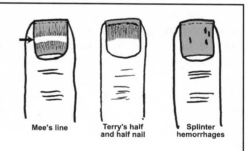

Figure 14. Abnormal Nail Colorations.
Any acute illness can produce transverse, milky, white lines called Mee's lines, if in the setting of arsenic poisoning and Reil's lines, in the setting of infection. Terry's half-and-half nails are pale at the base and dark red at the free edge. Terry's nails suggest chronic renal or liver disease. If there is a rust color line at the free edge, then consider renal disease as the cause; no brown discoloration suggests liver disease. Small, fat, red, longitudinal lines in the nail are called splinter hemorrhages, an important clue of infectious endocarditis and other conditions.

Table 5.6. Local discolorations of the nail

Discoloration	Possible associated illness
Transverse smooth white lines (Mee's lines)	• Significant illness, heavy metal toxicity, chemotherapy
Two transverse irregular lines (Muehrcke's lines)	• Hypoalbuminemia caused by edema of nail plate (these lines do not migrate)
White splotches (Leukonychia striae)	• Minor trauma to the nail matrix
Longitudinal brown lines	• Racial variation, Addison's disease, nevus at nail base, breast cancer, malignant melanoma (check for periungal pigmentation)
Splinter hemorrhages	• Infective endocarditis, systemic lupus erythematosis, trichinosis, pityriasis rubra pilaris, psoriasis, renal failure
Half white and half pink nails (Terry's half and half nails)	• Liver or renal disease (renal disease produces a brown discoloration at the free edge of the nail, while liver disease does not)

Transverse White Lines

Any acute illness can produce transverse milky white lines called Mee's lines, if in the setting of arsenic poisoning, and Reil's lines, in the setting of infection (see Figure 14). These lines should be distinguished from Muehrcke's lines which are two irregular parallel white lines caused by low serum albumin. Edema under the nail produces Muehrcke's lines which disappear when the albumin rises. Loss of the lunula reflects a low serum albumin and malnutrition.

Terry's Half-and-Half Nails

Terry's half-and-half nails are pale at the base and dark red at the free edge. Terry's nails suggest chronic renal or liver disease. If there is a rust color line at the free edge, then consider renal disease as the cause; lack of brown discoloration suggests liver disease. Terry also described a half-and-half nail where the lunula and lower half of the nail is red and the upper half is pale. These nails suggest congestive heart failure, severe lung disease or lymphoma. A completely pink nail suggests heart failure and occasionally vitamin C and B vitamin deficiencies. Lilac-colored nails may signify chronic congestive heart failure.

Splinter Hemorrhages

Small red longitudinal lines in the nail are called splinter hemorrhages, an important clue of infectious endocarditis. They should be differentiated from the black hair–like discolorations produced by trauma, in that they are wider and fuller. Transilluminating the digit can help to bring out the slightly fatter red splinters. Psoriasis can produce a reddish brown spot below the nail plate resembling an oil spot.

Yellow and White Nails

Yellow nails suggest lymphatic obstruction. Renal failure produces a brownish discoloration along the distal end of the nail just below the free margin of the nail. White nails suggest chronic liver disease or renal failure. (Look for the brown renal failure line at the distal nail margin to tell them apart).

Table 5.7. Generalized nail discoloration	
Nail discoloration	*Possible associated illness*
White nails	• Anemia, renal failure, cirrhosis, diabetes mellitus, chemotherapy, hereditary (rare)
Red or pink nails	• Polycythemia (dark red), systemic lupus erythematosis, carbon monoxide poisoning (cherry red), malnutrition
Brown or gray nails	• Topical agents, lichen planus, cardiovascular disease, diabetes mellitus, breast cancer, malignant melanoma, vitamin B12 deficiency, syphilis
Yellow nails	• Systemic amyloidosis, lymphedema and bronchiectasis (yellow nail syndrome), Median/Ulnar nerve injury, thermal injury, jaundice, diabetes mellitus
Green or black nails	• Topical preparations, chronic Pseudomonas infection, trauma

ABNORMAL FINGERS

Clubbing

Notice if the fingers are clubbed. In advanced clubbing they will be drumstick-like with the distal portion of the finger appearing slightly larger (see Figure 15). One of the earliest signs is that the nail loses its angle of in-

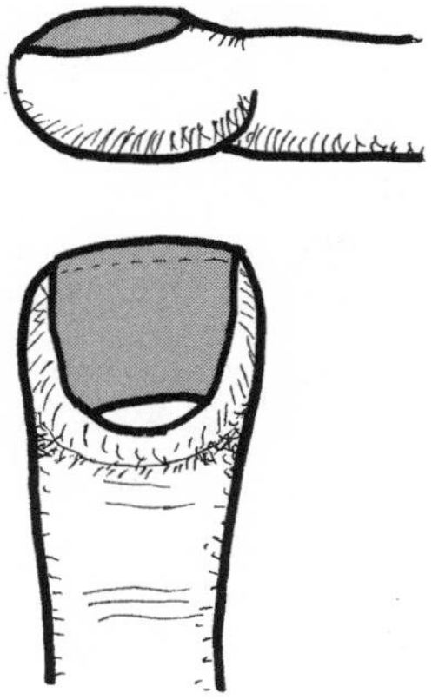

Figure 15. Clubbing.

This illustration shows advanced clubbing where the finger is drumstick-like, with the distal portion of the finger appearing slightly larger than the rest of the finger. Pulmonary and cardiovascular conditions account for 80% of clubbing.

sertion. To look for loss of this angle, check Schamroth's sign (see Figure 16) — have the patient place both forefinger nails together and look between them. If you can see a small diamond space between them, then the nails are not clubbed.

The mechanism of clubbing is not entirely clear (at least to me) although it may involve changes in autonomic control of the digital arterioles that help to modulate body heat. In addition, changes in vasomotor compounds such as kinins also affect blood flow through the fingertip. The mechanism for clubbing probably varies under differing conditions.

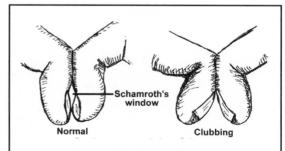

Figure 16. Schamroth's sign.

One of the earliest signs of clubbing is that the nail loses its angle of insertion. To look for loss of this angle have the patient place both forefinger nails together and look between them (Schamroth's sign). If you can see a small diamond space between them, then the nails are not clubbed.

Table 5.8. Possible causes of clubbing

Causes	Examples
Pulmonary disease	• Bronchogenic carcinoma • Alveolar cell carcinoma • Lung abscess (the condition Hippocrates first associated with clubbing) • Interstitial pulmonary fibrosis • Sarcoidosis • Beryllium poisoning
Cardiovascular illness	• Subacute bacterial endocarditis • Infected arterial grafts • Aortic aneurysm
Gastrointestinal conditions	• Inflammatory bowel disease • Sprue • Neoplasms (esophagus, liver, bowel)
Other	• Hyperthyroidism

The causes of clubbing are numerous and Table 5.8 is not exhaustive. Pulmonary causes include bronchogenic carcinoma, alveolar cell carcinoma, lung abscess (the condition Hippocrates first associated with clubbing), interstitial pulmonary fibrosis, sarcoidosis, and beryllium poisoning. Important cardiovascular causes are subacute bacterial endocarditis, infected arterial grafts, and aortic aneurysm. Gastrointestinal causes associated with clubbing are inflammatory bowel disease, sprue, and neoplasms (esophagus, liver, bowel). Hyperthyroidism can also produce clubbing.

Blunt Fingers

Large, blunt fingers suggest acromegaly. As mentioned earlier, the characteristic handshake is another clue. Small, blunt fingers can be seen in renal failure with secondary hyperparathyroidism. This condition can produce resorption of the terminal portion of the digit leading to fat, thin nails and fingers with blunt tips.

Spider Fingers, Slender Palm (Arachnodactyly)

While not often seen in old age, Marfan's syndrome sometimes produces arachnodactyly. Check Steinert's sign by having the patient make a fist over the opposed thumb; if the thumb extends beyond the base of the little finger, consider Marfan's syndrome. Significant overlap of the thumb and pinky when grasping the opposite wrist also suggests Marfan's syndrome (Wrist sign). Another cause of thin, spidery fingers is pulmonic valve stenosis.

Antoine Bernard-Jean Marfan (1858–1942) was the French father of pediatrics who first recognized the importance of skin tests for tuberculosis. In addition to describing the syndrome that bears his name, Marfan reported the spastic paraplegia of the lower extremities and mental retardation in children with congenital syphilis (Dennie-Marfan syndrome), Marfan's symptom of medial malleolar swelling in rickets, Marfan's sign of typhus (a red triangle on a furred tongue in a febrile child) and Marfan's law (which basically states that people who recover from childhood tuberculosis rarely get re-infected).

Slender, Delicate, Hyperextensible Fingers

Slender, delicate and hyperextensible fingers suggest a hypopituitary state.

Syndactylism

Abnormalities in the numbers of fingers are related to congenital malformations of the heart and great vessels. They can also be seen in normal individuals as an inherited trait.

Other Abnormal Finger Findings

Having the patient make a fist and then seeing a dimpled fourth knuckle can determine a foreshortened fourth metacarpal bone (Fuller Albright's sign). This suggests pseudo-hypoparathyroidism.

> *Fuller Albright (1900–1969) was the remarkable American endocrinologist who coined the term "Cushing's syndrome." Albright was an extensive clinical researcher, especially in the parathyroid gland, bone and mineral metabolism and abnormalities of sex hormones. He developed an elegant method of FSH measurement and distinguished several forms of primary amenorrhea including Klinefelter's syndrome. (He reportedly let Klinefelter be the first author on the paper.)*

A very short pinky suggests congenital syphilis (Du Bois' sign).

JOINT FINDINGS

Various arthritides can produce findings on the hands. These clues are well worth appreciating if they are present because musculoskeletal problems are common in elderly people.

Osteoarthritis

Osteoarthritis produces nontender bony nodules of the distal interphalangeal joints and proximal interphalangeal joints called Heberden's nodes and Bouchard's nodes, respectively. Involvement of the metacarpophalangial (MCP) joints should suggest another diagnosis.

> *William Heberden (1710–1801) quickly established himself as an outstanding physician. When he was asked to accept an appointment to the court of King George III as the personal physician to the Queen, Heberden initially was reluctant to accept because he feared that it might interfere with his usual work of visiting and treating the sick.*
>
> *He would record, in Latin, the historical and physical particulars, and outcome of all of his patients. Then, at the end of every month, he reviewed his records to try to draw more general conclusions from his observations. To take it a step further, he spent the last twenty years of his life organizing these notes into the publication* Commentaries on the History and Cure of Diseases. *Heberden was the first to describe angina pectoris, and described the features differentiating chickenpox from smallpox. He also observed the improvement in tuberculosis with pregnancy.*
>
> *The diarist Samuel Johnson lauded Heberden's scholarly approach and contributions to medical care. Heberden's virtue perhaps had even medical benefit, as he lived to age 91.*

Autoimmune Disease

Rheumatoid arthritis is a symmetrical small joint polyarthritis (sparing the DIPs) that produces swan neck deformities, boutonniere deformities, and ulnar deviation. It can produce fusiform swelling of the fingers during the acute phase of the illness. Remember that rheumatoid arthritis affects the ulna side of the wrist and tends to spare the radial side of the wrist. Synovial swelling of the PIP joints is called Haygart's nodes. Lack of ability to fold the hands in prayer suggests rheumatoid arthritis of the carpal joints (Plotz's sign).

Systemic lupus erythematosus can affect the hand in several ways. The joint findings are a symmetrical non-deforming polyarthritis with a rash that spares the knuckles. The rash is in contrast to dermatomyositis where there is a rash or ivory-colored (Gottron's) papules on the knuckles. Heinrich Adolf Gottron (1890–1974) was a German dermatologist who also described a variant of progeria (Gottron's syndrome).

Gouty Arthritis

Gout is evident by tophaceus deposits on the hands that appear as salmon-colored nodules.

Psoriatic Arthritis

Psoriasis tends to produce significant deformity affecting the DIP joints. Nail pitting and classical skin signs are usually present.

PHYSICAL FINDINGS IN THE PALM

Callus

Occupational and avocational causes of characteristic callus formation are shown in Table 5.9. Callosities on the non-dominant palm at the base of the fingers are sometimes seen in golfers. Calluses on the non-dominant fingertips sparing the thumb suggest a steel-string guitar player. (The nails will be shorter than the dominant nails). Circular blisters on the medial side of the thumb reflect a weekend gardener with raking or shoveling trauma. Writers using old-fashioned pencil and paper develop a callus on the medial portion of the middle finger where the writing utensil rubs the digit. If you see a callus ask the patient what activity produces the mark.

More extensive callus formation (actually palmar hyperkeratosis) is called tylosis and is associated with squamous cell carcinoma of the esophagus, lung cancer, and bladder cancer. Arsenical toxicity produces hyperkeratoses of the palms with a yellowish waxy feel. Check for Mee's lines on the fingernails.

Dupuytren's Contracture

Dupuytren's contracture is a fibrosis of the palmar tendons usually affecting the ring and little finger. Palpating along the tendon can sometimes identify the lesion more easily than it can be seen. Conditions associated with Dupuytren's contracture include diabetes mel-

Table 5.9. Calluses on the hand	
Location	Possible Cause
Non-dominant palm at the base of the fingers	• Golfing
Non-dominant fingertips sparing the thumb	• Steel-string guitar playing (the nails will be shorter than the dominant nails)
Circular blisters on the medial side of the thumb	• Gardening, raking or shoveling
Medial portion of the middle finger	• Writing, using old-fashioned pencil and paper (callus develops where the writing utensil rubs the digit)
Extensive palmar callus	• Squamous cell carcinoma of the esophagus, lung cancer, and bladder cancer (callus is called tylosis)
Waxy palmar hyperkeratoses	• Arsenical toxicity (check for Mee's lines on the fingernails)

litus, postmyocardial infarction, cirrhosis, and Raynaud's phenomenon, though it is sometimes associated with syringomyelia and seen in normal persons. Tenderness over the palmar MCPs suggests flexion tenosynovitis.

Baron Guillaume Dupuytren (1777–1835) was born impoverished and remained quite poor through medical school. It is said that he lived in a garret lit by a lamp that burned oil from the fat of cadavers in the dissecting room. As chief of surgery, he led the Hôtel-Dieu to a leading position in Europe. His ambition earned him the nicknames "Napoleon of Surgery" and "The Beast at the Seine." He was once described as "first among surgeons and last among men." Dupuytren was the first to correctly describe the pathology of the contracture that bears his name.

Dupuytren's very busy practice made him one of the wealthiest physicians of his time. He offered to give Charles X one million francs when the former king was dethroned and in need of money. This was actually out of character, as Dupuytren was generally considered quite parsimonious. In 1833, he suffered a stroke while giving a lecture but insisted on finishing the address. He lived only two years longer, and died in Paris at age 58.

Xanthomata

Xanthomas are deposits of fats and cholesterol. The presence of xanthomas raises the question of a familial disorder or hypercholesterolemia, especially type II and type IV. Apoprotein abnormalities can also produce xanthomas. Palmar xanthomas suggest diabetes mellitus, myxedema, renal failure, biliary cirrhosis (mainly in children), chronic pancreatitis, and cobalt chloride toxicity.

Palmar erythema

Red palms are often due to states that increase the amount of circulating estrogens. Conditions producing palmar erythema include cirrhosis (liver palms), alcoholism, hyperthyroidism (erythema and sweat), diabetes mellitus, vitamin B deficiency, beriberi, rheumatoid arthritis, polycythemia rubra vera, and

tuberculosis. Palmar erythema also occurs in 3–5% of normal persons.

Unusual Colors on the Palm

Blue palmar creases suggest the possibility of generalized purpura. Pale, silvery, or white creases that do not darken with hyperextension reflect hemoglobin below 7gm/100ml. Normally, hyperextending the palm causes the creases to turn a dark red color. Dark brown or black palmar creases raise the possibility of Addison's disease, but those are also a normal racial variation. Petechiae on the palm suggest blood dyscrasias, thrombocytopenic purpura, subacute bacterial endocarditis, and scurvy. Livedo reticularis over the palm raises the possibility of the anti-phospholipid antibody syndrome.

NEUROMUSCULAR CONDITIONS

General Painless Atrophy

Painless atrophy of the intrinsic muscles of the hand without sensory loss suggests central nervous system disease such as amyotrophic lateral sclerosis, Charcot-Marie-Tooth peroneal atrophy, syringomyelia (loss of heat, cold and pain sensation), and loss of function as in old rheumatoid arthritis. Occasionally neural leprosy can produce this finding.

General Painful Atrophy

Painful atrophy suggests peripheral neuropathy; extrinsic pressure on the nerves (cervical, axillary, supraclavicular or brachial); Pancoast's tumor in the pulmonary apex (look for Horner's syndrome); aneurysms of the subclavian arteries, axillary vessels, or thoracic aorta; cervical rib; degenerative arthritis of cervical spine; and herniation of a cervical intervertebral disc.

Table 5.10. Causes of atrophy of the intrinsic muscles of the hand

Painless atrophy (without sensory loss)	*Painful atrophy*
Diabetes mellitus	• Peripheral neuropathy
Charcot-Marie-Tooth peroneal atrophy	• Extrinsic pressure on the nerves (cervical, axillary, supraclavicular, or brachial)
Syringomyelia (loss of heat, cold, and pain sensation)	• Pancoast's tumor in the pulmonary apex
Loss of function, as in old rheumatoid arthritis	• Aneurysms of the subclavian arteries, axillary vessels, or thoracic aorta
Neural leprosy	• Cervical rib
Amyotrophic lateral sclerosis	• Degenerative arthritis of cervical spine
	• Herniation of a cervical disk

Possible Radial Nerve Palsy (Wrist Drop)

Check wrist extension and thumb extension (toward the radius) for signs of radial nerve damage. Weakness producing wrist drop can be caused by lead poisoning, alcoholism, polyneuritis, trauma, polyarteritis, and neurosyphilis. Since the radial nerve supplies the forefinger and the wrist extensors, inability to extend the forefinger can be a sign of radial nerve palsy even if the wrist extensors are normal. If you suspect radial nerve damage, check the sensation at the base of the thumb.

Possible Ulnar Nerve Palsy

Check finger abduction by asking the patient to spread fingers as wide as possible. Difficulty with this suggests ulnar neuropathy. Abduction of the fifth finger suggests ulnar nerve palsy (Wartenberg's finger sign). Another excellent maneuver (provided the median nerve is intact) is testing for Froment's sign. Have the patient pinch a piece of paper between the thumb and the radial aspect of the forefinger. If you can pull out the paper there is ulnar nerve weakness and Froment's sign is present.

If you suspect ulnar nerve palsy, look for hypothenar atrophy and interosseous atrophy. The sensation of the little finger and usually the ulnar side of the ring finger will be impaired. Also check for atrophy of the flexor carpi ulnaris in the forearm. (If you have forgotten the location of this useful muscle, flex and extend your ring and little fingers and observe the muscles that contract in your medial forearm.) No atrophy of the flexor carpi ulnaris suggests ulnar nerve entrapment at the wrist (ulnar tunnel syndrome). Atrophy suggests C8 radiculopathy or nerve entrapment at the elbow (cubital tunnel syndrome). Polyneuritis and trauma can produce ulnar neuropathy in addition to the entrapment syndromes. Anesthesia of the ulna nerve in the setting of neurosyphilis is Biernacki's sign.

Possible Median Nerve Palsy

One tip off to a possible median nerve problem is inability of the patient to flex the forefinger and sometimes the middle finger. (This posture is called the papal benediction hand.) To test for median nerve integrity check the "OK" sign. Have the patient make an "OK" sign by opposing the thumb and forefinger to make a ring. Check the strength of the "O" by trying to open it with your fingers. Weakness indicates a median nerve abnormality.

Have the patient make a fist, to test the finger flexors and to see if the forefinger can flex. Also look for thenar atrophy, which reflects median neuropathy. If these signs are present, then check for atrophy of the flexor carpi radialis. (If necessary, refresh your memory by making a fist and feeling the muscle contraction on the lateral forearm.) No atrophy of the flexor carpi radialis suggests entrapment at the wrist (carpal tunnel syndrome). Atrophy of the flexor carpi radialis suggests entrapment at the elbow (pronator syndrome due to entrapment by the ligament of the pronator teres).

If the findings suggest carpal tunnel syndrome, check Tinel's sign (see Figure 17) and consider rheumatoid arthritis, tenosynovitis of the wrist, amyloidosis, gout, myxedema, plasmacytoma, and acromegaly.

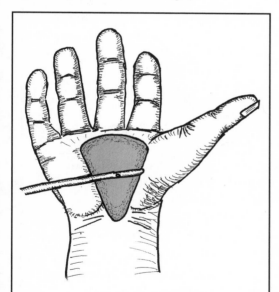

Figure 17. Tinel's Sign.
Jules Tinel (1879–1952) is remembered for his two signs that each involve tapping on a peripheral nerve trunk. One sign, illustrated in this figure, is tapping over the median nerve in the wrist and producing a tingling sensation in the setting of carpal tunnel syndrome. The other sign is tapping over any peripheral nerve trunk that has been damaged and noting the tingling sensation as a sign of nerve regeneration.

COLOR CHANGES IN THE HANDS

Cyanosis

Cyanosis of the hands suggests congestive heart failure, cor pulmonale, Raynaud's phenomenon, systemic lupus erythematosus, polycythemia, drug effects (including the Coumadin "purple fingers & toes syndrome" and phenolphthalein ingestion), arteriovenous aneurysm, myxedema, and syringomyelia (Morvan's disease).

Pallor

Pallor of the hands can reflect anemia, aortic insufficiency ("paradoxical pallor"), Raynaud's phenomenon, and vasospasm (consider tobacco abuse, Buerger's disease, anxiety, and vasomotor instability).

Rubor

A red, sunburned appearance on the dorsum of the hand suggests pellagra. Generalized rubor can be a sign of polycythemia, systemic lupus erythematosus (especially involving the fingertips), dermatomyositis, and chronic lymphocytic leukemia. Coldness, redness and edema of the hand suggest syringomyelia (Marinesco's sign).

Georges Marinesco (1864–1938) was a Romanian neurologist who published over 250 articles on a variety of topics, ranging from the bone changes in acromegaly to the patterns of body movement in health and disease. With colleagues, he published an atlas of pathological neurohistology. He described senile neuritic plaques and a case of parkinsonian tremor caused by a tumor in the substantia nigra. These observations led to Broussard's hypothesis that Parkinson's was caused by disease in the substantia nigra.

Miscellaneous Pigmentations

Pigmentation overlying the dorsum veins suggests lymphoma (especially Hodgkin's

Table 5.11. Hand findings: Alphabetic Listing of Useful Signs

Name of the Sign or Test	Description	Positive Finding	Interpretation
Dubois' sign		Very short pinky	Suggests congenital syphilis
Eichhoff–Finkelstein's sign	Have the patient make a fist over the opposed thumb and then flex and ulnarly deviate the fist.	Pain over the anatomic snuffbox or production of a painful click	Thumb dysfunction from de Quervain's tenosynovitis
Froment's sign	Have the patient pinch a piece of paper between the thumb and the radial aspect of the forefinger.	If you can pull out the paper, Froment's sign is present.	Ulnar nerve weakness
Fuller Albright's sign	Have the patient make a fist.	Dimpled fourth knuckle	Foreshortened fourth metacarpal bone, which suggests pseudohypoparathyroidism
Grind test	Grasp the patient's thumb and gently grind it like a peppermill.	Pain	Osteoarthritis of the thumb
Gubler's sign		Fusiform swelling of the dorsal wrist	Suggests chronic lead poisoning
Kanaval's sign		Passive extension of the digits produces pain on the dorsum of the hand.	Tenosynovitis
Maisonneuve's sign		Extreme hyper-extension of the hand	Suggests a Colles fracture
Millan's sign		Lilac discoloration along the free edge of the fingernail	Possible syphilis
"OK" sign	Have the patient make an "OK" sign by opposing the thumb and forefinger to make a ring. Check the strength of the "O" by trying to open it with your fingers.	Tests integrity of the median nerve	Weakness indicates median nerve abnormality.

Table 5.11. **Hand findings: Alphabetic Listing of Useful Signs (continued)**

Name of the Sign or Test	*Description*	*Positive Finding*	*Interpretation*
Pastia's sign		Pink or red transverse lines along the wrists, antecubital fossa, or groin that remain hyperpigmented	Suggests scarlet fever
Plotz's sign		Lack of ability to fold hands in prayer position	Possible rheumatoid arthritis of the carpal joints
Schamroth's sign	Have the patient place both forefinger nails together and look between them.	If you can see a small diamond space between them, then the nails are not clubbed. No diamond space, then clubbing is present.	Many pulmonary, cardiac, and gastric conditions can cause clubbing (see text). Hyperthyroidism can also cause clubbing.
Steinert's sign	Have the patient make a fist over the opposed thumb.	If the thumb extends beyond the base of the little finger, the test is positive	Possible Marfan's syndrome
Wartenberg's finger sign		Abduction of the fifth finger	Suggests ulnar nerve palsy
Watson's stress test	Pinch the patient's hand between your thumb at the anatomic snuffbox and your forefinger at the palmar base of the thumb, then, as you radially deviate the wrist, release your forefinger.	If you feel a click with your thumb, the test is positive.	Scapholunate sprain or dislocation
Wrist sign		Significant overlap of the thumb and pinky when grasping the opposite wrist	Possible Marfan's syndrome

disease). Diffuse melanosis can reflect Addison's disease or malignant melanoma. A slate-gray pigmentation to the hands suggests silver ingestion (argyria). Yellow palms can be a sign of pernicious anemia, carotinemia, or laborers' callus. Depigmentation raises the possibility of vitiligo, pinta, postdermatitis, scleroderma, and dermatomyositis. Purpura suggests subacute bacterial endocarditis, thrombocytopenic purpura, and blood dyscrasias. A rash of the palms and soles has a limited differential that includes Rocky Mountain spotted fever, secondary syphilis, and coxsackie infection. Pink or red transverse lines along the wrists, antecubital fossa, or groin that remain hyperpigmented suggest scarlet fever (Pastia's sign).

Ulcerative Lesions on the Hands

Hand ulcers have a fairly limited differential diagnosis. Conditions to consider include sporotrichosis (rose gardeners' disease), cutaneous anthrax, actinomycosis, coccidiomycosis, tuberculosis, tularemia, syphilis (the ulcer should feel like a coin under the skin because the margins of the ulcer are usually fibrotic), leishmaniasis, and blastomycosis.

SPECIAL CIRCUMSTANCES

Painful hands

A burning sensation of the hands suggests alcoholic neuritis, polyneuritis, diabetes mellitus (look for atrophy of the interosseous muscles), carcinoma of the lung (check for the thenar atrophy of a Pancoast's tumor), lymphoma, gastric carcinoma, chemical neuritis (look for antimony, benzene, bismuth, carbon tetrachloride, heavy metals, alcohol, arsenic, lead, or gold), ischemic neuropathy (sensory loss in fingers), compartment syndromes, B

vitamin deficiency, or hookworm infestation. Trousseau's sign (carpal digital spasm) with ischemic vasoconstriction of the fingers is the Kahn-Falta sign.

Arthridities can also produce hand pain, so check for tenosynovitis. If passive extension of the digits produces pain on the dorsum of the hand, then Kanavel's sign of tenosynovitis is present.

Shoulder-hand syndrome produces pain, stiffness, and swelling in the hand but spares the elbow. Miscellaneous causes of hand pain include myocardial infarction, Pancoast tumor, brain tumor, intrathoracic neoplasms, cervical spondylosis, vascular occlusion, hemiplegia, and herpes zoster.

Edema of the Hands

Edema of the hands can be associated with generalized anasarca, or hypoproteinemia. To tell whether the edema is protein-rich or hypoalbuminemic in origin, check the pit recovery time. Push into the edema fluid to produce a pit. Protein-poor fluid will spring back quickly (like pushing into a balloon filled with saline); protein-rich fluid will retain the pit for more than a minute. Protein-poor fluid suggests hepatic disease, renal disease or malnutrition. Protein-rich fluid suggests cardiac disease (congestive heart failure) or inflammation.

Vascular obstruction can also produce swollen hands. Superior vena caval syndrome can result from superior thoracic outlet tumor, mediastinal tumor or inflammation, pulmonary apex tumor, aneurysm of the ascending or transverse aorta or axillary artery, or pressure on the innominate or subclavian vessels.

Ischemic paralysis produces a cold, blue, swollen, numb hand. Lymphatic obstruction suggests lymphoma, axillary mass, metastatic tumor, abscess, leukemia, or postoperative lymphedema from radical mastectomy, hemiplegic hand, syringomyelia, Raynaud's phenomenon, myositis and trichiniasis.

CHANGE IN FUNCTION

Decreased Finger Range of Motion

Decreased range of motion of the fingers suggests arthritides, fracture, and collateral ligament sprain. (Look for medial or lateral PIP swelling.) Flexion tenosynovitis can present with intermittent "locking" (trigger finger), tenderness over the palmar tendons and a snap or click on flexion and extension. For diffuse tenosynovitis check Kanavel's sign (vide supra).

Decreased Thumb Range of Motion

Osteoarthritis of the thumb is very common. Check the grind test for osteoarthritis of the thumb. Grasp the patient's thumb and gently grind it like a peppermill. Pain on movement is a positive test.

Scaphoid fracture will show tenderness and depression over the anatomical snuffbox (see Figure 18). Ulnar collateral ligament tear will present as swelling at the base of the thumb, tenderness on the medial aspect, and excessive

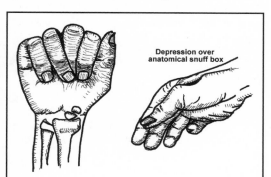

Figure 18. Scaphoid Fracture.
A scaphoid fracture is usually caused by a fall on an outstretched hand. There is tenderness and depression of the anatomical snuffbox and tenderness of the scaphoid tubercle. When the patient makes a fist the fingers should normally point to the scaphoid. Seeing the ring finger deviate toward the thumb in the setting of wrist pain suggests a fracture.

abduction to passive flexion and extension (>30 degrees and 10 degrees). Fracture can also limit the function of the thumb.

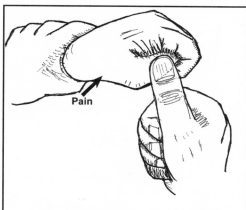

Figure 19. Finkelstein's Test.
Finkelstein's test is a way to check for de Quervain's tenosynovitis as a cause of thumb pain. Have the patient make a fist over the opposed thumb and then flex and ulnarly deviate the fist; pain over the anatomic snuffbox or producing a painful click is a positive test.

Another cause of thumb dysfunction is de Quervain's tenosynovitis. To test for this, check for Eichhoff-Finkelstein's sign (see Figure 19). Have the patient make a fist over the opposed thumb and then flex and ulnarly deviate the fist. Pain over the anatomic snuffbox or producing a painful click is a positive test.

Fritz de Quervain (1868–1940) was a Swiss surgeon with a special interest in the thyroid gland. He introduced an iodized tablet in the treatment of thyroid disease. He was one of the first clinicians to appreciate that some postoperative pneumonias were in fact caused by pulmonary emboli. In addition to the chronic tenosynovitis that bears his name, de Quervain also described subacute inflammation of the thyroid gland after viral illness (de Quervain's stuma), and a syndrome of male pseudohermaphroditism caused by complete testicular feminization (de Quervain's syndrome).

Wrist and Hand Problems

Ulnar swelling and ecchymoses suggest a boxer's fracture. Pushing on the extended fingers and gently palpating the area or visible deformity can sometimes diagnose fractures. Fracture of the little finger can result in a dropped knuckle when the patient makes a fist.

Diffuse tenosynovitis causes swelling of the wrists and can be seen in gout and pseudogout. Check for Kanavel's sign. Fusiform swelling of the dorsal wrist suggests chronic lead poisoning (Gubler's sign).

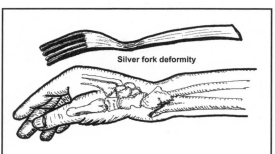

Figure 20. Colles Fracture.

Colles fracture is a transverse fracture of the distal radius where the distal fracture fragment is displaced superiorly. The lateral view of the wrist is often depressed, producing a silver fork deformity.

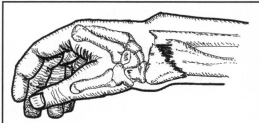

Figure 21. Smith's Fracture.

Smith's fracture is a fracture of the distal radius where the distal fragment is displaced toward the palm. This produces a marked drop-off at the wrist.

Colles fracture is a transverse fracture of the distal radius (see Figure 20). Extreme hyperextension of the hand suggests a Colles fracture (Maisonneuve's sign). The lateral view of the wrist is often depressed, producing a silver fork deformity. A very prominent ulnar head in the wrist suggests Smith's fracture where the radial segment is displaced toward the palm (see Figure 21).

Finally, consider scapholunate sprain or dislocation. To test for this, perform Watson's stress test. Pinch the patient's hand between your thumb at the anatomic snuffbox and your forefinger at the palmar base of the thumb, and as you radially deviate the wrist release your forefinger. If you feel a click with your thumb, the test is positive.

CHAPTER 6

The Upper Extremities

"Although nature commences with reason and ends in experience, it is necessary for us to do the opposite, that is to commence with experience and from this to proceed to investigate the reason."

— **Leonardo da Vinci**

"If the artist is obligated to communicate his meaning, the public in return should bear in mind that they are no less obligated to make an effort to understand what the artist is attempting to say to them."

— **Francis Henry Taylor**

The upper extremity examination is clinically important because upper extremity skills are essential in the performance of activities of daily living. The assessment mainly consists of careful examination of the elbow and shoulder. Elbow and shoulder problems are very common in elderly people.

ELBOW EXAMINATION

The elbow is a complex hinge with the basic range of motion being in a single plane. Pronation and supination of the forearm result from motion of the radius on the capitellum at the elbow and at the radioulnar articulation at the wrist.

> **Table 6.1. Sequence of the elbow examination**
>
> - Inspect the elbow for deformities and nodules
> - Check the passive and active range of motion
> - Feel for epitroclear lymphadenopathy and areas of tenderness
> - Search for nerve entrapment syndromes

INSPECTION

The elbow joint is fairly visible and many abnormalities can be uncovered by careful observation (see Figure 22). Most of the joint action is best observed from the side of the patient and from the back. The angle of full extension is called the carrying angle. It is about 10 degrees in men and slightly greater in women. Any significant increase or decrease in this angle indicates significant elbow pathology.

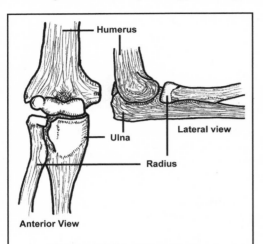

Figure 22. The Elbow Joint.
The elbow is a complex hinge consisting of articulations between three bones, the humerus, radius, and ulna. The elbow joint is fairly visible and many abnormalities can be uncovered by careful observation.

Bony Deformities

Elbow deformities usually result from previous trauma and may not be conspicuous when the elbow is flexed. Check for cubitus varus and cubitus valgus deformities with the forearm extended as straight as possible, but not hyperextended (see Figure 23). Varus deformity (sometimes called gunstock deformity) represents a decrease in the carrying angle and is usually caused by a previous supracondylar fracture. A cubitus valgus deformity is an increase in the carrying angle. It can be associated with chronic stretching of the ulnar nerve. Sometimes former throwing athletes, such as football quarterbacks or baseball players, will have an increase in the carrying angle on their dominant arm.

The epicondyles and the olecranon should form an equilateral triangle when viewed from the back (see Figure 24). Consider subluxation

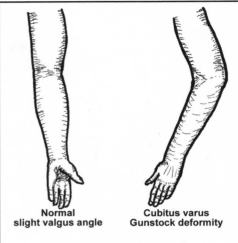

Figure 23. Carrying Angle.
The angle of full elbow extension is called the carrying angle. It is about 10° in men and slightly greater in women. Any significant increase or decrease in this angle indicates significant elbow pathology. Varus deformity (called a gunstock deformity) represents a decrease in the carrying angle and is usually caused by a previous supracondylar fracture.

if the triangle is not present or if there is extreme prominence of the olecranon. This finding is seen in rheumatoid arthritis.

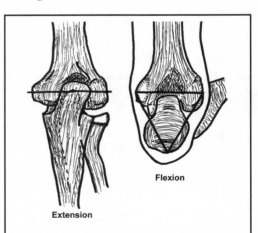

Figure 24. Posterior View of the Elbow.
When the elbow is extended and viewed from behind, the epicondyles and the olecranon form a straight line. On flexion to 90° the olecranon and epicondyles form an equilateral triangle. If the triangle is not evident consider subluxation or previous fracture.

Nodules and Swelling

Rheumatoid nodules are located on the medial aspect of the extensor surface of the elbow. An old clinical teaching was that the first rheumatoid nodule would be located exactly two inches distal to the elbow joint (possibly caused by minor trauma from sitting at a table, since the forearm usually contacts the table edge approximately two inches from the joint).

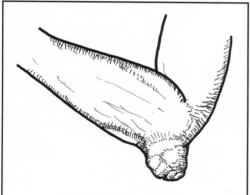

Figure 25. Gouty Tophi.

Tophaceous gout can appear around the elbow joint as irregular lumpy masses. The masses do not transilluminate, which helps to differentiate them from olecranon bursitis. Finding tophi on the hands, or feet (and occasionally on the pinna if the patient has lived in a cold climate) helps confirm the finding.

Tophi are also found around the elbow joint. The presence of other tophaceus deposits helps distinguish these nodules from other possibilities.

Swelling from an effusion can sometimes be appreciated on the side of the elbow, as a bulging in the olecranon groove.

Atrophy and Muscle Wasting

Careful inspection can also reveal scars from previous surgery or trauma, and muscle wasting or atrophy from ulnar or median nerve entrapment (see Figure 26).

Check for atrophy of the flexor carpi ul-

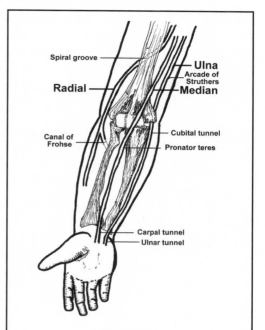

Figure 26.
Peripheral Nerve Entrapment Locations.

The radial nerve can be damaged or trapped in the spiral groove of the humerus, especially following medial humeral compression (Saturday Night Palsy). More distally, the posterior interosseus nerve can be trapped in the Canal of Frohse penetrating the supinator muscle. The ulna nerve can be compressed in the Arcade of Struthers in the upper arm or in the cubital tunnel at the elbow. More distally the ulna can be entrapped at the wrist in the ulnar tunnel. The median nerve is most often compressed in the carpal tunnel but can rarely be trapped in the pronator teres muscle. Redrawn from John Patton's *Neurological Differential Diagnosis*, 2nd Edition, 1995. Figure 16.1, page 283. Used with permission of Springer Science and Business Media.

naris in the forearm. (If you have forgotten the location of this useful muscle, flex and extend your ring and little fingers and observe the muscles that contract in the medial forearm.) Atrophy of this muscle suggests radiculopathy of the eighth cervical nerve root (C8) or nerve entrapment at the elbow (cubital tunnel syndrome). Polyneuritis and trauma can produce ulnar neuropathy in addition to the entrapment syndromes.

Atrophy of the flexor carpi radialis of the lateral forearm suggests entrapment of the median nerve at the elbow (also called pronator syndrome — due to entrapment by the ligament of the pronator teres).

ACTIVE RANGE OF MOTION

Elbow range of motion is critical to feeding, using a telephone and opening a door, so it is important to carefully assess passive and active mobility. Pain can produce a difference in the passive and active range of motion.

End Point Resistance

Joint abnormalities can change the feel of the movement and the nature of the feeling at the extremes of the range. For example, a rubbery endpoint suggests that something is inside the joint. A rock-hard endpoint at the extremes implies bone-on-bone limitation. Muscle contraction due to spasm or pain produces a fluid increase in resistance.

Elbow Flexion and Extension

Flexion and extension are key components of the elbow range of motion needed to perform daily activities. Limited range of motion suggests degenerative joint disease or previous fracture. Limited extension is an important sign of abnormality in the elbow joint because it is the first aspect of the range of motion to be influenced. Painful extension suggests the radial tunnel syndrome or lateral epicondylitis. Painful flexion suggests medial epicondylitis.

Supination and Pronation

Supination and pronation are not as critical for activities of daily living as flexion and

extension. Impairment suggests degenerative joint disease or previous radial fracture. Pain on supination and pronation suggests fracture of the radial head. Lead pipe rigidity to passive supination and pronation of the forearm suggests early Parkinsonism.

PALPATION

Epitroclear lymph nodes

The presence of epitroclear lymph nodes is always abnormal and suggests syphilis. An easy way to feel for them is to shake hands with the patient while you support the elbow in the palm of your other hand. Your supporting fingers will lie along the medial aspect of the upper arm in position to appreciate any nodules or swelling. This technique was called "the potential father-in-law's handshake" for obvious reasons.

Tenderness and Swelling Over the Olecranon

Tenderness and swelling over the olecranon suggests olecranon bursitis. Transilluminate the swelling to differentiate olecranon bursitis (which transilluminates) from gouty tophi, rheumatoid nodules or abscess, which allow no transillumination (see Figure 25). The olecranon bursa does not communicate with the joint; therefore, elbow range of motion may not be painful with this condition. A gelatinous mass with internal nodules suggests chronic olecranon bursitis. Consider diabetes mellitus, renal failure and systemic lupus erythematosus (SLE) as predisposing causes.

Tenderness Over the Medial Aspect of the Elbow

Tenderness over the medial aspect of the elbow is an important observation. Discomfort over the medial epicondyle suggests medial

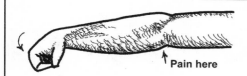

Figure 27. Golfer's Elbow Test.
Discomfort over the medial epicondyle suggests medial epicondylitis or golfer's elbow (a linguistic misfortune since the discomfort has little to do with playing golf). Characteristically there will be pain at the medial epicondyle on passive or resisted palmar flexion at the wrist.

epicondylitis or golfer's elbow. Characteristically there will be pain on resisted palmar flexion at the wrist (see Figure 27).

Check for a dimple next to the radial head, which suggests a severe medial collateral ligament tear. If present, test for stability by having the patient lie supine with their arm held perpendicular (straight up in the air) and the elbow flexed about 30 degrees to move the olecranon from its fossa. Stability can be assessed by gently moving the joint medially and laterally in both supination and pronation.

Also check for median nerve entrapment syndromes (see Chapter 5). Carpel tunnel syndrome is entrapment at the wrist. Check Tinel's sign (reproducing tingling paresthesias by tapping on the nerve in the middle of the wrist) and touching thumb to the fingertips to evaluate median nerve function. In addition, perform Phalen's maneuver by having the dorsal aspects of the hands touching to produce tingling on acute passive wrist flexion. The anterior interosseous syndrome is nerve entrapment between wrist and elbow.

Thumb weakness and thenar atrophy without Tinel's sign suggest the pronator syndrome with nerve entrapment at the elbow. The patient may have a claw hand with weakness of finger flexion, weak "OK" sign and thenar atrophy.

Jules Tinel (1879–1952) was a French neurologist born in a family with five generations of physicians. His teachers were some of the greatest

names in French medicine at the beginning of the twentieth century. He obtained his doctorate in 1910. During World War I he served as the head of the neurological center in Le Mans, France. After the war Tinel worked on the psychosomatic aspects of medicine. He was actively involved in the French resistance and was imprisoned. When he retired in 1945 he worked in the Boucicaut Hospital, Paris, France, and died of heart failure in 1952.

Tinel is remembered for his two signs: each involves tapping on a peripheral nerve trunk. One sign is tapping over the median nerve in the wrist, producing the tingling sensation of carpal tunnel syndrome. The other sign is tapping over any peripheral nerve trunk that has been damaged and noting the tingling sensation as a sign of regeneration.

Tenderness Over the Lateral Aspect of the Elbow

Tenderness to palpation over lateral epicondyle suggests lateral epicondylitis (tennis elbow). Pain can be demonstrated on resisted dorsiflexion of the wrist. Pain at the lateral epicondyle on passive pronation of forearm is called Mill's maneuver. Check Cozen's sign (flexing elbow against resistance with fist held in pronation).

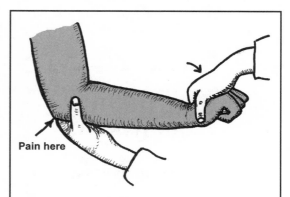

Figure 28. Cozen's Sign.
Cozen's sign is pain in the region of the lateral epicondyle when flexing the elbow against resistance with fist held in pronation. The sign suggests lateral epicondylitis or tennis elbow. Pain can be also be demonstrated on resisted dorsiflexion of the wrist.

Check for radial nerve entrapment by looking for decreased sensation over the dorsal hand and lateral forearm. Also look for painful finger extension with the wrist flexed and pronated. Another clue of radial nerve entrapment is tingling in the radial distribution with tapping over arcade of Frohse, which is present in over 60% of individuals and is located in the superior hiatus of the supinator muscle.

Tenderness of the medial aspect of the hand with palpation between the olecranon and medial epicondyle suggests cubital tunnel syndrome (ulnar nerve entrapment). The ulnar nerve can be trapped in several anatomic sites:

• The arcade of Osborne (the cubital tunnel under the two heads of the flexor carpi ulnaris), the most common location
• The arcade of Struthers (a thin band extending from the medial head of the triceps muscle to the medial intermuscular septum, located approximately 8 centimeters proximal to the medial epicondyle)
• The ulnar groove

Prolonged elbow flexion can stretch the nerve over the epicondyle (analogous to Phalen's test at the wrist) and sometimes reproduce the paresthesias associated with this syndrome.

SHOULDER EXAMINATION

Relevant Anatomy

A fibrous sheet of tissue surrounds the shoulder joint. There are no discrete ligaments and all structures are relaxed in the resting position. No structure remains tense throughout all joint movements. When the arm is abducted 90 degrees and externally rotated, there is a weak point in the anterior shoulder. In this

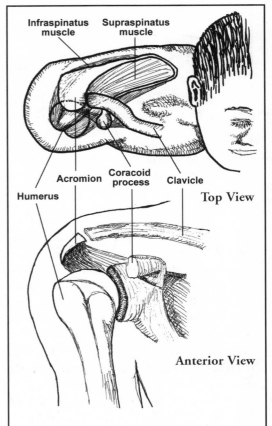

Figure 29. Shoulder Anatomy.
The shoulder joint is a shallow ball-in-socket joint that gives significant flexibility to upper extremity motion. The coracoid process and acromion, connected by the coraco-acromial ligament, produce support to the upper portion of the joint. This arch is protected by another arch produced by the clavicle and its attachment to the acromion. These arches protect the head of the humerus that articulates in the geno-humeral fossa. The supraspinatus and infra-spinatus muscles originate on the scapula and run under the arches to insert on the humeral head.

position the inferior glenohumeral ligament is the only structure that holds the head of the humerus. The rotator cuff muscles primarily stabilize the shoulder. In addition, there is a vacuum in the shoulder joint capsule that holds the humeral head in place. Puncturing this capsule can cause over a centimeter of humeral head displacement.

INSPECTION

Observe the patient standing from the front, side and back. Note the sloping contours of the deltoid muscles, bony prominences and any areas of asymmetry. A tuberculous lung abscess may change the shape of the deltoid to a shallower curve (Delmege's sign). A lowered axillary fold suggests shoulder dislocation (Bryant's sign).

Bony and Soft Tissue Abnormalities

A dropped shoulder suggests muscle injury or significant hypertrophy in a former athlete. Look for symmetry of the clavicles, sternoclavicular joints and the humeral head position. Bony enlargement of the medial portion of the right clavicle suggests congenital syphilis (Higoumenakis's sign). Visible swelling of the clavicle suggests clavicular fracture. Swelling of the lateral deltoid suggests subacromial bursitis. Anterior swelling at the coracoid process suggests a Baker's cyst. Winging of the scapula, where the scapula seems to be pulled away from the chest wall, suggests serratus anterior muscle weakness or damage of the long thoracic nerve (also called the external respiratory nerve of Bell). Congenital upward displacement of the scapula is Sprengel's deformity. A gap between the clavicle and the acromion suggests acromioclavicular separation.

Soft Tissue Atrophy

Atrophy of the supraspinatus or infraspinatus muscles suggests severe malnutrition.

Protected Arm Movements

Notice if the patient protects the arm when moving. If the patient holds the arm tight against his and her body, with the palm on the abdomen, this suggests posterior glenohumeral dislocation. If the patient has the arm held close to the body with contralateral hand supporting the elbow, this is the "dead arm" sign of either anterior glenohumeral dislocation or brachial plexus injury.

PALPATION

Start at the front and work around to the back. Begin by palpating the sternoclavicular joint along the clavicle to the acromioclavicular joint and the acromion. A painful sternoclavicular joint suggests sternoclavicular separation. Feel the greater and lesser tuberosity of the humerus and palpate for any gaps in the rotator cuff muscles. Move to the glenohumeral joint and palpate the anterior and posterior dimensions. Examine the biceps tendon and progress along the spine of the scapula. Pain along the biceps groove implies bicipital tendonitis. Localized contractions on tapping the biceps muscle suggest typhoid fever (Goggia's sign).

Muscle spasm over the posterior scapula suggests trapezius strain. Tenderness between the vertebra and the medial border of the scapula suggests rhomboid strain.

SHOULDER RANGE OF MOTION

If there is upper back or shoulder pain, always examine the cervical spine before testing the shoulder range of motion.

A useful functional screening test is to have the patient place both hands on the head and then touch the hands behind the back as if tying an apron. If these movements can be performed the functional capability of the shoulder is intact. Watch the rhythm of the movement and note any restricted range of motion. Have the patient perform this functional screen a second time while feeling for crepitus by placing your hands on the patient's shoulders during these movements.

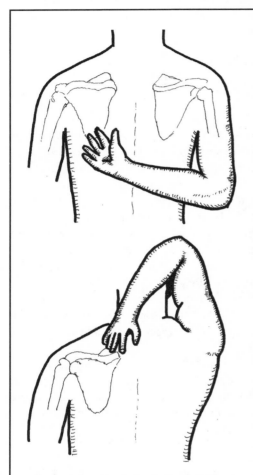

Figure 30. Apley's Back Scratch Test.
This test evaluates active shoulder range of motion. Ask the patient to bring his or her arm around to the back and reach up as if to scratch the back. Normally, a person can reach his or her thumbs up to T7 or T8 of the thoracic vertebra from the lower back, which is just about the lower border of the scapula. Inability suggests subscapularis tendonitis or rotator cuff tear. Next, have the patient reach down from the upper back. The normal range of motion from above is to level T4 or T5 of the thoracic spine (mid-portion of the scapula); limitation implies infraspinatus or teres minor tendonitis or tear.

Apley's Back Scratch Test

Apley's back scratch test is performed to more formally evaluate active range of motion. Ask your patient to bring the affected arm or shoulder around to the back and reach up as if to scratch the back. Normally, the patient can reach his or her thumbs up to around T7 or T8 of the thoracic vertebra from the lower back, which is just about the lower border of the scapula. If he or she cannot reach that high, consider subscapularis tendonitis or tear.

Next, ask the patient to reach down from the upper back. The normal range of motion from above is to level T4 or T5 of the thoracic spine. Comparing affected to non-affected arm, one thumb may not reach as far down as the other. If this is the case, consider infraspinatus, teres minor tendonitis or tear.

Limited Range of Motion

Loss of passive and active range of motion of glenohumeral joint suggests anterior dislocation, humeral head fracture, or frozen shoulder (if no pain). Painful active and passive abduction suggests supraspinatus tendonitis. Limited active but relatively full passive range of motion suggests supraspinatus tendon tear. If passive range of motion on lateral arm raising is less painful than active range of motion, this suggests rotator cuff tear.

GLENOHUMERAL JOINT

Check Osteophony

Tap each olecranon while listening over the manubrium with the bell of your stethoscope (see Figure 31).

Intact bone gives a bright, crisp tapping sound to percussion. Equal sound transmission on each side is normal. Unequal sound suggested by a muffled, distant quality on one side

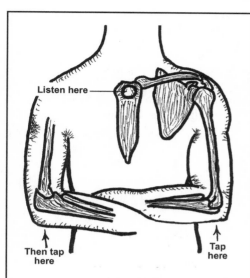

Figure 31. Heuter's Sign.
This useful sign to evaluate for a fracture tests the transmission of sound through bone. To look for an upper extremity fracture or dislocation, tap each olecranon while listening over the manubrium with the bell of your stethoscope. Intact bone gives a bright, crisp, tapping sound to percussion. Equal sound transmission on each side is normal. Hearing a muffled, distant sound on one side suggests fracture of the humerus or clavicle, or glenohumeral dislocation.

suggests humeral fracture or glenohumeral dislocation. This is Hueter's sign, sometimes called Auenbrugger's bone sign (not to be confused with Auenbrugger's sign which is an epigastric bulge produced by a large pericardial effusion).

Locate the Humeral Head

The humeral head is usually felt deep in the fossa under the deltoid. If the humeral head is not palpable, that suggests glenohumeral dislocation. The nature of the dislocation will depend on the location of the humeral head. If the humeral head is medial and below the coracoid process, then there is an intracoracoid glenohumeral dislocation. If the humeral head is inferior to the coracoid, there is a subcoracoid subluxation. If the humeral head is lateral to the coracoid, there is an extracoracoid

glenohumeral subluxation. Dugas' sign suggests shoulder dislocation rather than shoulder fracture. To perform this test, have the patient touch his or her opposite shoulder with the affected arm. If the person cannot bring the elbow in close to the body while touching the opposite shoulder, this is a positive Dugas' sign.

Check Neurovascular Function in the Hands and Wrists

See Chapter 5 for details of neurological testing in the hands and wrists.

ANTERIOR SHOULDER PAIN

For any of the painful shoulder presentations discussed below, always consider the possibility of referred pain (see Table 6.2).

Inspect and palpate basic shoulder landmarks as explained above. Then check Apley's back scratch test for range of motion and possible subscapularis tendonitis or tear.

Carefully search for pain or abnormality at the sternoclavicular joint. Tenderness here suggests sternoclavicular subluxation. A palpable step or separate edge suggests dislocation.

Check for pain or abnormality in the clavicle that would indicate a fractured clavicle. Listen for osteophony if you suspect a fracture.

Carefully palpate the acromioclavicular joint. No springing movement and no pain is normal. A springing movement and exquisite pain suggests a first-degree separation. Space between lateral clavicle and acromion suggests second- or third-degree separation.

Check for tenderness deep to the deltoid for subdeltoid bursitis. Swelling below the deltoid muscle suggests bursitis or a Baker's cyst. (The Baker's cyst will transilluminate.)

Table 6.2. Possible causes of referred shoulder pain		
Shoulder Location	*Referred Site*	*Examples*
Trapezius muscle	Near the diaphragm	Pericarditis, gallbladder disease, splenic infarct
Acromioclavicular joint	Below the diaphragm	Gallbladder disease
Upper left chest	Mediastinum	Cardiac ischemia, pericarditis
Lower scapula	Below diaphragm	Gallbladder disease
Between scapula	Cervical spine	Epidural abscess
Deltoid muscle	Shoulder joint and periarticular tissues	Bursitis, tendonitis

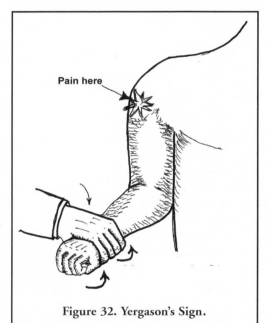

Pain here

Figure 32. Yergason's Sign.
Yergason's sign is tenderness over the biceps tendon when the patient "makes a muscle" and actively supinates the arm. You can accentuate the tenderness by resisting external rotation to isolate the biceps groove.

The next step is to look for bicipital tendonitis that will produce tenderness over the bicipital groove. Check for discomfort in the biceps groove with supination against resistance. Also see if Yergason's sign is present (see Figure 32). Yergason's sign is tenderness over the biceps tendon when the patient "makes a muscle" and actively supinates the arm. You can accentuate the tenderness by resisting external rotation to isolate the biceps groove. Speed's sign is tenderness over the biceps tendon when the patient pushes hands together over the abdomen.

Check the belly of the biceps muscle. A lump just below the deltoid suggests biceps tendon rupture. A large bruise and a lump suggest acute tendon rupture or fracture of the humeral head. Two lumps suggest biceps muscle rupture. Next, have the patient place both hands on his or her head; if you cannot palpate the tendon on the affected side, rupture of the biceps tendon is suggested (Ludington's sign). Biceps contraction that is stronger in pronation than in supination suggests possible rupture of the long head of the biceps. Pushing on the medial portion of the biceps and seeing the hand make a fist suggests hypocalcemia (Hochsinger's sign). This occurrence is similar to Trousseau's phenomenon, which is spasmodic contraction of a muscle (or tetany) when pressure is applied to the nerves enervating them.

A fleshy mass on the upper chest wall suggests pectoralis major rupture.

A PAINFUL LATERAL SHOULDER

Inspect and palpate basic shoulder landmarks as explained above.

Check range of motion with Apley's back scratch test. If the thumbs can reach T4-T5 from above, then the test is normal. If one thumb is higher than the other, then consider infraspinatus, teres minor tendonitis or tear.

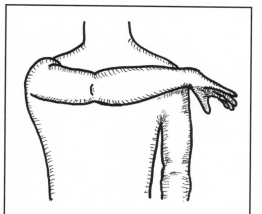

Figure 33. Scarf Test.

The scarf test evaluates the acromioclavicular joint. The patient actively places the arm on the opposite shoulder as if putting on a scarf. Pain with this maneuver suggests a problem in the joint. This test is sometimes called the crossover test.

Have the patient grasp the opposite shoulder to perform the crossover test, also known as the Scarf test. Also check the acromioclavicular compression test (see Figure 33).

Tenderness in the acromioclavicular joint suggests acromioclavicular separation. Tenderness in the subacromial area suggests rotator cuff tear, bursitis, or supraspinatus tendonitis.

Look for the Hawkins-Kennedy subacromial impingement sign. With the arm forward elevated at 90 degrees, internally rotate the arm. Tenderness on this maneuver suggests nerve impingement, rotator cuff tear, subacromial bursitis, or supraspinatus tendonitis. Direct shoulder palpation causing pain, and pain relief with arm abduction, suggests subacromial bursitis (Dawbarn's sign). Pressure on the inner portion of the humerus (compressing

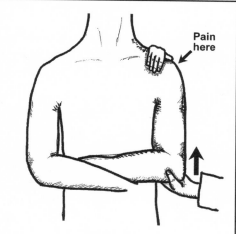

**Figure 34.
Acromioclavicular Compression Test.**

This test evaluates the acromioclavicular joint as a possible cause of shoulder pain. The examiner places one hand on the trapezius and the other under the patient's elbow. Firm downward and upward pressure between the two hands normally should not produce pain. If pain is caused by this test, then further examination of the acromioclavicular joint is indicated.

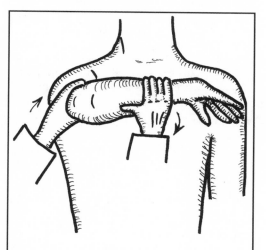

Figure 35. Hawkins-Kennedy Test.

This is a test to look for possible subacromial impingement. With the patient's arm forward, elevated at 90°, internally rotate the arm. Tenderness on this maneuver suggests nerve impingement, rotator cuff tear, subacromial bursitis, or supraspinatus tendonitis.

the circumflex nerve) causing pain in the deltoid suggests bursitis (Brickner's sign).

Have the patient write a sentence. If he or she needs to use the contralateral hand to pull the paper, then there is an infraspinatus, teres minor or subscapularis tear.

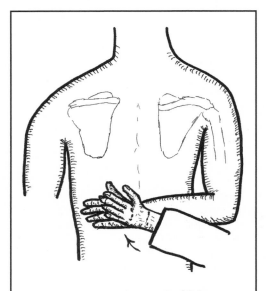

Figure 36. Gerber's Lift-off Test.
Have the patient place his or her hand on the lower back (palm facing away from the body). Place your hand on the palm and have the patient lift the hand off the back against your gentle resistance. If he or she cannot push your hand away from that position, subscapularis tear is suggested.

Check Gerber's lift-off test. Have the patient place a hand on the lower back (palm facing away from the body). If he or she cannot push your hand away from that position, subscapularis tear is suggested. Check the drop test by passively abducting the arm to 90 degrees, then have the patient slowly adduct the arm. A sudden drop in the arm suggests supraspinatus tear. Similarly, check for Codman's sign, which looks at the degree of active versus passive abduction. If the passive and active ranges of motion together are less than 90 degrees, then this suggests supraspinatus tendonitis. Shoulder pain on releasing the

passively abducted shoulder suggests ruptured supraspinatus tendon (Codman's sign). Limitation of active range of motion but nearly full passive range of motion suggests supraspinatus tear. You may also see atrophy of the supraspinatus and infraspinatus muscles creating a prominent scapular spine.

Ernest Armory Codman (1869–1940) is remembered today mostly as a crusader for the reform of hospital standards, a zealous effort that cost him his faculty position at Harvard Medical School. Codman graduated from Harvard Medical School in 1895 and subsequently completed his internship at the Massachusetts General Hospital. He joined the surgical staff of the hospital and became a member of the Harvard faculty, but lost his staff privileges there in 1914 when the hospital refused to institute his plan for evaluating the competence of surgeons.

Basically shunned by his colleagues, Codman was forced to develop his own private hospital in order to test his management concepts. Around the time that he presented his "End result system of hospital standardization," the American College of Surgeons was founded. His work in quality assessment eventually led to the founding of what is now the Joint Commission on Accreditation of Health Care Organizations (JCAHO).

Codman invented a number of surgical instruments (drill, sponge, vein stripper, wire passing drill), and is remembered for numerous eponyms: Codman's tumor of connective tissue, Codman's radiographic triangle in osteosarcoma, Codman's sign in rupture of the supraspinatus tendon, and Codman's exercises in shoulder injury.

Next, search for Jobe's sign. Passively abduct the arm to 90°, then passively lower the arm to 0° and ask the patient to actively abduct the arm to 30°. If the patient can abduct to 30° but no further, then suspect deltoid muscle paresis. Pain in the lateral shoulder with this maneuver suggests supraspinatus tendonitis. If the patient cannot get to 30°, but if passively placed at 30° can actively abduct the arm further, think supraspinatus tear. If the patient uses the hip to propel the arm from 0° to beyond 30°, then suspect supraspinatus injury.

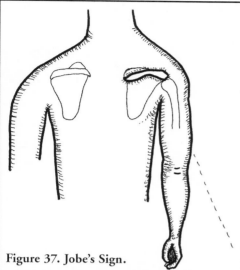

Figure 37. Jobe's Sign.

Jobe's sign helps to localize the site of shoulder dysfunction. Passively abduct the arm to 90° to check for mechanical limitation and passively lower the arm to 0°. Ask the patient to actively abduct the arm. If the patient can abduct to 30° but no further, deltoid muscle paresis should be suspected. Pain in the lateral shoulder with this maneuver suggests supraspinatus tendonitis. If the patient cannot get to 30°, but if passively placed at 30° can actively abduct the arm further, think supraspinatus tear. If the patient uses the hip to propel the arm from 0° to beyond 30°, then suspect supraspinatus injury.

NECK AND UPPER BACK PAIN

If the patient presents with the neck tilted and spasm of the trapezius then suspect torticollis.

The next step is to palpate the neck muscles. Tenderness over the trapezius suggests trapezius muscle strain or referred pain from below the diaphragm. Tenderness over the paraspinal muscles suggests muscle strain, as does tenderness over the rhomboid muscles.

Palpate and percuss the spinous processes to check for bony lesions producing pain with percussion, such as epidural abscess, metastatic disease or vertebral compression fracture.

Next palpate the supraclavicular fossa while the patient tries to place contralateral ear on the corresponding shoulder to stretch the brachial plexus. Pain along the involved shoulder or arm suggests a brachial plexus injury, or cervical radiculopathy.

Check Spurling's test by placing one hand on the patient's head and compressing the neck by passively extending the neck, rotating the head toward the side of discomfort, and gently pushing down on the head. Pain radiating down the arm suggests cervical radiculopathy.

Roy Glenwood Spurling (1894–1968) served for two years as surgical house officer at Peter Bent Brigham Hospital. His experience there with Harvey Williams Cushing (1869–1939), professor at Harvard and Surgeon-in-Chief at the Peter Bent Brigham Hospital, influenced him to direct his high intellect and boundless energy to neurosurgery. In 1925 he became the neurosurgical consultant at the Louisville General Hospital while still a resident surgeon, and his practice became heavily weighted toward surgery of the brain and spine. In 1931 Spurling took the initiative to form the organization that became the Harvey Cushing Society, now the American Association of Neurological Surgery. He was also one of the founders of the American Board of Neurological Surgery.

During World War II, working at the Walter Reed General Hospital, Washington, D.C., Spurling became the hospital's first Chief of Neurosurgery and organized neurosurgery for the entire army. When he was posted in London in March 1944, he became responsible for all neurosurgical services in the European theater. On his way home to Louisville in December 1945, in response to a request from Mrs. Patton, he was summoned back to Europe to attend to General George Patton, Jr., following the auto accident that was to take the general's life.

Have the patient do a standing push-up while beside a wall. Observe the scapula for winged scapula with posterior displacement.

Check for a cervical rib (thoracic outlet syndrome). Auscultate over the subclavian artery for a bruit and feel for a decrease in the radial pulse. Provocative tests include Adson's sign (where the pulse disappears when the head is extended and rotated toward the side being tested) and having the patient lying supine raising the arms over the head and squeezing a tennis ball. Another test is to have the patient sit and move the shoulders back and down. Hearing a systolic bruit over the brachial artery suggests aortic aneurysm (Glasgow's sign).

Alfred Washington Adson (1887–1951) became a pioneer of neurosurgery while working at the Mayo Clinic. He was one of the first to use sympathectomy for the treatment of hypertension, and cervical sympathectomy for Raynaud's syndrome. Adson invented a new forceps and a new retractor, and is remembered for his maneuver to test for thoracic outlet syndrome.

CHAPTER 7

The Head

"It has been said that until a person is 40, his face belongs to his forbears, because its appearance is principally determined by his genes. After that time, the face mirrors the establishment of a human being distinct from the generations preceding him; it is a reflection tempered and altered by the sum total of the unique happenings that compose his life's experience."

— **Robert N. Butler**

"'As a rule,' said Holmes, 'the more bizarre a thing is the less mysterious it proves to be. It is your commonplace, featureless crimes which are really puzzling, just as a commonplace face is the most difficult to identify.'"

— **Sir Arthur Conan Doyle**

There is no part of the human body more closely examined than the roughly twenty-five square inches that comprise the face. From birth to death our emotional and psychological feelings are reflected in facial expression. Faces are a central focus of our attention and we are intimately attuned to the nuances of those expressions (like joy, fear, pain, anger, sadness, and surprise) that can change with the subtlest movements of the facial muscles.

The basic challenge for us is to be able to transcend our usual and preconditioned way of looking at the individual nuances of the patient's face to appreciate the individual's nature as well as inner state of health. In addition, specific conditions may alter the head and face in characteristic ways that occasionally can lead to a spot diagnosis.

Pay careful attention to the eyes, the periorbital tissues, and the mouth and surrounding muscles. These parts of the face participate disproportionately in facial expression and communication. Disease predilection also seems to favor these areas.

INSPECTION

Facial Abnormalities

The first part of the examination is to appreciate obvious facial abnormalities. Does the

Table 7.1. The findings of classic facies

Condition	Description of Facial Findings	Other Visible Clues to Aid Diagnosis
Acromegaly	Prominent jaw; enlarged facial features, especially lips and nose which project away from the head	Large hands with enveloping, pillow-like feel to the handshake
Amyloidosis	Periorbital purpura (raccoon eyes) just after rapid increase in venous pressure from coughing, for example, or, classically, after proctoscopy	Note: raccoon eyes can also be a sign of basilar skull fracture.
Cushing's syndrome	Moon face where the buccal fat pads obscure the ears from the front view	Red cheeks, easy bruising
Depression	Worn, weary look; poor eye contact; smile, if present, forced	Appearance of sadness, loss of pleasure
Klippel-Feil syndrome	Exaggerated forward head position from congenital abnormalities of the cervical vertebrae	Congenital abnormality of cervical spine
Mitral stenosis	Flushed cheeks, drawn look to the face making nose seem prominent	Exertional dyspnea, atrial fibrillation
Myxedema	Coarse facial features; full, coarse, dry, brittle hair; periorbital edema with little sacs of fluid; facial puffiness; dull, lethargic expression may be present	Slow movements, large tongue, elbows with dirty-appearing hyperkeratosis
Nephrotic syndrome	Periorbital puffiness, dullness, lassitude	Grayish, sallow pallor if renal failure is present
Paget's disease	Bossing of the forehead causing a large, "Mr. Magoo" shaped head	Possible hearing aides from deafness
Parkinson's disease	Expressionless, mask-like face; slow facial movements; dull eyes peering from upper half of the orbit.	Bent posture; in men, several days of beard growth under the neck because of inability to see this area in a mirror
Polycythemia rubra vera	"Man-in-the-moon face"—concave facial profile resembling a nutcracker	Ruddy complexion
Scleroderma	Small, tight mouth that may not be fully closed; small oral opening; narrow, pinched nose; shiny skin with minimal wrinkles	Tightening of the fingers, loss of the finger pad and transverse creases
Seborrhea	Dermatitis may be evident in the eyebrows or across the bridge of the nose	Abrupt onset of severe disease suggests HIV infection
Smoking addiction	Excessive facial wrinkles; thin, vertical cracks along the lips; hollow cheeks	Nicotine stains on fingernails
Stroke	Facial asymmetry, facial droop leading to loss of nasolabial fold (droop may include lip)	Upper extremity hemiparesis may be present
Tuberculosis	Temporal wasting, malar sweat, loss of the buccal fat pad	Sunken yet bright-appearing eyes

patient exhibit the classic facies of a recognizable illness? Spot diagnosis is notoriously treacherous, however, so be careful not to overcall your findings. Nonetheless, sometimes the weight of observational evidence is so compelling that a diagnostic impression congeals into an epiphany of recognition (see Table 7.1).

Head Movements

A variety of tremors, including essential and familial, can cause rhythmic head movements. Aortic insufficiency (AI) can produce head-bobbing (de Musset's sign), which is a manifestation of the collapsing pulse of AI. Head bobbing from side to side suggests severe tricuspid regurgitation. Sinuous orofacial movements suggest tardive dyskinesias from medications. Jerky head movements raise the possibility of chorea.

Facial Expression

After noting any classical facies or head movements, consider the overall facial expression:

- Is the face animated or flat and masked?
- Are the facial movements symmetric or asymmetric?
- Does the patient seem to be in pain?
- How does the patient use his or her eyes? More material on the use of the eye is contained in Chapter 8.

Normally the forehead shows long wrinkles when the person looks up or when the eyebrows raise; absence of this forehead wrinkling suggests thyrotoxicosis. Cosmetic surgical scars may be visible behind the ear.

General Complexion

The patient's complexion can provide clues to underlying illness (see Table 7.2).

The carcinoid flush has 3 different presentations:

- Facial edema, swollen eyes, lacrimation, and parotid enlargement suggesting bronchial carcinoid
- Bright red face suggesting gastric carcinoid
- Vascular fine purple malar rash suggesting ileal carcinoid metastatic to the liver.

The wearing of makeup suggests either well-being or camouflage. Notice what parts are being hidden or accentuated.

Obvious Facial Skin Lesions

Some skin lesions commonly appear on the face and may be visible on simple inspection. Basal cell carcinoma has a pearly rounded appearance.

Acne rosacea, actinic changes, pigmented lesions such as melanoma and the malar rash of systemic lupus erythematosus present on the face and are necessary to keep in mind.

Table 7.2. Complexion as a clue to underlying illness

Complexion	Possible cause
Pallor	Anemia
Cyanosis	Hypoxemia
Jaundice (bronze-yellow color)	Liver disease or hemolysis
Sallowness (gray-yellow color)	Renal failure
Gray discoloration (argyria)	Contact with or ingestion of silver salts
Hyperpigmentation (excessive suntan)	Addison's disease, melanoma, HIV
Ruddiness (rubor)	Hypertension, alcoholism, gastric carcinoid

Perioral lesions can be seen in nutritional deficiency states (for example, zinc deficiency) and candidiasis.

Signs of Trauma

A bruise over the mastoid process is called Battle's sign and reflects basilar skull fracture (see Figure 38). It appears days after the trauma.

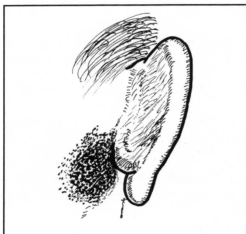

Figure 38. Battle's Sign.
A bruise over the mastoid process is Battle's sign and usually signifies a basilar skull fracture.

Raccoon eyes suggest basilar skull fracture or amyloidosis. Superficial trauma can also involve the ear or the adjacent parietal area and produce a bruise that appears immediately after the trauma. If this sign is present, stabilize the spine and check for cerebrospinal fluid (CSF) rhinorrhea and cervical spine trauma. In a fracture of the zygomatic arch there is a change in the angle of two straight edges placed vertically at the outer margin of the eyes (Rockley's sign). While scalp wounds bleed vigorously, the wound should not gape open; if it does, then a compound skull fracture is likely.

William Henry Battle (1855–1936) was an English surgeon who developed the vertical incision for the appendectomy with temporary medial retraction of the rectus muscle. He also created a surgical operation for femoral hernia. Battle researched concussion and described the sign of a bruise over the mastoid process as clue to basilar skull fracture.

Hair Quantity and Distribution

Another area to inspect is the hair quantity and distribution. Especially note any areas of hair loss. The patient may wear a wig if the hair loss is significant. Diffuse hair loss suggests:

- Endocrine abnormalities like thyroid dysfunction or panhypopituitarism
- Alopecia totalis
- Medication effect — for example, cancer chemotherapy, heavy metals, or Hepatitis B vaccine

Frontal balding, oily skin and loss of the lateral eyebrows (Hertoghe's sign) suggests heavy metal poisoning or syphilis.

Scattered hair loss suggests alopecia areata if the scalp appears normal. Scalp conditions that affect hair distribution include tuberculosis, syphilis and sarcoidosis. In cases of extreme malnutrition there is a band of hypopigmented hair during recovery called the Flag sign.

Hair Texture

Coarse, straw-like hair texture can be a normal variant or it may be a result of chemical dyes, hypothyroidism, or poverty. Fine hair suggests hyperthyroidism. Rarely patients with other hypermetabolic states will have fine hair. Color is not generally significant, as the hair color of most elderly people is gray or a salt and pepper color. The ingenuity of cosmetic manufacturers and power of vanity significantly broaden the range of artificially tinted hair color. Blue-tinted hair suggests cataracts in an older woman who dyes her own hair. (The cataract acts as a yellow filter masking the true color to the user.)

Infestations like head lice, or scalp infections such as tinea capitis, should be searched for and noted if present.

PALPATION OF SCALP AND FACE

After inspecting the hair it is useful to palpate the scalp and skull. Start along the vertex of the skull and systematically work around the skull until you have surveyed the entire area. Palpable lumps can represent old trauma or metastatic disease. Burr holes will occasionally be felt, representing previous neurosurgical encounters.

Lymph Nodes
(see also Chapter 11)

Preauricular lymph nodes suggest lymphoma, Romana's syndrome (with unilateral palpebral edema and pink eye due to American trypanosomiasis) or Leptothrix infection. Posterior cervical nodes imply scalp infection or seborrheic dermatitis. Postauricular nodes are sometimes seen in old toxoplasmosis infection and posterior scalp infections. Occipital nodes suggest HIV infection. Submental nodes are felt in mandibular dental infection.

Areas of Warmth or Tenderness

As you palpate the skull, note any areas of warmth or tenderness. Paget's disease of the skull can produce a distinctive warm feeling over the involved bone; a vascular bruit may also be heard there.

Discomfort over the occiput suggests a tumor in the posterior fossa, while pain along the temple may be seen in temporal arteritis. Pain over the frontal sinuses or maxillary sinuses suggests possible sinusitis. Obstruction of the frontal sinus produces palpable tenderness in the superior and medial aspect of the orbit near the frontal sinus (Ewing's sign). Bilateral maxillary pressure producing elbow flexion suggests meningitis (Brudzinski's cheek sign).

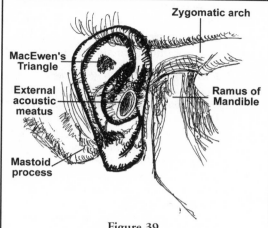

Figure 39.
MacEwen's Suprameatal Triangle.

This triangle is a little depression in the temporal bone located just behind the pinna in the eleven o'clock position for the right ear and the one o'clock position on the left ear. It is above the mastoid process and posterior to the zygomatic arch. Tenderness in this location suggests mastoiditis. External otitis media will not produce tenderness at this site.

An important place to check is the suprameatal triangle of MacEwen. This triangle is a little depression located just behind the ear in the eleven o'clock position for the right ear and the one o'clock position for the left ear (see Figure 37). Take a moment and feel this area on your own ear. Tenderness in this location suggests mastoiditis. External otitis media will not produce tenderness at this site. Tenderness posterior to the ear with inflammatory swelling on the end of the mastoid (Bezold's sign) suggests mastoiditis. If it is accompanied by dysphagia, dyspnea, nuchal rigidity, this suggests Bezold's abscess.

Friedrich Bezold (1842–1908) was a German otologist who developed an approach to evaluating deafness using a tuning fork. In 1877, he gave the first clear description of mastoiditis. Bezold's triad for otosclerosis is diminished perception of low frequency tones, reduced bone conduction and a negative Rinne's test.

Edematous swelling posterior to the mastoid process suggests thrombosis of the transverse sinus (Griesinger's sign). The sensation of exquisite tenderness over the mastoid process with no change in degree of pain on palpation suggests myocardial infarction (Libman's sign).

Wilhelm Griesinger (1817–1868) was a German neurologist and psychiatrist. He succeeded Moritz Heinrich Romberg (1795–1873) as head of the polyclinic in Berlin. Griesinger introduced pathological anatomy to clinical psychiatry and reformed the mental health system. He also described two forms of muscular dystrophy and an Egyptian tropical disease that usually appears in barefoot workers operating in damp soil. It is caused by infestation with the nematode Ancylostoma duodenale and Necator americanus.

Another area to palpate is the temporomandibular joint while the patient opens and closes his or her mouth (see Figure 40). Place your forefinger and middle finger just in front of the tragus on each side during this maneu-

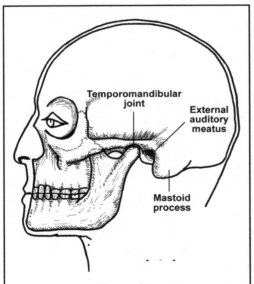

**Figure 40.
Temporomandibular Joint.**

The temporomandibular joint is located just in front of the external auditory meatus. Palpate the temporomandibular joint while the patient opens and closes his or her mouth. Place your forefinger and middle finger just in front of the tragus on each side during this maneuver. If there is tenderness in this location, consider rheumatoid arthritis. Crepitus with this movement suggests osteoarthritis.

ver. If there is tenderness in this location consider rheumatoid arthritis. Crepitus with this movement suggests osteoarthritis.

PERCUSSION

The skull is not usually percussed unless you are checking for vertebral metastasis. If so, percussing the skull may produce discomfort that localizes to a distant vertebra (diseased or damaged from infection, compression, or malignancy). With brain abscess there is sometimes a more resonant percussion note and a cracked pot sound just above the ear (MacEwen's sign).

Guarino's Auscultatory Percussion for Intracranial Masses

This amazing technique to determine intracranial masses is fully described in the *British Medical Journal* in 1982. An abbreviated description is included here. The technique is subtle but worth the effort to learn. It is potentially very useful especially in nursing home and bedfast patients.

Place the diaphragm of your stethoscope over the left ear and percuss in midline of the forehead about two inches above the bridge of the nose. Then listen over the right ear while tapping in the same midline location. Compare the tapping sound on each side. Move posteriorly in one to two centimeter increments, again comparing the quality and volume on each side.

Move up the skull toward the vertex, again comparing each side. A mass lying in the path of the percussed note will produce a dullness or distinct increase in the sound. Be careful to consider the plane of the mass in relation to where you are listening and where you are tapping. You can change your tapping location to better triangulate the coordinates of the mass. A tuning fork may also be used. (I suggest 512 Hertz.)

AUSCULTATION

Auscultation of the skull is not usually performed but can sometimes provide useful information (see Table 7.3). If the clinical situation warrants (for example, if the patient has a bruise on the head or a black eye) listen over the mastoids, temples, forehead and occiput. Hearing increased breath sounds over the skull suggest, Paget's disease or osteolytic metastasis.

Table 7.3. Causes of vascular bruits over the skull

- Paget's disease
- Transmitted aortic valvular murmur
- Carotid artery stenosis
- Carotid artery-cavernous sinus fistula (bruit decreasing in intensity or disappear with jugular vein compression)
- Intracranial angioma
- Intracranial tumor encasing an artery
- Vascular meningioma
- Arteriovenous malformation (produces a coarse, machinery-like sound)

SPECIAL TESTS

Transillumination of sinuses

To transilluminate the frontal sinuses, shine a bright light into the supraorbital notch and check the glow of the forehead. Seeing an air-fluid level suggests infection (see Figure 41).

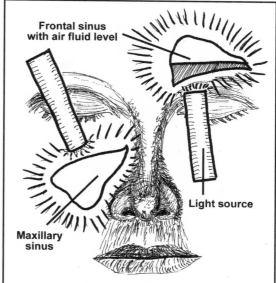

Figure 41. Sinus Transillumination.

Transillumination is best performed in a darkened room. To transilluminate the frontal sinuses shine a bright light into the supraorbital notch and check the glow of the forehead. Seeing an air-fluid level, as shown in the illustration, suggests infection. To transilluminate the maxillary sinuses put the bright light under the eye and look along the malar area and in the patient's open mouth (which regrettably is not open in the illustration). Alternatively place the light in the mouth and check for a glow of lower eyelids. Also check for the red reflex coming from pupils. A lack of glow in a maxillary sinus is always abnormal (Davidsohn's sign).

To transilluminate the maxillary sinuses, put the bright light in the mouth and check for a glow of lower eyelids. Also check for the red reflex coming from pupils. A lack of glow in a maxillary sinus is always abnormal (Davidsohn's sign).

CHAPTER 8

The Eyes

"The common eye sees only the outside of things, and judges by that, but the seeing eye pierces through and reads the heart and the soul, finding there capacities which the outside didn't indicate or promise, and which the other kind couldn't detect."
— **Mark Twain**

"An animal will always look for a person's intentions by looking them right in the eyes."
— **H. Powers**

"Why does the eye see a thing more clearly in dreams than the imagination when awake?"
— **Leonardo da Vinci**

A considerable amount of useful information can be obtained by careful examination of the patient's eyes. According to the late mythologist Joseph Campbell, the eyes are the messengers of the heart. They search for what the heart seeks to possess. The eyes are the most compelling feature of expression and together with the oral musculature communicate an infinite variety of inner states.

BULGING OR PROMINENCE

Eye prominence is called proptosis. If the prominence is unilateral (at least a 3mm difference between eyes) then consider hyperthy-

---

Table 8.1.
Sequence of the eye examination

- Notice any bulging or prominence (proptosis)
- Measure the visual acuity
- Check the patient's glasses
- Examine the eyelids
- Examine the sclera
- Assess the conjunctiva
- Examine the lacrimal duct
- Evaluate the cornea
- Examine the iris
- Check the pupils and pupillary reflexes
- Evaluate the anterior chamber
- Examine the extraocular eye movements
- Check the visual fields
- Evaluate the fundus

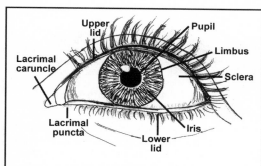

Figure 42. Normal Left Eye.
This illustration shows the basic external features of the eye. The white portion of the eye is the sclera while the colored portion is the iris with the pupil in the center. The junction of the iris and sclera is called the limbus. The tear duct apparatus (the lacrimal caruncle and puncta) is shown in the corner of the eye.

roidism, neoplasm (such as metastatic cancer), lymphoma, or melanoma. Neural tumors and basilar skull fracture can also produce unilateral proptosis. If the bulging is pulsating then suspect a carotid artery cavernous sinus fistula and look for prominent facial veins, periorbital edema, and ophthalmoplegia, as well as listening for a bruit over the eyeball.

Bilateral proptosis suggests a systemic process such as hyperthyroidism, lymphoma, Wegener's granulomatosis, or fungal infection.

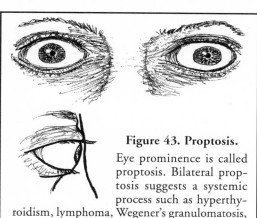

Figure 43. Proptosis.
Eye prominence is called proptosis. Bilateral proptosis suggests a systemic process such as hyperthyroidism, lymphoma, Wegener's granulomatosis, or fungal infection. If the prominence is unilateral (at least a 3mm difference between eyes) then consider hyperthyroidism, neoplasm such as neural tumor, metastatic cancer, lymphoma, or melanoma or basilar skull fracture.

A recessed eye in the orbit caused by the loss of periorbital fat is called enophthalmos. Weight loss and dehydration produce bilateral enophthalmos, while trauma can create unilateral eye recession.

MEASURE THE VISUAL ACUITY

The next consideration is to test visual acuity using a standard eye chart. A Snellen card held 14 inches away checks central vision. Test the vision in each eye one at a time. If the patient is illiterate, or in cases of severe visual impairment, have him or her count your fingers held 12 inches away. If there is visual difficulty, repeat the test with the patient looking through a pinhole punched in an index card. Improvement looking through a pinhole suggests a refractive problem.

Herman Snellen (1834–1908) was a Dutch ophthalmologist who focused his attention solely on visual problems. Snellen did comprehensive work on glaucoma, astigmatism, inflammation, diseases of the retina and connective tissue. He also concerned himself with the calculations of eyeglasses, as well as eye surgery. Snellen is best remembered for the Snellen chart. Test types were invented in 1843 by Heinrich Kuechler (1811–1873) and were improved by the Vienna oculist Eduard Jaeger Ritter von Jaxtthal (1818–1884) in 1854. Herman Snellen invented his chart of square-shaped letters that soon gained international acceptance.

CHECK THE PATIENT'S GLASSES

If the patient wears glasses, then look at an object through the upper portion of the patient's glasses. If the object is smaller than normal, then the person has myopia. (The eye is too long, so the lenses in the glasses have to stretch or shrink the image.) If the image is larger than normal, then the eye is too short, so the image must be shortened (hypermetrope). Loss of accommodation with age is called presbyopia and may be inferred by bifocals with the lower lens being a magnifying lens. Some progressive lens bifocals will not show a discrete line, so note any change in the image size as you look from the top of the lens to the bottom (where the magnifying lens is).

EXAMINE THE EYELIDS

The key eyelid observations include coloration, blinking, ptosis, retraction, or periorbital edema. Various colorations to note are excessive eye makeup (perhaps as a sign of vanity), the heliotrope rash of dermatomyositis, and the buttery colored xanthelasmas of hyperlipidemia.

Blinking

Also notice the nature of the blinking of the eyes. Normally the blinking is no more than once every three seconds (twenty times a minute). A decrease in the blinking suggests reduced corneal sensitivity (first division of Cranial Nerve V) such as from herpes infection or Bell's palsy. If the reduced blinking is bilateral consider Parkinsonism or thyrotoxicosis if there is also proptosis (Stellwag's sign). Increased monocular blinking suggests foreign body or other mechanical irritation in the eye. Increased bilateral blinking suggests nervousness or eye dryness (consider Sjogren's syndrome).

Ptosis

Drooping of the eyelids from failure to fully open them is called ptosis (see Figure 44). One tip-off is that the upper lid covers part

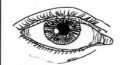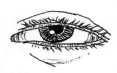

Figure 44. Left Eye Ptosis.
Drooping of the eyelids from failure to fully open them is called ptosis. Note that the upper lid covers part of the left pupil. Bilateral ptosis suggests myasthenia gravis or prior encephalitis while unilateral ptosis suggests a cranial nerve III disorder or Horner's syndrome.

or all of the pupil. Sometimes a squint can mimic the drooping of ptosis. The basic way to tell ptosis from a squint is to have the patient look up and watch the corresponding eyelid movement. Normal upward movement of the eyelid suggests a squint. Bilateral ptosis suggests myasthenia gravis or prior encephalitis, while unilateral ptosis suggests a cranial nerve III disorder or Horner's syndrome. The pupil size can help you to differentiate these conditions. If the pupil is large and nonreactive, then consider cranial nerve III compression. A normal reactive pupil suggests central cranial nerve III infarction from hypertension, diabetes mellitus or vasculitis. A small nonreactive pupil implies Horner's syndrome. Uncommonly a patient may be able to elevate a ptotic eye by moving the mandible away from the side of the ptosis (the Marcus Gunn jaw reflex). The retraction of sunken eyes suggests dehydration or malnutrition. Facial nerve disorders such as Bell's palsy can cause lid retraction by affecting the obicularis oculi muscle.

Johann Friedrich Horner (1831–1885) was a Swiss ophthalmologist remembered as a great clinical teacher. A capable surgeon, he performed some 2,000 cataract and glaucoma procedures and it has been estimated that he treated 100,000 patients during his medical career. Horner established that a man with a red-green color blindness transmitted this anomaly to his male grandchildren through his daughter who was not color blind, similar to hemophilia, i.e. sex-linked transmission.

Horner's syndrome was first described in 1727 by François Pourfour du Petit, after the dissection of the nerves in the necks of dogs. In 1852, Claude Bernard offered a more complete description of the syndrome and, in 1864, three American army physicians influenced by Bernard's work described a clinical case of Horner's Syndrome in which a man was shot through the throat. In 1869, Horner described a woman in her forties who developed the classic symptoms of the syndrome.

Periorbital Edema

Periorbital edema suggests renal failure (especially nephrotic syndrome), myxedema (no indentation with pressure is one clue), trichinosis, allergic reactions and angioedema. Redness, swelling and inflammation suggest periorbital abscess. Patients treated with imatinib mesylate for chronic myeloid leukemia can also develop periorbital edema.

Redness or Swelling

Note any redness, swelling or masses around the eye as signs of inflammation. Focal erythema involving the nasal portion of the upper lid suggests infection or inflammation of the adjacent frontal sinus. Redness of the lateral (temporal) portion of the upper lid can be a sign of lacrimal gland inflammation called dacryoadenitis. Focal edema with redness and pain suggests obstruction and subsequent infection of the parafollicular glands of Zeis producing a hordeolum (also called a sty). A painless lid mass along the lid margin is a chalazion due to an obstructed meibomian gland. Also remember that a mass on the medial portion of the lower lid could be a basal cell carcinoma. "Black eye" appearance below the eyes suggests chronic allergies. Localized cyanosis of the eyelid implies orbital vein thrombosis, aneurysm or malignancy. Bulging of the lower lid when the eye looks down suggests cornea swelling (Munson's sign). Swelling of the lower lid suggests CHF, myxedema, nephritic syndrome, or liver failure.

Eyelashes and Eyebrows

Also examine the nature of the eyelashes including their distribution and any signs of scaling. Oily flakes around the base of the eyelashes suggest seborrhea. Absent eyelashes suggest secondary syphilis or may be a component of the alopecia totalis complex. Decreased resistance to opening the buried eyelids suggests facial paralysis of central origin (Legendre's sign). A fine line in the skin along the lower eyelid suggests atopic dermatitis (Dennie's sign). Loss of the lateral third of the eyebrow (Queen Anne's sign) suggests myxedema.

Lid Retraction

Retraction of the upper lid showing more of the superior sclera suggests hyperthyroidism (Dalrymple's sign). Lid lag on downward gaze is von Graefe's sign of hyperthyroidism. Many of the hyperthyroid eye signs are easier to elicit with the patient supine. If the patient is sitting, make sure your eyes are below the patient's eye level to appreciate subtle lid movement abnormalities.

Friedrich Wilhelm Ernst Albrecht von Graefe (1828–1870) was a German physician who is considered to be the father of ophthalmology and the most important ophthalmologist of the nineteenth century. He was known as a fine teacher and attracted students from around the world, including Douglas Moray Cooper Lamb Argyll Robertson and Theodore Billroth, who noted the teacher's "great personal kindness and his great humility." The clinic was founded in the same year Herman Ludwig Ferdinand von Helmholtz introduced his new invention the "eye mirror" which later became known as the ophthalmoscope.

Despite having grown up in a family of wealth, von Graefe treated the poor without charge and performed more than 10,000 eye operations on all ranks of people. Von Graefe described optic retinitis and acute visual loss due to retinal artery embolism, and was one of the first physicians to successfully treat glaucoma. He also pioneered the iridectomy for cataracts and invented a special knife that is still used in cataract surgery.

Table 8.2. Eye signs of hyperthyroidism

Sign	Description
Abadie's sign	Spasm of the levator palpebrae superioris muscle
Ballet's sign	No voluntary eye movements but normal papillary reflexes
Boston's sign	When the eye looks down there is a stop and shudder, then continued movement.
Cowen's sign	Irregular, ratchet-like, consensual contractions to papillary stimulation
Dalrymple's sign	Upper lid retraction and widening of the palpebral fissure
Dunphy's sign	Conjunctival redness adjacent to the insertion of the lateral rectus muscle
Enroth's sign	Prominence of the upper lids
Gifford's sign	Difficulty in everting the eyelid
Graefe's sign	Eye moves downward slowly and upward quickly
Griffith's sign	Lower lid lag on upward gaze
Jellinek's sign (Tallais' sign)	Brown pigmentation of the lower margin of the upper lids
Joffroy's sign	Lack of forehead wrinkling with sudden upward gaze
Knie's sign	Unequal pupillary dilation
Kocher's sign	Slow retraction of the upper lid when the eye fixes on an object
Mann's sign	Eyes that do not seem to be on the same level
Mean's sign	Lag of the globe on upward gaze
Mobius' sign	Difficulty in maintaining convergence during accommodation due to myopathy of the medial recti
Riesman's sign	Hearing a bruit over the eyeballs
Roesnbach's sign	Fine tremor of the closed eyelids
Stellwag's sign	Infrequent blinking and retraction of the upper eyelid
Wilder's sign	Ratchet movement to horizontal eye movement

At the age of only 42, he succumbed to a reactivation of tuberculosis.

Compression of the Orbits

Gently pressing on the patient's closed eyes can sometimes yield useful information. The technique is to carefully place both forefingers on the patient's closed upper lid. One finger gently presses the globe of the eye while the other finger perceives the degree of outward pressure. Compression of the eyes normally slows the pulse (Aschner's sign); a paradoxical increase (Cantelli's sign) suggests autonomic (vagal) insufficiency. Loss of pain to digital compression of the eye (Haenel's sign) suggests syphilis, however compression of the globe to the point of discomfort is not recommended. The eyeballs feel soft in dehydration (Riesman's soft eye sign). A rock-hard orbit suggests glaucoma.

EXAMINE THE SCLERA

The color of the sclera can be an important clue to systemic illness.

White and Blue Patches

White spots on the temporal side of the eye suggest severe vitamin A deficiency (Bitot's spots). Blue patches are signs of atrophy and suggest connective tissue diseases (Eddowes' sign), iron deficiency anemia, scleromalacia or a result of corticosteroid therapy.

Muddy Sclera

Muddy sclera have a brownish color that is not to be confused with scleral icterus. The muddy color is common in southerners who spent their childhood outside in dry, dusty conditions. To confirm the scleras are indeed muddy, have the patient look up and examine the inferior portion of the sclera. The portion that is not normally exposed will be a more normal white color.

Scleral Icterus

The bright yellow discoloration of scleral icterus is an important sign of an elevated bilirubin. If possible, use direct sunlight to illuminate the eye. The better the light, the more accurately you can estimate the serum bilirubin, and with practice you can get pretty good at estimating the bilirubin level. Bilirubin may bind to the elastin in the scleral tissues, so, with rapid changes, your estimate may lag the changes noted by the laboratory.

Bright Red Hemorrhage

Large bright red hemorrhage can be caused by a number of local and systemic conditions (infra vide). Sometimes they are idiopathic or due to local trauma. Other possibilities include vasculitis (always with other signs of vasculitis), thrombocytopenia, clotting disorders, diabetes mellitus, or hypertension.

Other Pigmentation

Additional areas of pigmentation can be seen in certain situations. Senile hyaline plaques are noted at the insertions of the medial and lateral rectus muscles. They tend to be square or rectangular.

ASSESS THE CONJUNCTIVA

Vessels and Vascularity

The next step in the eye evaluation is to check the conjunctiva. First note the vessels and the nature of the vascularity. Redness or other signs of inflammation require that you examine both the upper and lower palpebral conjunctiva.

To flip the upper lid and examine the superior conjunctiva, evert the upper lid over a

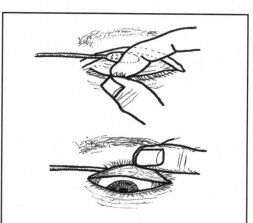

Figure 45. Examining the Upper Eye Lid. Have the patient look down throughout the examination and gently place a cotton swab on the closed upper eyelid. Pull out on the eyelid and with your other hand gently push down on the upper lid with the cotton swab. The swab acts as a pivot. After your inspection is complete, have the patient look up to restore the lid.

cotton swab placed on the closed upper eyelid (see Figure 45). With the patient looking down throughout the examination, gently pull out on the eyelid and with your other hand push down on the upper lid with the cotton swab. The swab acts as a pivot. After your inspection is complete, have the patient look up to restore the lid.

Signs of vascular sludging can be seen especially on the inferior bulbar conjunctiva. Note the nature of the vessels and look for comma forms, angular forms, and corkscrew vessels. These vascular abnormalities are classically seen in sickle cell disease. Venous dilatation can also be appreciated.

The Lower Palpebral Conjunctiva

The lower palpebral conjunctiva can enable an estimate of the hematocrit by appreciating the degree of pinkness. Practice looking at the pinkness, estimating the hematocrit, then checking the value in the patient's chart. (This technique is especially helpful to practice in hospitalized patients where there is relatively simultaneous determination of the hematocrit in the patient's medical record.) After practicing from ten to twenty times, you can regularly get to within two points of the hematocrit. (Your attentive and focused eye is really that sensitive.) Hemorrhages on the lower palpebral conjunctiva can suggest bacterial endocarditis.

Conjunctival Edema

Conjunctival edema (chemosis) can be appreciated when you examine the lower lid and notice a thick, cobblestone appearance to the conjunctiva (see Figure 46). Chemosis is caused by local or systemic inflammation, hypersensitivity reactions, increased venous pressure (increased right heart pressure or superior vena caval syndrome), thyroid disorders (both myxedema and hyperthyroidism), and infection (consider early meningitis). Unilateral chemosis in a trauma setting suggests anterior basilar skull fracture.

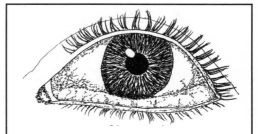

Figure 46. Chemosis.
Chemosis is conjunctival edema producing a thick, cobblestone appearance to the conjunctiva. Chemosis is caused by local or systemic inflammation, hypersensitivity reactions, increased venous pressure, thyroid disorders, and infection. Unilateral chemosis in a trauma setting suggests anterior basilar skull fracture.

Conjunctival Hemorrhage

Conjunctival hemorrhage is often dramatic and painless. A large bright red hemorrhage may appear spontaneously during sleep or after coughing and sneezing. For many elderly people the cause is unknown but may be due to capillary fragility. Local trauma can produce bleeding, but if the head trauma was one or two days earlier you must consider basilar skull fracture. Systemic causes include vasculitis (always with other signs), thrombocytopenia, clotting disorders, diabetes mellitus or hypertension. If the bleeding does not clear over several days, then consider Kaposi's sarcoma.

Small petechial hemorrhages may signify bacterial endocarditis.

EXAMINE THE LACRIMAL DUCT

Note the opening of the lacrimal duct (the puncta) and the lacrimal sac. The lacrimal duct is a medially located little tube in the corner of the eye. The lacrimal sac is located on the lower border of the conjunctiva, while the lacrimal glands are located above the lacrimal duct. Unilateral swelling of the lacrimal sac suggests infection or tumor. Bilateral swelling

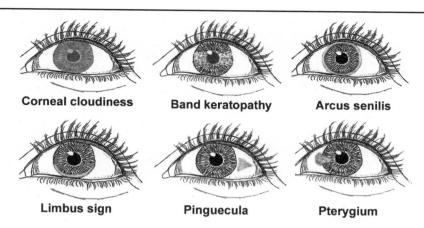

Corneal cloudiness **Band keratopathy** **Arcus senilis**

Limbus sign **Pinguecula** **Pterygium**

Figure 47. Corneal Opacities.

Cloudiness of the cornea suggests eye problems, previous corneal damage, hypercalcemia, or rheumatic diseases. Band keratopathy appears as a fine frost-like cloudiness. Usually the sun-exposed part of the cornea is affected so that the more normal transparent cornea can be appreciated above and below the cloudiness. It is caused by hypercalcemia. Arcus senilis is a milky deposit of lipid that is commonly seen in elderly people. It is not associated with illness. Unilateral arcus implies ipsilateral carotid obstruction (on the side without the arcus) or a prosthetic eye. Dystrophic calcification (Limbus sign) can produce a milky white ring around the limbus that resembles arcus senilis but tends to accumulate more heavily along the inferior margin of the limbus. A pinguecula is a triangular discoloration representing a collection of fat that is medial or lateral to the iris. It never crosses the limbus. A pterygium is a fan-shaped, wing-like, yellow area of fibrous tissue, usually on the medial portion of the eye, that may invade the cornea and affect vision.

suggests sarcoidosis or Sjogren's syndrome. A ropy, cobblestone appearance of the lacrimal duct suggests local inflammation.

Schirmer's Test

The function of the lacrimal tissue (producing moisture) can be measured by Schirmer's test. This test measures the amount of tear production using a standardized strip of filter paper placed at the palpebral and scleral conjunctiva, but avoiding the cornea. The paper is removed after five minutes and the amount of moisture is measured. The normal value is 10mm or more of tear moisture. Less than 5mm is definitely abnormal. Schirmer's test also evaluates cranial nerve VII (facial) function, which mediates the tearing reflex. (Nasal stimulation produces tearing.)

Rudolf Schirmer *(1831–1896) was a German ophthalmologist who trained under Albrecht von Graefe (1828–1870). Early glaucoma in the*

Sturge-Weber syndrome is sometimes called Schirmer's syndrome.

EVALUATE THE CORNEA

Note the reflection of light off the cornea. Normally the cornea is glistening and transparent, and its light reflection is sharp. A defect in the cornea suggests corneal abrasion or herpetic keratitis. Stain the cornea with a fluorescein dye to highlight the defect by touching a fluorecein strip to the lower conjunctival sac.

Corneal Cloudiness

Cloudiness of the cornea suggests eye problems, previous corneal damage, hypercalcemia, or rheumatic diseases. Eye disorders producing cloudiness are glaucoma (steamy appearance) and uveitis, among others. Previous corneal damage is usually the result of mechanical trauma or exposure to the toxic fumes of heavy metals. Rheumatic diseases that produce corneal cloudiness include juvenile rheumatoid arthritis, discoid lupus, rheumatoid arthritis (rare), and gout (very rare).

Hypercalcemia produces band keratopathy that appears as a fine frost-like cloudiness. Usually the sun-exposed part of the cornea is affected so that the more normal transparent cornea can be appreciated above and below the cloudiness. This change does not reflect the level of the serum calcium and can be seen for a long time after the calcium value normalizes. Causes of hypercalcemia to consider include primary hyperparathyroidism, sarcoidosis, multiple myeloma, and lymphoma.

Corneal Opacities

Corneal opacities suggest herpetic infection, pterygium, pinguecula, dystrophic calcification, and arcus senilis. Herpes simplex infection produces a fine lacy corneal opacity. A pinguecula is a triangular discoloration representing a collection of fat that is medial or lateral to the iris. It never crosses the limbus. A pterygium is a fan-shaped, wing-like yellow area of fibrous tissue, usually on the medial portion of the eye, that may invade the cornea and affect vision.

Dystrophic calcification (Limbus sign) can produce a milky white ring around the limbus that resembles arcus senilis, but tends to accumulate more heavily along the inferior margin of the limbus. Arcus senilis is a milky deposit of lipid that is commonly seen in elderly people. It is not associated with illness although there may be a weak association with vascular disease. Unilateral arcus implies ipsilateral carotid obstruction (on the side without the arcus) or a prosthetic eye. Some older forms of cataract surgery can produce an irregular white line along the limbus. Transient corneal opacities can be seen in febrile illness (Brunati's sign).

EXAMINE THE IRIS

The next step in the external evaluation of the eye is to examine the iris. The purpose of the iris is to control the pupil size. The iris may seem to jiggle if the patient has undergone lens replacement surgery. Defects in the iris can be seen after lens replacement surgery. A small triangular defect is an iridectomy scar, while a laser produces a small circular defect. A cloudy lens suggests a cataract.

Nodules in the Iris

Nodules in the iris are usually significant. Nodules that seem to invade the pupil are Koeppe's sign and suggest sarcoidosis, tuberculosis, or uveititis. Elevated dark pigmentations may be malignant melanomas.

Pigmentation

Clumps of copper-colored pigmentation suggest neurofibromatosis (Lisch sign). A bronze ring at the limbus superiorly and inferiorly suggests Addison's disease. Copper-green-colored ring at the limbus in both eyes suggests Wilson's disease (Kayser-Fleischer ring). Pure white dots are Brushfield spots (hypoplasia of the iris) and are sometimes seen in Down syndrome. A small black ring in the iris next to the pupil suggests tuberculous meningitis (Skeer's sign).

Bernhard Kayser (1869–1954) was a German physician who worked for two years as a ship's physician and general practitioner in Brazil before settling on ophthalmology as a career. Bruno Fleischer (1874–1965) was also a German ophthalmologist, born in Stuttgart where Bernhard Kayser established his ophthalmologic practice. They are remembered for gray-green or brownish ring in the deep epithelial layers at the outer border of the cornea near the limbus. It is a pathogonomic eye sign of Wilson's disease.

Red Blood Vessels in the Iris

Red blood vessels in the iris suggest rubeosis iridis. This condition results from neovascularization and is often associated with diabetes or glaucoma.

Blood in the Anterior Chamber

Seeing blood in the anterior chamber indicates hyphema, *an ophthalmologic emergency.* Trauma is the most common cause of hyphema, although it may be caused by benign or malignant intraocular tumors. Neovascularization of the iris or ciliary body may also result in hyphema. This neovascularization can be caused by posterior segment ischemia, which usually is associated with microvascular disease in diabetes, or retinal arterial or venous occlusion.

Pus in the Anterior Chamber

Pus in the anterior chamber indicates a hypopyon, *another ophthalmologic emergency.* This condition is most often seen after penetrating trauma to the eye.

PUPILS AND PUPILLARY REFLEXES

The pupils should be equal and round. Any abnormality in shape is important. Pupil dilation with pinching the neck over C6 suggests meningitis (Parrot's sign). Unilateral pupillary dilation and an elevated upper lid (Roque's sign) suggest cervical sympathetic dysfunction. Inability to close one eye without closing both eyes together suggests central hemiplegia. The pupil changes size when the orbicularis muscle is tapped (Piltz's sign). Visual improvement with head bowing suggests retinitis pigmentosa (Gould's sign).

Joseph Marie Jules Parrot (1829–1883) was a French physician who initially studied cardiovascular disease and wrote a number of papers on cardiac murmurs and vascular bruits, especially in the neck. Eventually he decided to devote himself to pediatrics and became one of the pioneers in that field. Parrot described and classified numerous disorders of the newborn and devoted considerable attention to the development of the brain and the effects of hereditary syphilis, both on the nervous system and other body organs, including the bones, liver and lung. He wrote the first report on the pneumococcus in 1881 with Louis Pasteur and in 1876 was first to describe the Ghon lesion. Parrot was an enthusiastic anthropologist and one of the founders of the French Society of Anthropology.

Irregularly Shaped Pupils

Irregularly shaped pupils suggest syphilis (Argyll Robertson pupil), Berger's sign or post-ophthalmic surgery. A unilateral Argyll Robertson pupil can be seen in severe Vitamin D deficiency (Frenkel's eye sign). Scalloped pupils suggest rupture of the sphincter caused by amyloidosis. Oval pupils are seen in syphilis, glaucoma or Adie's pupil. Adie's pupil neither reacts nor accommodates and is associated with absent ankle jerks and a segmented palsy of the iris sphincter. Teardrop pupils are usually a post-surgical or neurological finding, or suggest prior trauma. The point of the teardrop indicates the location of the trauma.

Small Pupils

If both pupils are small (miosis) this suggests narcotic use or hyperopia (farsightedness). Pupil size tends to decrease with aging.

Unilateral miosis suggests Horner's syndrome. (The small pupil is the abnormal one and does not relax when the light is removed.) Also check for ipsilateral ptosis, enophthalmos, and absence of sweating. Check the ipsilateral hand for thenar atrophy, and inability to oppose the thumb and little finger, signs of Pancoast's syndrome. The differential diagnosis of Horner's syndrome includes Pancoast's syndrome, brain stem tumor, cervical spinal cord tumor, mediastinal tumor, posterior inferior cerebellar artery (Wallenberg's syndrome), carotid artery aneurysm and demyelinating disease.

Table 8.3. Pupillary findings		
Pupillary Reaction	**Small Pupils**	**Large Pupils**
Reactive to light	Normal aging	Anxiety
	Horner's syndrome	Brain stem damage
		Medication effect
Nonreactive to light	Pontine hemorrhage	Adie's pupil
	Argyll Robertson pupils	Medication effect
	Medication effect	

Douglas Moray Cooper Lamb Argyll Robertson (1837–1909) became a noted Scottish ophthalmologist and eye surgeon. Apart from his status in the medical arena, his social skills and "party talents" also impressed his peers. He won the golfing gold medal of the Royal and Ancient Club of St. Andrews five times.

In 1863 he published his findings on the Calabar bean (Physostigma venenosum), a plant native to eastern Nigeria. Argyll Robertson described the plant's effects on the human eye. Instilling an extract of Calabar into his own eye, Argyll Robertson found that the solution makes the pupil contract and foresaw "an agent that will soon rank as one of the most valuable in the ophthalmologic pharmacopoeia."

Large Pupils

If both pupils are large (mydriasis) then consider myopia (nearsightedness), use of sympathomimetics, or brain stem damage. Obviously, death produces fixed and dilated pupils. Rhythmic pupillary dilation coincident with the pulse suggests aortic insufficiency (Landolfi's sign).

Unilateral mydriasis suggests acute glaucoma, unilateral instillation of medication to eye, blindness, carotid artery aneurysm, neurosyphilis, or neurological illness.

Anisocoria

More than half a millimeter difference in pupil size is anisocoria. The differential diagnosis of anisocoria in an elderly person is broad, but consider previous trauma, neurological illness (masses or infections), and vascular conditions, including subdural hematoma, carotid artery disease, or carotid sinus thrombosis. Acquired anisocoria in the setting of dementia suggests neurosyphilis (Baillarger's sign). Note any clouding of the lens, which suggests a cataract.

Pupillary Response to Light

Shine light into the eyes and note the direct response. (The pupil constricts with direct stimulation.) Rapid papillary oscillation may be a sign of neurosyphilis (Gower's sign). Next, note the consensual response. Shine the light in one eye while observing for constriction in the contralateral eye. Optic tract damage anterior to the geniculate bodies produces a hemiopic pupillary response so that half of the retina produces a pupil reaction and half does not (Wernicke's sign). Very sluggish pupillary reactions can be a sign of Addison's disease (Arroyo's sign).

If the direct response is absent but the consensual response is present, then consider neurosyphilis, acute glaucoma or medication effect. Reappearance of the light reflex when the patient is in a dark room suggests neurosyphilis (Saenger's sign).

If both direct and consensual responses are absent in one eye, this suggests monocular blindness (an efferent problem on the nonreactive side). If both responses are absent bilaterally, this suggests a brain stem lesion or bilateral blindness.

Swinging Flashlight Test

Next, perform the swinging flashlight test (see Figure 48). Swing the light from one eye to the other eye and note whether the direct or the consensual response is more vigorous. Dilation to the direct response (following a consensual constrictive response) implies an afferent defect in that eye (Marcus Gunn pupil). Sometimes the patient will notice that the light seems brighter to the affected eye. Conditions that produce a Marcus Gunn pupil in elderly people include demyelinating disease, multiple sclerosis, unilateral macular degeneration, retinal disease, and severe unilateral cataract.

Robert Marcus Gunn (1850–1909) was a Scottish ophthalmologist who was influenced by Joseph Lister (1827–1912), and Douglas Moray Cooper Lamb Argyll Robertson. He introduced the sterile procedure to cataract surgery by applying Lister's principles. He enjoyed outdoor life, spent his holidays collecting fossils, and later donated his large collection to the British Museum.

Gunn is immortalized in four eponyms: the Marcus Gunn pupil where the consensual response is stronger than the direct response; Gunn's syndrome of ptosis in which chewing or lateral movement of the jaw causes elevation of the eyelid; Gunn's sign of crossing of an artery over a vein, with compression of the underlying vein in the fundus of the eye as a sign of hypertension (AV nicking); and Gunn's dots (drusen) which are minute white dots on the retina of the eye, close to the macula.

Pupillary Accommodation

Note pupillary accommodation by having the patient focus on your finger held about eighteen inches away. Slowly move your finger toward the patient's nose. As the eyes begin to cross, the pupils will normally constrict. Loss of

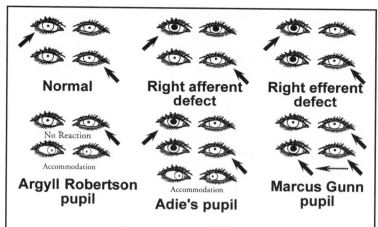

Figure 48. Pupillary Reactions.

Seeing both pupils constrict (direct and consensual responses) is normal. No direct or consensual response when shining the light in the right eye, but with normal responses when shining the light in the left eye, suggests a right afferent defect. A right efferent defect is suggested when the right eye does not show direct or consensual responses but the left eye shows normal responses. Irregularly shaped pupils that do not react but show accommodation are called Argyll Robertson pupils and indicate possible neurosyphilis. Adie's pupil does not react but may accommodate sluggishly in a darkened room. Dilation to the direct response (following a consensual constrictive response) implies an afferent defect in that eye, called a Marcus Gunn pupil. Conditions that produce a Marcus Gunn pupil in elderly people include demyelinating disease, multiple sclerosis, unilateral macular degeneration, retinal disease, and severe unilateral cataract.

accommodation suggests Adie's pupil or Wernicke's encephalopathy. Pupils that accommodate vigorously but do not react are called Argyll Robertson pupils. While Argyll Robertson pupils are classically associated with neurosyphilis, they can be seen in a number of metabolic (alcoholism or diabetes mellitus), infectious, vascular (cerebral aneurysms, hemorrhage) and neoplastic lesions. Tachycardia with extreme gaze convergence is Ruggeri's reflex.

William John Adie (1886–1935) was an Australian physician and neurologist who learned German from hanging around sailors, and used it to study neurology in Germany. In World War I he saved numerous soldiers by devising an emergency gas mask of urine-soaked cloth. He was an excellent teacher and diagnostician, treating his students as colleagues. Adie described narcolepsy and the dilated sluggish pupil that bears his name. He died of a myocardial infarction at the age of 48.

Hippus

Note the speed of hippus, which is the normal rhythmic oscillation of pupil at 60 beats per minute or faster. You can bring out the oscillation by shining your light so that just one-third of the pupil is illuminated. Normal oscillation rules out significant autonomic dysfunction to the level of the cervical ganglion. Hippus slows in autonomic dysfunction of any cause. Common etiologies include medications, diabetic neuropathy, Horner's syndrome, and increased intracranial pressure.

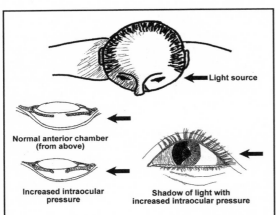

Figure 49. Evaluating the Anterior Chamber.
Have the patient look at your nose and check the corneal angle by shining your light from the temporal side of the eye across the cornea, as shown in the upper part of the illustration. The entire iris should light up immediately when the light hits the limbus. A small triangular shadow from the pupil that points toward the nasal side and away from the light source (right side of the illustration) suggests anterior displacement of the lens (left side of illustration) caused by increased intraocular pressure.

EVALUATE THE ANTERIOR CHAMBER

Have the patient look at your nose and check the corneal angle by shining your light from the temporal side of the eye across the cornea. The entire iris should light up immediately when the light hits the limbus. A small

triangular shadow from the pupil that points toward the nasal side away from the light source suggests increased intraocular pressure. Likewise, a small crescent shadow on the nasal side of the iris near the limbus suggests anterior lens displacement and increased risk for acute narrow angle glaucoma.

Estimate intraocular pressure by gently pressing on the patient's closed eyes with your thumbs. Normal eyes are soft like ripe grapes. Dehydrated patients have very soft, over-ripe grape-feeling eyes. Increased ocular pressure makes the affected eye feel firm and hard.

EXTRAOCULAR EYE MOVEMENTS

Shine a light at the patient from two to three feet away so that the light reflects in both eyes. Note the point of reflected light in each eye for symmetry (Hirschberg's test). Each millimeter of deviation of the reflected point of light suggests seven degrees of eye deviation. (The reflected point of light will move opposite to the direction of deviation.) Deviation suggests strabismus, gaze palsy or orbital displacement.

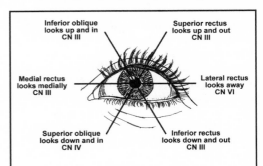

Figure 50. Cardinal Points of Gaze.
The cardinal positions are horizontal, upper right to lower left, and upper left to lower right. Note that vertical is not a cardinal gaze position. The primary muscle and cranial nerve innervation is labeled for each of the cardinal positions.

Move the light in a large circle while the patient follows the light, and trace the six cardinal gaze positions. The cardinal positions are horizontal, upper right to lower left, and upper left to lower right. Note that vertical is not a cardinal gaze position.

Note any deviation of the light in each eye. (Normally the reflection will be in the exact center if the patient is looking right at the light.) Pay particular attention to the edge of each gaze position, since weakness may appear here first. Unilateral dilation of the abducting eye (Tournay's sign) is normal. Also notice the yoking of gaze, in that the eye movements are together and conjugate.

Strabismus

If one eye deviates from the other producing dysconjugate gaze, then that is called strabismus. In nonparalytic strabismus, each eye can move in all of the cardinal gaze directions. Crossed eyes which both look medially are esotropia. Laterally deviated (wall) eyes are called exotropia. An upwardly deviated eye is called hypertropia while a downward eye is hypotropia. Sometimes vision in the deviated eye is poor due to cortical factors that tend to reduce the vision to avoid diplopia. If the patient has a flash photograph of their face, unilateral loss of a red eye reflex suggests strabismus.

Paralytic strabismus (where one or both eyes cannot move in all six cardinal points of gaze) suggests a cranial nerve or ocular palsy. No eye movement except laterally suggests a third cranial nerve palsy called internuclear ophthalmoplegia. No or limited lateral eye movement suggests a sixth cranial nerve defect or a lateral rectus palsy.

Abnormalities in Extraocular Movements

Classical abnormalities in extraocular eye movements are shown in Figure 51. If the eye moves down and nasally but gets stuck (Brown's syndrome), this suggests inferior oblique tenosynovitis sometimes seen in rheumatoid arthritis. The patient senses vertical diplopia and feels a click or ratcheting sensation. There is no true inferior oblique palsy. Some schol-

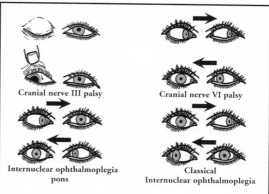

Cranial nerve III palsy   Cranial nerve VI palsy

Internuclear ophthalmoplegia pons

Classical Internuclear ophthalmoplegia

Figure 51.
Abnormal Extraocular Eye Movements.
The upper panel shows a right cranial nerve III palsy with ptosis and a dilated pupil that rotates downward with external elevation of the lid. Loss of this subtle rotation suggests coexistent cranial nerve IV palsy. The upper right panel shows a right cranial nerve VI lesion with loss of lateral gaze. The lower two panels show internuclear ophthalmoplegias at the level of the pons and, classically, where the medial longitudinal fasiculus is impaired between the opposite third nerve nucleus above and the sixth nerve nucleus below. (Consider demyelinating disease as the most likely cause.)

ars believe that Alexander the Great had Brown's syndrome (probably from a battle wound) because he always walked with his chin elevated and his nose in the air looking to the right.

If the eye cannot move down nasally this suggests cranial nerve IV palsy or a superior oblique problem. Note that the head tilts away from the side of the lesion (Bielschowsky's sign) and if you gently move the head to tilt in the opposite direction, the affected pupil will elevate. Consider a superior oblique palsy in patients with torticollis. One eye that cannot look upward and nasally suggests inferior oblique palsy.

Confirm subtle movement abnormalities by having the patient gaze at a distant object. Cover one eye and watch for any movement of the uncovered eye. Any movement at all suggests a subtle defect requiring the eye to reposition itself. Next cover the other eye and again watch for any movement in the uncovered eye. In Bell's palsy, the eye with the facial paralysis rolls upward and outward on attempted closing. In extreme increased intracranial pressure, the eyes may roll down (Setting Sun sign).

Nystagmus

Nystagmus is primarily a neurological sign that reflects a structural or metabolic problem in the oculomotor, cerebellar or vestibular connections. The slow movement is the vestibular component, while the fast movement is the central nervous system component. Nystagmus is normally present in extreme lateral gaze. The rapid movement is in the direction of the gaze, and is never more than three beats. True nystagmus appears very early in lateral eye movement, so going to the extremes of gaze is unnecessary.

These eye movements should not be confused with saccadic eye movements that are normal in elderly people. Saccadic movements are generally a jerky pursuit movement with no fast or slow component.

In abnormal or pathological nystagmus, the rapid movement is always in the same direction regardless of gaze, and the abnormality can be appreciated in the middle of the visual field, not just at the extremes of gaze. End point horizontal nystagmus suggests problem in the vestibular system, brain stem or cerebellum. Horizontal nystagmus when fixed on an object suggests severe cerebellar disease. Vertical nystagmus suggests Wernicke's encephalopathy, progressive supranuclear palsy, or a midline central nervous system process. Downbeating nystagmus suggests severe brain stem dysfunction or injury due to phenytoin or lithium toxicity, magnesium deficiency, alcoholic cerebellar degeneration, paraneoplastic syndromes, or encephalitis. If nystagmus increases with following the examining finger, that suggests a central cause; if the nystagmus decreases, that suggests congenital nystagmus (Bard's sign). Nystagmus in demyelinating disease is Uhthoff's sign.

CHECK THE VISUAL FIELDS

Screen the visual fields by having the patient sit across from you and stare at your opposite eye. The patient's right eye looks at your left eye and the patient's left eye is covered (see Figure 52). For bedfast patients, lean over the bed, keeping the distance constant during the testing. If the patient's vision is too poor to see your eye, have him or her look at your face. Hold a small bright-colored item in your left hand and extend your left arm. Ask the patient

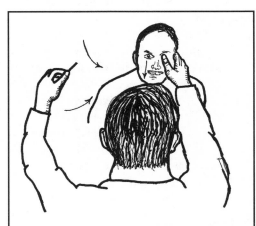

Figure 52. Visual Field Testing.
Have the patient sit across from you and stare at your opposite eye; for bedfast patients, lean over the bed, keeping the distance constant during the testing. Hold a small, bright-colored item in your left hand and extend your left arm. Ask the patient to tell you when he or she sees the object. Quickly move the object in an arc from your upper left quadrant to the center. Compare when the patient sees the object with when you see it. Do the same test starting from your lower left quadrant, arcing up to the center. Repeat the test on the opposite side, covering the patient's right eye and testing the superior arc and then the inferior arc. The text includes interpretations of the various findings. Redrawn from John Patton's *Neurological Differential Diagnosis*, 2nd Edition, 1995. Figure 3.1, page 18. Used with permission of Springer Science and Business Media.

to tell you when he or she sees the object. Quickly move the object in an arc from your upper left quadrant to the center. Compare when the patient sees the object with when you see it. Do the same test starting from your lower left quadrant, arcing up to the center. Repeat the test on the opposite side, covering the patient's right eye and testing the superior arc and then the inferior arc. If the patient has a limited visual field on one side (both arcs less than your field of vision), consider a homonymous hemianopsia, optic tract disease, or monocular blindness. If the patient has limited vision on all four arcs, consider bitemporal hemianopsia due to disease in the sella tursica.

An upper outer quadrantanopsia (only one of the superior arcs) suggests temporal tumor or infarction, while a lower outer quadrantanopsia (missing one of the inferior arcs) suggests a parietal tumor or infarction. A midline defect implies heteronymous hemianopsia.

FUNDOSCOPIC EVALUATION

The serious fundoscopic examination requires dilating the pupils with 1% Mydriacil or 0.5% tropicamide. Make sure the patient has transportation home because the dilating agent may not completely wear off for hours and he or she may not be able to drive. Have the patient seated comfortably, focusing on a specific point on the wall, looking slightly over your shoulder of the arm holding the ophthalmoscope (see Figure 53). This will allow you to zero in on the optic disc later and will not be as uncomfortable for the patient. The red (negative) numbers of the ophthalmoscope will help in examining the optic fundus and nearsighted patients. (You did check the patient's glasses.) The black or green (positive) numbers will help you examine the anterior chamber.

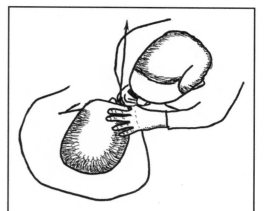

Figure 53. Positioning for the Fundoscopic Examination.

Have the patient seated comfortably and focusing on a specific point on the wall, looking slightly over your shoulder of the arm holding the ophthalmoscope. This positioning will allow you to zero in on the optic disc later and the bright light will not be as uncomfortable for the patient. Notice that the examiner and the patient are almost cheek to cheek, and that the examiner uses the right eye to look into the patient's right eye and vice versa. Redrawn from John Patton's *Neurological Differential Diagnosis*, 2nd Edition, 1995. Figure 4.1, page 40. Used with permission of Springer Science and Business Media.

To determine the appropriate black and red number setting for you, perform the following tests. Hold your left forefinger tip approximately one inch away from the ophthalmoscope which is held in your right hand while you look through it. Turn the dial until your fingertip is in perfect focus. Note the black or green number. That will be the setting you use to examine the anterior chamber. To determine the correct red number, look across the room through the ophthalmoscope and focus on a distant object such as the light switch. Turn the dial until the object is in focus and you have your red number. These numbers will be constant for you unless your vision significantly changes.

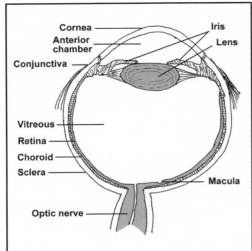

Figure 54. Top View of the Eye.
This illustration shows the cross-sectional anatomy of the eye as seen from above. The basic structures are labeled.

Examining the Anterior Chamber and Vitreous

With the ophthalmoscope on your black number, begin by shining the light into the eye to obtain the red reflex. Next, examine the anterior chamber by moving close to the patient, almost cheek to cheek (see Figure 53), looking at the anterior and posterior cornea. You should be able to see a faint reflection of the light on the lens. (The brightest reflection is off the corneal tear film.) Haziness of the anterior cornea suggests interstitial keratitis. Check for lens opacities such as cataracts. Round gray spots on the posterior cornea are mutton fat bodies and suggest sarcoidosis, tuberculosis, candidiasis or other fungal disease.

You can tell anterior from posterior corneal opacities by looking at the center of the pupil with the ophthalmoscope. Slowly move up while you keep the light on the center of the pupil. Anterior opacities will tend to move up as well, while posterior opacities will move down or below your visual axis.

Once you have examined the anterior chamber, focus through the vitreous to see if there are any lesions (see Figure 54). Vitreous

hemorrhage is not subtle. Occasionally you will see white or glassy spheres (Asteroides hyalosis), which are a benign finding.

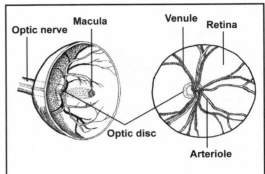

Figure 55. Optic Fundus.
This illustration shows an angled view of the optic fundus on the left panel and how it looks to the examiner on the right. The optic nerve head is the optic disc, with the arterioles and venules exiting from it and the fibers leading to the macula. The venules are darker than the arterioles because the wall of the venule is transparent, allowing the blood to be seen more clearly.

Examining the Optic Disc

The next step of the fundoscopic examination is to change to your red number on your ophthalmoscope (and reduce the light intensity) and to systematically evaluate the optic disc. Follow the vessel branches to the disc, as they will point to the disc. A decrease in the number of arterioles suggests optic atrophy (Kestenbaum's sign). An apparent loss of temporal vessels, so that they appear to come only from the nasal side, suggests glaucoma.

Carefully notice the disc color. It is usually slightly paler on the temporal side. A bone-white disc with normal vessels is optic atrophy caused by vascular conditions (temporal arteritis, thrombosis of the retinal vein or artery, or aneurysm), toxic or metabolic states (Vitamin B12 deficiency, nutrient deficiency, carbon monoxide poisoning, or alcohol, methanol or ethylene glycol ingestion), optic neuritis, tabes dorsalis, neoplasm or glaucoma. A red disc (hyperemia) suggests neovascularization, papilledema, retinal vein thrombosis, retinal ischemia, or polycythemia. Flame hemorrhages and exudates around the disc suggest papilledema. Chunks of yellow gelatinous material on the disc are hyaloid or colloid bodies of the disc and can cause wedge-shaped visual field defects.

Also pay careful attention to the disc margins. The nasal border may not be as sharp as the temporal border. Loss of the disc margins suggests papilledema. Normally, the disc cup appears as a pale circle in the center of the disc. Having the cup appear vertically oval suggests glaucoma. Also note the size and depth of the cup in relation to the disc. Normally the cup is less than one-half the size of the disc. Enlargement of the cup or deepening of the cup suggests glaucoma.

Venous Pulsations

Note venous pulsations by finding a fat vein that exits the disc and focusing on the pulsations that are normally present. These pulsations occur because the intraocular pressure is normally less than venous pressure. (If it were higher we would not see the veins at all.) The arterial pulse pressure plus the intraocular pressure is enough to collapse the veins. When the pulse pressure drops, the veins can refill and we perceive a "venous pulse." These are important observations because seeing these pulsations rules out increased intracranial pressure. The absence of venous pulsations may signify increased intracranial pressure, since the veins cannot refill.

Examining the Retinal Vessels

After carefully looking at the disc, systematically examine the vessels. Follow each vessel from the disc outward going as far as possible.

Arteries are red or copper in color and the reflection of light along the vessel is normally a thin white streak. Atherosclerosis does not affect the optic fundus, so arteriolar scle-

rolosis with eosinophilic hyaline cause the arteriolar changes to be seen. Copper wire color suggests hypertension and hypertrophy of the vascular wall. Seeing a glistening diamond-like sparkle within an artery suggests cholesterol emboli (Hollenhorst plaque). Noticing increased retinal artery pulsations (Becker's sign) suggests hyperthyroidism or aortic insufficiency.

Veins are a dark burgundy color and are normally larger than the arteries. The darkness is due to the lack of a muscular wall in the more transparent vein. Note any venous engorgement, which would suggest retinal vein occlusion, increased venous pressure (Superior Vena Cava syndrome, tricuspid insufficiency, congestive heart failure, cardiac tamponade), increased plasma viscosity (Waldenstrom's macroglobulinemia, multiple myeloma, cryoglobulinemia, hemoglobinopathies), diabetes mellitus or hematologic malignancy. In lateral sinus vein thrombosis, compression of the contralateral jugular vein provides visible swelling of the retinal veins (Crowe's sign).

While examining each vessel check the vascular crossings for AV nicking (Gunn's sign). These need to be seen more than two disc diameters from the disc to be significant, and there must be a clear zone separating the artery from the underlying vein. This is an important finding because hypertensive elderly patients with these vascular changes (AV nicking) will also have left ventricular hypertrophy. Also look for any segmental vascular narrowing. Vascular sausaging suggests hyperviscosity.

Another thing to look for is tortuous vessels. Tortuosity suggests chronic hypertension, so this can help distinguish normal aging from chronic hypertension. Tortuous vessels near soft exudates suggest neovascularization. Also look for the microaneurysms of diabetes mellitus.

Carefully check for vascular sheathing, which looks like parallel white lines along vessels. Venous sheathing is seen in diabetes mellitus, hypertension, and infection (candidiasis, tuberculosis, fungi). Arteriolar sheathing suggests hypertension, polyarteritis nodosa and leukemia.

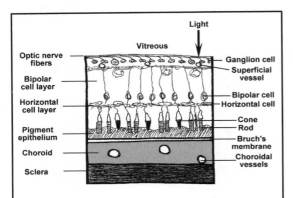

Figure 56. Cross-Section of the Retina.
The most superficial layers of the retina are parallel layers of optic nerve fibers, including the ganglion cells, bipolar cell layer, horizontal cell layer and the rods and cones. Bleeding within these layers will be red and flame-shaped, and infarction of these layers will produce fluffy, cotton wool spots. Bleeding below the pigment epithelium layer will look black rather than red. Bruch's membrane is the location where Drusen and angioid streaks occur. The choroidal and scleral layers lie below Bruch's membrane.

Retinal lesions

After examining the vessels, the next set of observations involve the retina. Normally the retina is a pale, orange color. A very pale retina compared to the retina of the other eye suggests central retinal artery occlusion. A change in the retinal shape, with vascular irregularities in the superior temporal field, suggests retinal detachment.

Note any lesions in the retina. Hemorrhages are always abnormal but not specific diagnostically for any particular disease. Small hemorrhages (one millimeter) suggest hypertension, or vasculitis. A small hemorrhage with a white spot in the center, due to deposited fibrin (Roth's spot), suggests bacterial endocarditis, acute leukemia, pernicious anemia, neurological disorders, scurvy, carbon monoxide poisoning, vasculitis, or post–cardiac bypass

surgery. Small blot hemorrhage suggests hypertension, diabetes mellitus, infection, sarcoidosis, Waldenstrom's macroglobinemia, leukemia, multiple myeloma, TTP, severe anemia, or collagen vascular disease. Large hemorrhages suggest hypertensive retinopathy, intracranial hemorrhage, central retinal vein occlusion, and increased intracranial pressure.

Moritz Roth (1839–1914) was a Swiss pathologist and anatomist. Roth wrote a number of articles related to medical history. His book on Andreas Vesalius is a standard historical reference text. Roth is remembered for his Roth spot, a white, round spot in the retina close to the optic disk, often surrounded by oval areas of hemorrhages.

A large hemorrhage with a pocket shape (straight line top) suggests a subhyaloid hemorrhage in an upright patient.

Red dots are usually microaneurysms and suggest diabetes mellitus or hemoglobinopathy.

Exudates

Hard exudates have hard distinct borders with a shiny quality. They are never normal and imply disruption of the blood-brain barrier so that protein can be deposited. Conditions to consider include severe proteinuria, renal disease, diabetes mellitus, collagen vascular disease (polyarteritis, SLE, dermatomyositis), multiple myeloma, leukemia, pernicious anemia, infections, and lead poisoning.

Soft exudates have fluffy borders and are not near vessels. They result from retinal infarction and are never normal. Causes of soft exudates include severe hypertension, severe anemia (hemoglobin less than 8mg/dl), malignancy, collagen vascular disease, or embolization (fat, cardiac bypass surgery, SBE).

Single large soft exudates in the periphery, with satellite lesions, suggest toxoplasmosis chorioretinitis. Multiple soft exudates suggest histoplasmosis or CMV infection.

Other Light-Colored Retinal Lesions

Drusen (Gunn's dots) are small distinct yellow dots in clusters that are usually a clue to old macular degeneration. Sometimes they can be seen in chronic leukemia. Sarcoidosis can produce ocular granulomas that are distinct but with fluffy margins, so they are technically not hard exudates. Myelinated nerves have a soft, feathery edge.

Acute chorioretinitis from numerous infections can produce light-colored retinal lesions. If you are not sure if a retinal lesion is significant, note it and obtain additional help. Some important conditions with retinal clues to consider include fungi, bacteria, parasites, rickettsia, viruses, leukemic infiltrates, metastatic disease, and old laser therapy.

Pale lines radiating from the discs are angioid streaks. Angioid streaks are defects in Bruch's membrane and appear to run under the vessels. They look like vessels and resemble the vapor trail of jet aircraft in the sky. In elderly people the most common cause is Paget's disease, although they are classically associated with pseudoxanthoma elasticum and hemoglobinopathies. Lines not radiating from the discs are pseudoangioid streaks and suggest choroidal atrophy or retinal detachment.

Hyperpigmented Retinal Lesions

Dark pigmented soft exudates around the disc suggest tuberculosis. Large dark, black lesions with sharp borders suggest old chorioretinitis. Malignant melanoma may appear more gray or light brown than black if it is below the retinal layer in the choroids. It sometimes appears raised or nodular.

Choroidal hemorrhage can appear as a dark retinal lesion, but the retinal vessels are on top of the pigmentation, so the vessels travel over the hemorrhage. Conditions that can produce choroidal hemorrhage include diabetes mellitus, TTP, pernicious anemia, and leukemia.

Multiple small, dark, circular spots suggest previous laser therapy. Multiple brown, oval spots bilaterally suggests Gardner's syndrome. (The elderly patient will have had previous colectomy since the colon cancer rate associated with this condition is 100%.)

Examining the Macula

After examining the retina it is important to examine the macula. The macula is usually two disc diameters lateral to the disc. It appears as a rounded blush about one disc diameter wide. Look for the light reflection around the rim. A glistening spot in the center of the macula is the fovea. Radiations from the macula (macular star) suggest papilledema. Pigmented rings around macula (bull's eye macula) suggest drug-induced macular degeneration. A bright, cherry-red macula suggests retinal artery occlusion, temporal arteritis, cryoglobulinemia, severe hypertension, or quinine toxicity.

SPECIAL TESTS

The Cover Test

The cover test is helpful in evaluating the patient with double vision. Have the patient stare at an object about two feet away. Cover one eye and then move the cover to the other eye, noting any movement of the eye being uncovered. Any eye motion on uncovering is abnormal and suggests strabismus.

SPECIAL CIRCUMSTANCES

The Elderly Patient with a Red Eye

The basic differential is acute narrow angle glaucoma, acute iritis, or acute conjunctivitis. Beware; the patient may have more than one condition.

♦ CAREFULLY INSPECT THE EYE

A dilated pupil, perilimbal fine vascularity and diffuse red, swollen conjuctiva with redness extending into the limbus suggest acute glaucoma. Acute iritis often presents as redness along the limbus. The causes of acute iritis are SLE, adult juvenile rheumatoid arthritis, polyarteritis, sarcoidosis, Behcet's syndrome and inflammatory bowel disease. Red, tender papules on the sclera, not touching the limbus, suggest episcleritis. Acute conjunctivitis often shows visible pus and is caused by Reiter's syndrome, bacterial infection, viral infection (check for palpable preauricular lymph nodes), and chlamydia. A bright, red, obviously hemorrhagic area suggests subconjunctival hemorrhage. Subconjuctival hemorrhage around the limbus suggests Apollo disease caused by picornavirus.

♦ CHECK THE CORNEAL ANGLE

The next step is to check the corneal angle by shining the light from the temporal side (see Figure 49). The entire iris should light up. Seeing a shadow from the pupil suggests increased intraocular pressure. Also, a crescent shadow on nasal side of the iris suggests acute narrow angle glaucoma in this setting.

♦ PERFORM THE AU-HENKIND TEST

The third step in evaluating an elderly person with a red eye is to perform the Au-Henkind test to differentiate iritis from conjunctivitis (highly sensitive and specific). To perform the Au-Henkind test, have the patient close the red eye and lightly cover the eye with a hand. Shine a bright light into the open eye. If the consensual response produces pain in the closed eye, then the Au-Henkind test is positive indicating iritis. The pain is caused by the pupillary contraction of the consensual response.

♦ EXAMINE THE CORNEA AND ANTERIOR CHAMBER

Step four is to carefully examine the cornea and the anterior chamber. Areas of corneal cloudiness suggest corneal abrasion, corneal ulcer, acute keratitis, and chronic hypercalcemia (band keratopathy). Anterior chamber cloudiness with vascular dilation suggests anterior uveitis.

♦ CHECK FOR DISCHARGE UNDER THE LIDS

The final step is to check for discharge under the eyelids. Seeing a purulent discharge suggests bacterial conjunctivitis, while a ropy discharge and general redness suggests atopic conjunctivitis. A clear discharge suggests viral conjunctivitis, and you should confirm by palpating a preauricular lymph node. Refer the patient to an ophthalmologist immediately for slit lamp and additional evaluation.

CHAPTER 9

The Ears, Nose, Mouth and Throat

"Wisdom ceases to be wisdom when it becomes too proud to weep, too grave to laugh, and too selfful to seek other than itself."

— **Kahlil Gibran**

"He should observe thus in acute diseases: first, the countenance of the patient, if it be like those of persons in health, and more so, if like itself, for this is the best of all; whereas the most opposite to it is the worst, such as the following: a sharp nose, hollow eyes, collapsed temples; the ears cold, contracted, and their lobes turned out; the skin about the forehead being rough, distended, and parched; the color of the whole face being green, black, livid, or lead-colored."

— **Hippocrates**

The ears, nose and mouth form the middle and lower third of the face. In contrast to the eyes and mouth, the nose has minimal impact on our emotional response and contributes relatively little to facial expression. The mouth has no fixed attachment to the skull and has an infinite variety of expressions. The rounded curves of the mouth represent a continuity of the surrounding structures. The nasolabial fold separates the cheeks from the upper lip and deepens with age. The lower lip tends to be fuller but lighter in color and less distinct in its inferior margin than the more sharply defined upper lip. The upper lip has a central notch (the filtrum) with two ridges on each side.

EARS

Inspection

Inspect the external ear and note the ear position. Ears that have their upper level below the level of the pupils suggest a congenital abnormality such as Down's syndrome. Basal cell cancers, squamous cell cancers, solar keratoses and other skin lesions may appear on the ear. Also look for symmetry of the ears. A unilateral painful rash with vesicles on the lower ear suggests Ramsey Hunt syndrome (herpes zoster of the geniculate ganglion). *Be sure to check for this in any patient who presents with facial paralysis.* A unilateral, bright, red, swollen ear suggests external otitis. Red, lax or floppy ears suggest relapsing polychondritis. In superficial skin infections the ears can be involved, but subcutaneous infections spare the ear (Millian's sign). Long ear hairs suggest normal androgenic function (Hamilton's sign).

James Ramsay Hunt (1872–1937) was an American neurologist who studied abroad before returning to New York to practice. His major research interest was neuroanatomy, and disorders of the corpus striatum and the extra-pyramidal system. He is best known for first describing a syndrome of herpes zoster involving the geniculate ganglion with lesions of the external ear and oral mucosa. Ramsay Hunt syndrome II is commonly seen in the elderly population, with equal distribution between men and women. In 1907 Ramsay Hunt first described this combination of symptoms as a syndrome that he separated into 4 forms:

1) Herpes zoster without neuralgic signs
2) Herpes zoster with facial paresis
3) Herpes zoster with facial paresis and hearing symptoms
4) Ramsay Hunt's syndrome — auricular herpes zoster syndrome

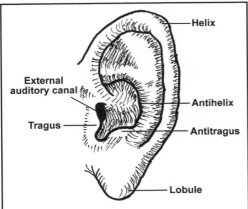

Figure 57. Normal External Ear.
The main portion of the outer ear is the helix, with the most dependent portion called the lobule or ear lobe. The inner ridge of the ear is the antihelix. The firm area just anterior to the external auditory canal is the tragus, while the corresponding portion on the opposite side of the canal is the antitragus.

Congenital abnormalities of the ear may be associated with congenital abnormalities of the kidneys, heart, and great vessels. Kidney lesions tend to be ipsilateral to the ear abnormality.

Traumatic abnormalities to the ear often present as a thick, rubbery painless deformity. A diagonal ear lobe crease suggests increased risk of coronary artery disease. Tender chalky nodules on the pinna suggest gouty tophi in a person who has lived in a cold climate, since lower temperature reduces the solubility of uric acid. Single nontender nodule on the helix since birth suggests a Darwinian tubercle.

Movement of the ear lobe coincident with the pulse suggests tricuspid insufficiency (Paul Dudley White's winking ear lobe sign).

Palpation

Stiffness of the earlobe suggests Addison's disease, while stiffness of the pinna and auricular cartilage suggests other endocrine abnormalities, such as hyperthyroidism, acromegaly, diabetes mellitus, and hypopituitarism. A crusted ulcer on the pinna suggests squamous cell cancer.

Painful ears on tugging the pinna or finding a tender tragus suggest external otis media. If the patient has diabetes, this could be a serious problem because of progression to osteomyelitis involving the temporal bone. In this case check for mastoiditis by palpating the suprameatal triangle of MacEwen, which is the depression at 11 o'clock on the right ear and 1 o'clock on the left ear (see Figure 39). Find these little depressions on yourself. This area is not tender in external otis media, so tenderness in MacEwen's space suggests co-existent mastoiditis.

Screening for Hearing Loss

Some patients thought to be demented or psychiatric may actually have hearing loss as the explanation of their odd behavior. While standing behind the patient (for me, usually during the back or lung examination) give a simple command such as "raise your right arm" to see if he or she can follow your command. This approach (of not providing a visual cue) is a useful initial screening test. The challenge is to remember to do it when you get to the pulmonary examination.

♦ THE FINGER FRICTION TEST

Another useful screening test is the finger friction test. Put your forefinger and thumb of each hand at the external auditory canal of each ear and ask the patient to tell you when they hear the sound. Rub the finger and thumb together on one side and then the other. Note if the patient can hear the sounds.

Sir Herman David Weber (1823–1918) was the son of a German father and Italian mother. He entered medical school in Marburg, Germany, and received his doctorate in Bonn in 1848. In Marburg he had the opportunity to work with several well-known physicians of that time, among them Sir James Simpson, the Scottish physician who introduced chloroform as a pain reliever in 1847. Weber obtained a position at Guy's Hospital in London and became a member of the Royal College of Physicians in 1855. He retired as a hospital physician in 1890, but remained the German Embassy physician in London. Weber was a great advocate of healthy exercise and advised his patients to take their vacation in the Alps, as he did.

♦ THE WEBER TEST

This test relies on the observation made by Weber in 1834 that sounds will be louder in an occluded ear canal than an open ear canal if the neurological function is intact. To test this, use a 512 Hz tuning fork because this frequency is in the middle of the normal conversational voice range.

Place the vibrating tuning fork in the middle of the patient's head and ask if he or she hears the sound (not feels the vibration). If the patient cannot hear the sound then he or she has bilateral sensorineural hearing loss and probably cannot hear your voice. If the patient does hear the tone, then ask in which ear he or

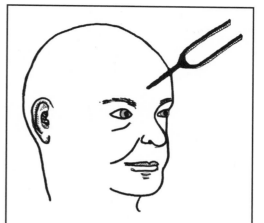

Figure 58. Weber Test.
Place a 512 Hz vibrating tuning fork in the middle of the patient's head and ask if he or she hears the sound (not feels the vibration). If the patient hears the tone, then ask in which ear he or she hears the sound. Hearing the sound in both ears or in the midline of the head is normal. If one ear is occluded, then the sound will localize to the *bad* ear. (The occluded side will sound louder.) If there is sensorineural hearing loss on one side, then the Weber test localizes to the good ear. In this case slowly move the tuning fork toward the bad ear until the sound is in the midline. Now occlude the good ear (furthest from the tuning fork) and see if the equality of sound changes. If the sound is now louder in the occluded good ear, then you have localized the hearing loss to the affected side.

she hears the sound. If one ear is occluded, then the sound will localize to the *bad* ear. (The occluded side will sound louder.)

Hearing the sound in both ears or in the midline of the head is normal. If there is sensorineural hearing loss on one side, then the Weber test localizes to the good ear. In this case slowly move the tuning fork toward the bad ear until the sound is in the midline. Now occlude the good ear (furthest from the tuning fork) and see if the equality of sound changes. If the sound is now louder in the occluded good ear, then you have localized the hearing loss to the affected side. If the patient does not appreciate any change when the canal is occluded, then he or she is responding to the vibration of the tuning fork, not the loudness of the sound.

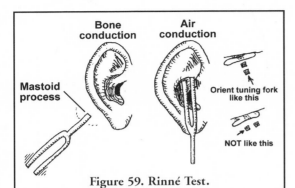

Figure 59. Rinné Test.

Place the vibrating 512 Hz tuning fork on the patient's mastoid process and ask the patient to tell you when the sound disappears. As soon as it disappears, shift the tuning fork to the external auditory canal and ask if he or she can hear the sound now. Hearing the sound is a normal test, since air conduction should be greater than bone conduction. Note that the tines of the tuning fork should both point toward the ear for the maximum vibratory sound, as shown in the illustration. Sometimes you can ask, "Which is louder, this?" (placing on the mastoid), "or this?" (placing at the external auditory canal). Obviously the canal should be louder than the mastoid. Not hearing the sound louder with air conduction suggests a conduction hearing loss on that side.

♦ THE RINNÉ TEST

This hearing test depends on the acoustic phenomenon that air conduction should be greater than bone conduction. To test this, place the vibrating tuning fork on the patient's mastoid process and ask the patient to tell you when the sound disappears. As soon as it disappears, shift the tuning fork to the external auditory canal and ask if he or she can hear the sound now. Hearing the sound is a normal test. Note that the tines of the tuning fork should both point toward the ear for the maximum vibratory sound. Not hearing the sound return suggests a conduction hearing loss on that side. Sometimes you can ask, "Which is louder, this?" (placing on the mastoid), "or this?" (placing at the external auditory canal). Obviously the canal should be louder than the mastoid.

♦ LOW FREQUENCY HEARING TEST

Have the patient listen for the dial tone on the telephone. If low frequency hearing is intact, Ménière's disease is ruled out.

♦ CHANDLER'S TEST OF RECRUITMENT

Lightly hit a tuning fork and present it back and forth between each ear. Hit the tuning fork hard and see if the affected ear now hears as well or better than the good ear. If so, then recruitment is present.

Friedrich Heinrich Adolf Rinné (1819–1868) was a German ENT surgeon who spent time working in an asylum.

♦ SCHWABACH'S TEST

Schwabach's test compares the patient's bone conduction with the examiner's bone conduction. Perform the first part of the Rinné test. When the patient can no longer hear the bone conduction, place the tuning fork on your own mastoid. If the patient has sensorineural hearing loss you will hear the sound longer than the patient does.

Dagobert Schwabach (1846–1920) was a German otologist who published numerous articles on hearing tests, deaf mutism, and the statistics of deaf mutism.

♦ POLITZER'S TEST

If a patient has unilateral hearing loss, then check Politzer's test. Place the vibrating tuning fork in front of the nose and ask the patient to swallow, to open the Eustachian tube. The patient will localize the sound to the good side if there is unilateral hearing loss, but only when they swallow. Politzer's maneuver is compressing the air in the external canal with the atomizer and noting nystagmus or vertigo. This is due to chronic inner ear infection and the development of a fistula in the horizontal semicircular canal.

Adam Politzer (1835–1920) was an Austrian otologist with great artistic talent. He trained in Vienna under Josef Skoda (1805–1881), Johann Ritter von Oppolzer (1808–1871), and Carl Ludwig (1816–1895). Oppolzer popularized bedside teaching and Ludwig interested Politzer in otology. Polizer developed innovative approaches to treat ear conditions and created a renowned clinic. At his retirement over 500 physicians came to the celebration. The light reflex on the tympanic membrane is sometimes called Politzer's luminous cone of light.

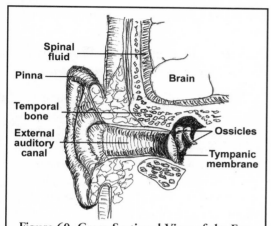

Figure 60. Cross-Sectional View of the Ear.
This illustration shows the relationships between the external and internal ear structures. Note the proximity between the ossicles and the brain.

Examination of the Inner Ear

Examine the right ear first by gently pulling up and back on the pinna with your left hand to straighten the external auditory canal. Introduce the otoscope under direct visualization using the largest speculum you can comfortably insert.

The External Auditory Canal

First note the skin of the external auditory canal. A red canal with white, cottage-cheese–like exudates suggests external otitis media. A red tender spot is a furuncle. Brown debris suggests a cerumen impaction. Blood in the external canal suggests local trauma from a foreign body (such as a toothpick), or furuncle. In the appropriate setting (such as after a fall, with head trauma) blood in the external canal can be a clue to fracture of the temporal bone. Bony exostoses that appear as

dome-shaped nodules (resembling a torus manibularis in the mouth) suggest the patient has been a cold-water swimmer.

Gently touch the posterior auditory canal and note any hypesthesia. Hypesthesia of the posterior auditory canal (Hitselberger's sign) suggests an acoustic neuroma.

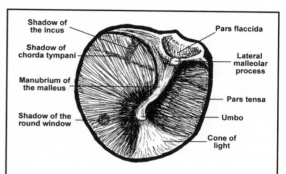

Figure 61. Tympanic Membrane.
The landmarks of the right tympanic membrane are shown in this illustration. The membrane seems to drape over the manubrium of the malleus. The end of the malleus is the umbo, with the light reflex appearing in the inferior nasal part of the eardrum. Just anterior to the light reflex is the pars tensa. The upper portion of the tympanic membrane is called the pars flaccida, a key place to look for subtle perforations or masses. Rarely shadows can be appreciated from the incus, chorda tympani or round window.

The Tympanic Membrane

Once you have examined the auditory canal, focus your attention on the tympanic membrane (see Figure 61). The normal color is a pale shiny gray. Diffuse erythema suggests otitis media, but be careful in interpreting redness since your touching of the posterior canal can produce a vascular flush that looks like a lacy, reticular net along the handle of the malleolus. Seeing serous or bloody vesicles on the eardrum suggests bullous myringitis from mycoplasma pneumonia. Sometimes herpes virus infection will produce serous vesicles (Ramsay Hunt syndrome).

Note the normal concave shape of the eardrum. Bulging is often a sign of infection. Blood behind the eardrum suggests basilar skull fracture (Laugier's sign). Retraction of the eardrum implies Eustachian tube obstruction. The umbo will be prominent and the tympanic membrane will drape posteriorly like a circus tent seen from the air (Dumbo's view of the umbo). If there are bubbles behind the eardrum, they suggest serous otitis media, and an air-fluid level may be seen.

The next part of the ear examination is to carefully look for perforations in the eardrum. Check all along the border (annulus) of the tympanic membrane. Defects along this margin can suggest cholesteatoma. Cholesteatoma looks like a shiny basal-cell-like lesion looking pearly gray or white. Next, examine the bony landmarks: look at the anterior orientation of the light reflection, and then examine the malleus. Look at the umbo or central point of the eardrum and the handle or manubrium of the malleus. Anesthesia of the tympanic membrane suggests otosclerosis (Itard's sign).

Jean Marc Gaspard Itard (1774–1838) entered medicine by deception. He got a position at a bank after formal education but had to leave this comfortable position to join the army. He presented himself as a physician and was employed as an assistant physician to a military hospital in Soliers. His brilliance, hard work and enthusiasm allowed him to acquire the necessary knowledge. He focused on the ear, and otology owes to him the invention and improvement of several surgical instruments and techniques, as well as the design of hearing aids. Among his pioneering achievements was the invention of the Eustachian catheter (Itard's catheter). Itard served as editor of several medical journals. His most important work on otology appeared in 1821, containing the results of his scientific research based on more than 172 detailed cases.

The Pars Flaccida

The pars flaccida is just above the malleus in the superior portion of the tympanic membrane. This area is hard for a tall physician to see because you have to get lower than the patient's ear to look up, but it is a key place to look because a defect or a pearly lesion here suggests cholesteatoma. This is an important place to look if the patient has a facial paralysis. (In fact, any patient with facial paralysis should be checked for cholesteatoma.)

Complete the internal ear examination by checking the eardrum motion. Simply have the patient hold his or her nose and swallow while you watch the tympanic membrane.

Evaluating the Patient Who Hears a Rushing or Clicking Sound

Hearing an unusual rushing sound may be due to a fistula involving the carotid artery. To check for this, auscultate the artery for a bruit. If present, pressing on the artery should change the quality of the sound perceived by the patient. Patients with a ventriculoperitoneal shunt (for low pressure hydrocephalus) may hear a flowing sound. Patients with myoclonus may hear clicking sounds. Inadvertent catherization of the internal jugular vein with subclavian line placement can produce a bubbling sensation in the patient's ears. Inflammation of the Eustachian tube can produce a bright clicking sound to the physician and tinnitus to the patient (Leudet's sign). In otitis media the patient may hear their own breath sounds. Tinnitus that improves at high altitude, such as on an airplane in flight, suggests Meniere's disease (Bigger's sign).

NOSE

The goal of the nasal examination is to obtain valuable information on the patient's general health status and to provide information needed to identify specific systemic diseases. In addition, this examination provides information on the part of the respiratory system that warms, moistens, and filters inhaled air, and also serves as the sensory organ for smell.

The nose is shaped like a triangle and is composed of the bridge, tip, nares, vestibule, columella, and ala. The bridge is the superior part of the triangle, the tip is the outer corner of the triangle, the nares are the oval openings at the base of the triangle, the vestibule is the widened area just inside each nares, the columella divides the nose into two nares and is continuous with the nasal septum, and the ala is the lateral outside wing of the nose on either side.

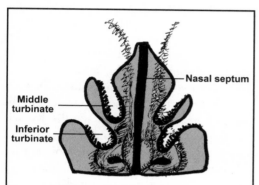

Figure 62. Nasal Cavity.

The nasal cavity has a medial wall composed of the septum that divides the nasal cavity into two oval air passages. The lateral walls have turbinates that project into the nasal cavity and add surface area for warming, moistening, and filtering inhaled air. The inferior and middle turbinates can be seen on examination, but superior turbinate cannot be seen. Under each turbinate is a meatus.

The nasal cavity has a medial wall composed of the septum that divides the nasal cavity into two oval air passages. The lateral walls have turbinates that project into the nasal cavity and add surface area for warming, moistening, and filtering inhaled air. The inferior and middle turbinates can be seen on examination, but superior turbinate is not accessible to examination (see Figure 63). Under each turbinate is a meatus.

The paranasal sinuses are air-filled areas in the skull bones that serve as resonators for sound production, and provide mucus that lubricates the nasal cavity. The frontal sinus is in the lower forehead just above and medial to the eyes. The maxillary sinuses are in the maxilla along the sidewalls of the nasal cavity. The

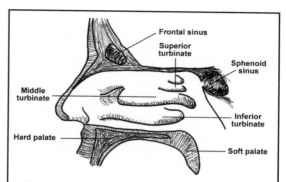

Figure 63. Lateral View of the Nasal Cavity.

The paranasal sinuses are air-filled areas in the skull bones that serve as resonators for sound production, and provide mucus that lubricates the nasal cavity. The frontal sinus is in the lower forehead just above and medial to the eyes. The maxillary sinuses are in the maxilla along the sidewalls of the nasal cavity. The ethmoid sinuses are in between the eyes. The sphenoid sinus is just anterior to the pituitary gland in the sphenoid bone. This view shows why the superior turbinates cannot be seen on routine examination.

ethmoid sinuses are in between the eyes. The sphenoid sinus is just anterior to the pituitary gland in the sphenoid bone.

Prepare the patient for the examination by explaining the procedure in simple terms. The patient should be sitting up straight with head at eye level.

Inspecting the External Nose

Inspect the external surface of the nose from all angles. Normally the skin is intact and similar in color to the face. The surface should be smooth and uniform. Check the nasolabial folds for skin lesions such as basal cell carcinoma and note any external features. Pay special attention to areas of redness, pigmented lesions, lumps, crusts, scaliness, visible vascular pattern, discharge from the nares, and flaring of the nares with respiration. Pulsation of the nasal arteries is increased in thoracic aortic aneurysm (Bozzolo's sign).

Camillo Bozzolo (1845–1920) was an Italian physician who studied the metastasis of cancer through the blood vessels, and particularly by

*spreading through the lymphatics. He reported on
pulse conditions such as the flushing of the nasal
arteries with thoracic aortic aneurysm, wrote
about the nature and treatment of pneumonia,
and made original observations on meningitis.*

Swelling over the bridge of the nose with
bloody discharge suggests nasal fracture. (Palpate for instability of the nasal cartilage.) Indentation and erythema with a turned-up appearance suggests Wegener's granulomatosis.
An enlarged thickened nose suggests acromegaly or rhinophyma (with erythema and telangiectasias). Multiple mucosal telangiectasias
suggests Osler-Weber-Rendu syndrome. Asymmetry suggests infections, trauma, neoplasm or
leprosy. Nasal flaring is an important sign of
respiratory distress. It is sometimes seen in
upper abdominal inflammation. Excessive
nose picking can be seen in early meningitis
(Lafora's sign).

Nasal Discharge

Clear nasal discharge suggests allergic
rhinitis, viral infection, or basilar skull fracture
if the patient has raccoon eyes. (Check the glucose of the fluid, usually above 30mg/dl, for a
clue to a CSF leak.)

Purulent discharge suggests bacterial infection.

If there is bloody nasal discharge in the
setting of trauma such as a fall, see if the blood
clots. If it does not clot consider a CSF leak.
Another useful test is to place a drop of the
bloody fluid on a white paper towel or piece of
filter paper. Seeing a clear wet ring around a
red dot suggests basilar skull fracture.

Evaluate Nasal Patency

Check the patency of each nares by standing directly in front of the patient and occluding the patient's left nares with the index finger
of your right hand. Ask the patient to breath
normally through his or her right nares. Repeat
by occluding the patient's right nares with the
index finger of your left hand and ask the patient to breathe through his or her left nares.
Normally the patient will be able to exhale
through the unoccluded nares. Nasal obstruction is present if the patient is unable to exhale
through the nares.

Evaluating the Nasal Septum

Inspect the nasal septum, by holding the
light and standing directly in front of the patient. Gently press the tip of the patient's vestibule with the thumb of your left hand. Shine
the light onto the patient's vestibule with your
right hand aiming the light parallel to the floor.
Normally the nasal septum is pink in the midline, and intact. The vascular network in the
anterior medial nasal septum is called Kiesselbach's plexus, the most common location of
nosebleeds. Common deviations from normal
findings include a red, pale, or bluish-gray
septum, a nasal septum deviated from midline or a perforation in the septum. Red and
swollen mucosa suggests acute allergic rhinitis. Pale and boggy mucosa suggests allergy.
Red and dry mucosa suggests decongestant use
or anticholinergic effect.

The next step is to transilluminate the
nasal septum to look for perforations. To do
this, shine the light on one side and look in
the other. Try to avoid contact with the very
sensitive nasal septum. Light shining through
to the other side suggests a septal perforation.
Common causes of septal perforations include
nose picking, infection, syphilis, TB, collagen
vascular disease, Wegener's granulomatosis,
SLE, RA, toxic exposure, old cocaine use, and
chromium poisoning. Look for nasal septal
deformities. (Plowshare deformities are common after vaginal delivery.)

Examining the Turbinates

Identify the inferior and middle turbinates. The inferior and middle turbinates, and
the middle meatus between them, should be
pink, intact, smooth, and moist. The area
should be free of foreign bodies. Note any

deviations from normal, such as a red, pale, or bluish-gray color, bogginess, dryness, fissures, crusts, exudate, edema, polyps, ulcers, watery discharge (rhinorrhea), mucopurulent discharge, or bloody discharge. Drainage and polyps are abnormal. Purulent mucus suggests upper respiratory infection or sinusitis. Bloody discharge suggests local trauma or a platelet abnormality. Polyps are usually nontender and a sign of allergy. Consider aspirin sensitivity if the patient also has asthma. Note any masses.

MOUTH AND THROAT

Note the symmetry of the mouth and note any perioral lesions. See if there is any shift in jaw when the patient opens his or her mouth. A soft swish of air coincident with the pulse can be heard through the open mouth in thoracic aortic aneurysm (Drummond's sign). Soft wheezing over the open mouth suggests foreign body in the bronchus (Jackson's sign).

Breath Odors

Next, note the breath for unusual odors. This sensory component is very useful because there are a number of characteristic odors of important conditions (see Table 9.1). If you feel uneasy, just take your time and move in from a distance. Have the patient say name and address while you smell the breath. If there is poor oral hygiene, have the patient breathe through his or her nose with mouth closed.

The Temporomandibular Joint

If the patient has jaw pain, place your forefinger of each hand on each temporomandibular joint (just in front of the ear) and have the patient open and close mouth (see Figure 40). Normally the patient's mouth should open wide enough for three of his or her fingers to be inserted vertically. A small oral opening suggests scleroderma, temporomandibular joint arthritis, or tetanus. Exquisitely painful opening with fever and drooling suggests peritonsillar abscess. Crepitus on movement suggests TMJ arthritis. Jaw aching or claudication suggests temporal arteritis.

Perioral Lesions

After examining the oral opening and the temporomandibular joint, check the lips. Fissures in the corners of the lips suggest candida infection, Vitamin B deficiency, folic acid deficiency, or drooling. Vertical cracking along lower lip suggests cheilitis. Cheilitis can be caused by alcoholism, Vitamin B deficiency, iron deficiency, malnutrition, and Crohn's disease. Rarely, old syphilis (rhagades) can produce permanent cracks that are epithelialized and radiate from the corners of the mouth. Congenital syphilis can produce lines radiating from the mouth (Krisovki's sign).

Red macular lesions resembling cherry angioma suggests Osler-Weber-Rendu syndrome, while freckles on the lips suggests Peutz-Jegher's syndrome. A blue, purple nodule on the lip border suggests a mucocele. Vesicles around the lip suggest herpes simplex virus. Petechiae may sometimes be seen, suggesting platelet abnormalities. A painless ulcer on the lower lip suggests squamous cell cancer. A hard nodule on the lower lip suggests epidermoid carcinoma. Swelling of the upper lip suggests angioedema. Swelling of the upper and lower lips with hemorrhage suggests Stevens-Johnson syndrome. Pallor around the mouth in a febrile patient suggests scarlet fever (Filatov's sign).

Nil Feodorovich Filatov (1847–1902) was a Russian pediatrician who described infectious mononucleosis as well as the small, irregular, bright red spots with blue-white centers, occurring on the inside of the cheek in measles (Koplik's spots), and the condition now called roseola.

Table 9.1. Possible causes of some unusual breath odors

Character of breath odor	Possible cause
Fishy ammonia (urine-like)	Renal failure
Fishy sweetness	Liver failure
Musty ammonia	Liver disease (fetor hepaticus)
Fruity chewing gum or acetone	Diabetic ketoacidosis
Fruity apples	Chloroform or salicylate ingestion
Fruity grapes	Pseudomonas infection
Fruity yeast	Alcohol ingestion
Fresh baked bread	Typhoid fever
Stale or musty (sourdough) bread	Pellagra (severe niacin deficiency)
Fresh meat	Yellow fever
Stale beer	Mycobacteria scrofula
Landfill or garbage dump, putrid (anaerobic infection)	Oral infection, bronchiectasis esophageal diverticulum, gastroparesis
Very putrid	Lung abscess
Stale smoke	Cigarette smoking
Burning rope	Marijuana smoking
Shoe polish	Nitrobenzene ingestion
Bitter almonds	Cyanide ingestion
Garlic	Arsenic, organo-phosphorus, or tellurium ingestion
Metallic	Iodine ingestion
Solvent	Hydrocarbon ingestion
Violets	Turpentine ingestion

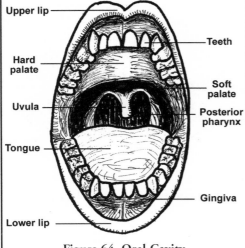

Figure 64. Oral Cavity.

This illustration shows the key landmarks on examining the oral cavity.

Lesions on the Mucous Membranes

The next part of the oral examination involves inspecting the mucous membranes. For this exam you will need a bright light and a tongue blade. First, notice the color of the mucosa. This is one of the most sensitive places to look for hyperpigmentation. Brown spots suggest Addison's disease or a racial variation (especially if opposite the molars). Next, estimate the amount of moisture. If the tongue blade sticks to the mucosa, it is too dry. Lack of moisture is xerostomia. No saliva under the tongue in the oral vestibule or between the gums and cheek is a key sign of dehydration.

After checking the degree of moisture, look carefully for mucosal lesions (see Table 9.2).

Table 9.2. Lesions on mucous membranes

Lesion	Possible Cause	Comments
Painless ulcer	Squamous cell cancer	
Multiple painful small round ulcers	Aphthous stomatitis	Consider autoimmune processes, stress, systemic lupus erythematosis, Vitamin B12 deficiency, inflammatory bowel disease, or Behcet's syndrome.
Ulcers with irregular borders	Systemic lupus erythematosis, pemphigus, viral illness	
Unilateral painful vesicles	Herpes zoster	Scattered painful vesicles and pustules suggests herpes simplex.
Painful ulcers on posterior pharynx	Coxsackie A virus (herpangina)	
Mucosal bulla	Pemphigus, pemphigoid, erythema multiforma, or lichen planus	Skin bulla are usually present; when in doubt, treat for pemphigus.
Red nodule	Malignancy, pyogenic granuloma	
White spots	Measles, Coxsackie A-16, ECHO 9 virus	
White plaque with ulceration	Squamous cell cancer	White plaque is called leukoplakia.
White coating on red base	Oral candiasis	
Irregular line on posterior buccal mucosa	Minor trauma	Called linea alba
Lacy white patches on inner cheek	Lichen planus	Called Wickham's sign
Dark patch adjacent to tooth filling	Dental amalgam pigmentation	
Pigmentation with ulceration	Malignant melanoma	
Pigmentation adjacent to front teeth	Smoker's gingiva	
Small red spots with central blue-white dot	Measles	Koplik's sign

Louis Frédéric Wickham (1861–1913) was a French internist who studied dermatology and the therapeutic use of radium, particularly to treat malignancies. He developed treatments for keloids, angiomas, and skin cancers. In 1888 he was commissioned to report on the methods of teaching dermatology in England. Wickham's stria are fine lacy lines or dots (usually white) over a patch of lichen planus.

Stenson's Duct

Check Stenson's duct on the lateral cheeks. Excessive redness or purulent drainage suggests a stone in the duct. A red spot sometimes appears on Stenson's duct in mumps (Tresiliah's sign). Parotid pain on tasting vinegar suggests parotid gland inflammation (Mirchamp's sign). Tenderness at the angle of the jaw also suggests parotid gland inflammation (Hatchcock's sign).

Gingival Lesions

The next step in the oral examination is to examine the gums. Red and swollen gingival tissue suggests gingivitis. Seeing an opening at the base of a decayed tooth suggests a periapical dental abscess. Gingival swelling suggests phenytoin effect, acute monocytic leukemia (M5), and, with gingival bleeding, Vitamin C deficiency (but never in edentulous patients). Gingivitis resembling a mulberry suggests Wegener's granulomatosis. Blue-gray dots along the gums suggest lead poisoning (Burton's sign). Pale purple discoloration along the gum line near the teeth suggests copper poisoning (Corrigan's sign). Gingival bleeding suggests platelet abnormalities but not coagulopathies.

Sir Dominic John Corrigan (1802–1880) was an Irish physician, born in Dublin. He conducted a series of pioneering experiments that have become famous for his descriptions of symptomatic heart disease, including aortic insufficiency. In addition, he described the purple line on the gingiva that is a pathognomonic sign of copper toxicity. Corrigan was five times elected president of the Irish College of Physicians, an

unprecedented honor. From 1870 to 1874 he served as a Member of Parliament for the city of Dublin. Corrigan was responsible for the improvement of Dublin's water supply. One of his quotations is especially appropriate to geriatric physical diagnosis: "The trouble with doctors is not that they don't know enough, but that they don't see enough."

The Teeth

After examining the gums, look carefully at the teeth. Lipstick on the teeth suggests xerostomia since saliva reduces the adhesion of lipstick. Poor dental hygiene may predispose to aspiration pneumonia. In fact, an edentulous state reduces the likelihood of aspiration pneumonia. Lung abscess may be due to an aspirated tooth, so count the teeth and check for a missing one. Erosion on a tooth suggests dental caries or wear and tear. Increased space between the teeth suggests acromegaly. (Patient may complain of food sticking between the teeth.) Dead teeth look darker gray compared to other teeth.

Stains on the teeth can be informative. Greenish teeth suggest the patient had jaundice as an infant. Fluoride toxicity in childhood can cause dark brown pits. Chewing tobacco stains the teeth in a predictable manner. Chalky white debris along gingival margin is calculus. A small protrusion lingual to the mesial portion of the first maxillary molar is Carabelli's tubercule. Seeing long teeth suggests periodontal disease with retraction of the gums. In a patient with fever of unknown origin, gently tap each tooth to check for the increased tenderness of an apical abscess.

Tongue Abnormalities

Note the tongue after checking the teeth. Seeing a large tongue (macroglossia) should suggest hypothyroidism, acromegaly, pemphigus vulgaris, or amyloidosis. Amyloid may also produce palpable stiffness with the enlargement. A soft nodule resembling a skin tag on the tongue suggests a papilloma, which is a

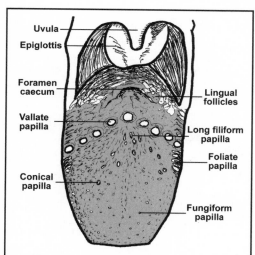

Figure 65. Top View of the Tongue.
The tongue forms the visible floor of the oral cavity, extending from the tip, behind the front teeth, to deep in the posterior pharynx. Taste buds are prominent in the vallate and fungiform papillae. The anterior two-thirds of the tongue is supplied by the facial nerve (cranial nerve VII) while the posterior third receives its neurological supply from cranial nerve IX.

premalignant lesion. A soft red mass at the base of the tongue may represent a lingual thyroid.

Tongue inflammation is called glossitis. Early glossitis produces papillary hypertrophy. The next phase of inflammation produces papillary flattening. If the inflammation progresses, the tongue develops atrophy and becomes smooth and shiny. Glossitis is caused by iron deficiency, Vitamin B deficiency, alcoholism, malnutrition, amyloid, and carcinoid syndrome. Tongue discolorations and lesions are shown in Table 9.3.

Being able to easily touch the tip of the nose with the tongue suggests Ehlers-Danlos syndrome (Gorlin's sign).

Involuntary tongue movements or tremors are also instructive. Fine tremor of the tongue suggests hyperthyroidism or trypanosomiasis (Castellani-Low sign). To check for chorea, ask the patient to stick out their tongue and keep it out. The tongue cannot stay protruded in chorea. Inability of patient to voluntarily

protrude the tongue suggests shortened frenulum, oral carcinoma, or louse-borne typhus (Malcz-Sterling-Okuniewskii sign).

Wladyslaw Sterling (1877–1943) was a Polish neurologist whose father was a conductor and musical composer. Sterling was multitalented and reportedly had a phenomenal memory. In 1943 the Gestapo killed him and his wife in their bed.

Yakov Leontievich Okuniewskii (1877–1940) was a Russian expert in infectious disease who spent much of his career studying disinfectants. He was in charge of teaching the courses in disinfectants for the Russian military.

Another useful technique is percussing the tongue for myotonia. Place a tongue blade across the lower teeth and have the patient drape the tongue over the blade. Tapping the tongue may produce myotonic jerking. In hypocalcemia, tapping the tongue causes the lips to protrude (Escherich's sign) or may cause a curved distortion of the tongue (Schultze's sign).

Friedrich Schultze (1848–1934) was a German neurologist who studied tetanus, cholera, multiple sclerosis, progressive muscular atrophy, poliomyelitis, basilar meningitis and forms of syringomyelia. Schultze also described a vasomotor disorder (Schultze's syndrome) characterized by tingling, numbness, stiffness, anesthesia or pain in the upper extremity. Symptoms occur especially along the pathway of the ulnar nerve and only during sleep, while the patient is in a recumbent position.

The Oral Vestibule

An important place to look is under the tongue just behind the lower front teeth. Pooling of secretions occurs there, so it is a prime site for oral tumors. Dilated sublingual veins are seen in increased central venous pressure. A translucent mass seen near the frenulum is a cyst of the sublingual salivary gland, called a ranula, while an opaque, white-colored mass is most likely a sublingual dermoid cyst. A blue-colored translucent mass is a mucus gland retention cyst.

Table 9.3. Tongue discolorations and lesions		
Lesion or Discoloration	*Possible Cause*	*Comments*
Red, shiny surface	B vitamin deficiency	Vitamin B12 deficiency and pellagra
Red with white exudate	Thrush	
Strawberry or raspberry	Scarlet fever	
Magenta cobblestone	Riboflavin deficiency	
Pale tongue	Giant cell arteritis	
Pale areas on tongue	Bacterial endocaritis	
Pale half of tongue	Air embolism	Liebermeister's sign
White hairy plaques	Hairy leukoplakia	EB virus in HIV patient
Black coat	Aspergillus niger colonization	
Nodularity from neuromas	Sipple's syndrome	
Transverse fissures	Congenital condition	
Longitudinal fissures	Dehydration, syphilis	
Irregular fissures	Not significant	Called geographic tongue
Shiny red tip on furred tongue	Typhoid fever	Marfan's sign
Posterior lateral ulcers	Malignancy	
Ragged ulcers under tongue	Behcet's syndrome	
Midline ulcers	Tuberculosis or histoplasmosis	Usually not malignant
Multiple painful ulcers	Tuberculosis	Almost always with pulmonary tuberculosis
Ulcer on tip	Syphilis	

The Hard Palate

After the tongue examination, focus your attention on the hard palate. A nontender lump on the hard palate is a torus palatinus, which is a benign normal variant. An arched palate can suggest Sipple's syndrome, Marfan's syndrome and homocystinuria. Defects or ulcers in the hard palate are seen in infection, radiation therapy, or neoplasm.

The Soft Palate

The next step of the oral examination is to examine the soft palate. The juncture of the hard and soft palate is often a place to see petechiae. Edema of the soft palate suggests gamma heavy chain disease.

The Posterior Pharynx

The final step of the oral examination is to check the posterior pharynx. Look for symmetry of the tonsillar pillars and the AP and lateral dimensions. Significant asymmetry suggests peritonsillar abscess. Diminished area (particularly in the horizontal plane) suggests a predisposition for obstructive sleep apnea. White plaques that bleed when scraped suggest candida infection, while exudate suggests bacterial infection. A dark red color to the anterior and inferior pillars of the posterior pharynx suggests syphilis (Biederman's sign).

The Uvula

A bifid uvula suggests a submucosal cleft palate. Flushing (Stone's sign) or pulsation (Mueller's sign) of the uvula suggests aortic insufficiency. Swelling suggests infection, obstructive sleep apnea, or gamma heavy chain disease. Redness of the uvula is seen in viral infection or bacterial infection. Seeing the epiglottis suggests acute epiglottitis. Note the elevation of the uvula by having the patient say the familiar "Ahhhh." Asymmetry suggests neurological disease or peritonsillar abscess.

CHAPTER 10

The Neck

"When I heard the learn'd astronomer,
When the proofs, the figures, were ranged in columns before me,
When I was shown the charts and diagrams, to add, divide, and measure them,
When I, sitting, heard the astronomer where he lectured with much applause in the
    lecture-room,
How soon, unaccountable, I became tired and sick,
Till rising and gliding out I wander'd off by myself,
In the mystical moist night-air, and from time to time,
Look'd up in perfect silence at the stars."

— Walt Whitman

"No man was ever wise by chance."

— Seneca

The neck, linking the head to the body, is a large conduit for vascular flow, neurological transmission, respiratory gases, and gastrointestinal nutrition (see Figure 66). It is the residence of numerous glands (parotid, thyroid and parathyroid) and chains of lymph nodes. Skin changes here (especially wrinkling) can be an early sign of aging. Usually sandwiched between the more extensive examinations of the head and chest, the neck examination can be under-appreciated.

Careful attention to this examination is always rewarding. Information can be gained about congenital abnormalities, right heart function, relative right and left intrathoracic pressures, risk of obstructive sleep apnea, signs of infection or malignancy (sometimes occult), glandular enlargement, and cervical spine structure and function.

INSPECTION

Asymmetry and Head Tilts

The first step of the neck examination is to look for asymmetry in the vertical axis and of the sternocleidomastoid muscles. A tilted neck suggests torticollis. Many conditions can produce this, including sleeping in an awkward position, but consider early Huntington's dis-

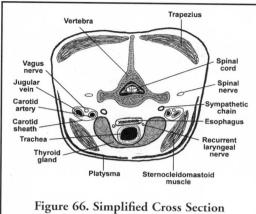

Figure 66. Simplified Cross Section of the Neck.

The neck is a conduit linking the head to the body. This illustration shows the relationships among some of the major structures.

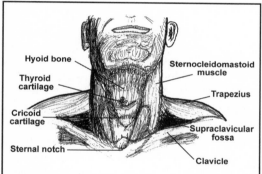

Figure 67. Surface Anatomy of the Neck.

The neck is bounded by the sternocleidomastoid muscles laterally and the trapezeus posteriorly. The clavicle, supraclavicular fossa and sternal notch are prominent anterior landmarks. The "voicebox" is the thyroid cartilage, with the hyoid bone above it and the cricoid cartilage below. The basic position of the thyroid gland is shown in the lower neck.

ease, and dystonic drug effects from phenothiazines (including some of the older anti-emetic agents) and L-dopa. Also, an isolated CN IV palsy can produce a head tilt, as can pneumothorax, cervical spine abnormalities (especially consider atlano-axial subluxation if the patient has rheumatoid arthritis), and tumors in the posterior fossa (check for Horner's syndrome).

Atrophy of the sternocleidomastoid muscle (SCM) produces a sharp jaw line and the appearance of the neck being slightly extended. If you see SCM atrophy, consider cervical spondylosis or tumor involving the foramen magnum or upper cervical cord. (Look again for Horner's syndrome.) Weakness of the hyoid muscles producing an angle between the larynx and chin suggests bulbar polio (Rope sign). Spasm of the sternocleidomastoid suggests inflammatory lymphadenopathy (Sternocleidomastoid sign). Weakness of the neck muscles in the setting of hemiplegia is Babinski's neck sign. A patient with severe neck weakness will hold head in hands when moving from a supine to a sitting position (Rust's sign). A sudden jerking of the shoulder on turning the neck suggests tuberculosis (Binda's sign).

Skin Discoloration

After noticing the symmetry of the neck, examine the skin for discoloration, scars or edema. Redness along the anterior neck is Maroni's sign of hyperthyroidism. Venous compression by a substernal goiter can produce venous dilation of the superficial veins of the neck. Another cause of redness is abscess. Dermatomyositis and acanthosis nigricans can also produce discolorations along the neck. Surgical scars can show evidence of previous thyroidectomy. In addition, scars can result from old sinus tracts, herpes zoster or cutaneous anthrax.

Neck Edema

Edema of the neck suggests Ludwig's angina. Angina is from *anchone*, the Greek word for strangulation, and was taken to connote throat pain and infection. At that time, the condition was almost always fatal. In Ludwig's angina there is tender swelling and redness in the submental area and along the anterior neck. Mediastinal tumor, aneurysm and SVC syndrome can all produce neck swelling and edema. Neck swelling with Valsalva's maneuver suggests laryngocele.

Wilhelm Friedrich von Ludwig (1790–1865) was a German obstetrician and surgeon who gained recognition by the German royal family as a gifted physician. He suffered with cataracts and renal stones, and when he died left the majority of his fortune to found a hospital for the poor in Württemberg. The description of Ludwig's angina was his only notable clinical observation. In 1836 he described five patients with marked swelling of the neck that progressed rapidly to involve the tissues covering the muscles between the larynx and the floor of the mouth. His first patient was Queen Catherine of Württemberg.

Webbed Neck or Short Neck

Congenital abnormalities can persist into old age. Seeing a webbed neck and a low hairline in a short female suggests Turner's syndrome. Patients with the Klippel-Feil syndrome have a characteristic short neck, low hairline in the back, and a cervical spine abnormality that makes the head appear to be placed low and forward on the neck. If the neck is large and short, consider coexistent obstructive sleep apnea. (The collar size in men is usually 18 or higher.)

Maurice Klippel (1858–1942), a French neurologist and psychiatrist, was a prolific writer. His name is associated with several syndromes and congenital deformities. Maurice Feil (1884–?) was also a French neurologist.

The syndrome that bears their names is a congenital anomaly characterized by a reduced number of cervical vertebrae or multiple hemivertebrae fused into a single mass, producing a short and wide neck with limited motion. A low hairline is another constant characteristic. The etiology is unknown. It was probably first described in 1893 by Sir Jonathan Hutchinson (1828–1913) with Klippel and Feil giving a comprehensive interpretation in 1912.

Neck Pulsations

Neck pulsations are due to arterial pulses, venous waves or vascular aneurysms. This topic will be covered in detail in Chapter 16.

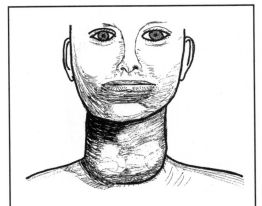

Figure 68. Multinodular Goiter.
Thyroid enlargement suggests multinodular goiter, hyperthyroidism, or thyroiditis. Having the patient look up at the ceiling can bring out the fullness. The large, irregular, lumpy fullness in the illustration suggests multinodular goiter.

Neck Masses

Look carefully for any masses in the neck. Fat pads suggest obesity or Cushing's syndrome (buffalo hump). Seeing thyroid enlargement suggests multinodular goiter (see Figure 68), hyperthyroidism, or thyroiditis. Having the patient look up at the ceiling can bring out the fullness. Another cause of neck masses is head and neck malignancy and enlarged lymph nodes. These will be discussed in Chapter 11.

Unilateral Neck Swelling

Unilateral neck swelling is often due to enlargement of the parotid and submandibular glands (conditions generally affect these glands together). Parotid tumor can present with unilateral enlargement. Also check for a stone in Stensen's duct (parotid gland). The duct is located on the cheek adjacent to the second molar on each side. Look for pus or decreased saliva. (Have patient bite a piece of lemon to increase salivary flow.) Also look for a stone in Wharton's duct (submandibular glands). Wharton's duct is located under the tongue near the frenulum. Look for pus or decreased saliva (have the patient bite a piece of lemon to increase salivary flow). Sometimes actinomycosis infection can produce unilateral neck swelling. Also consider head and neck malignancy.

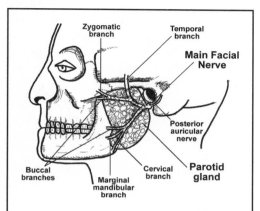

Figure 69. The Relationship Between the Parotid Gland and the Facial Nerve.
The facial nerve exits the skull through the stylomastoid foramen. The main body of the facial nerve supplies the muscles of facial expression. All of the main branches pass through the substance of the parotid gland. Facial nerve paralysis in the setting of a parotid tumor suggests malignancy until proven otherwise. Uveitis or facial nerve involvement in the setting of parotid enlargement due to sarcoidosis is Heerfordt's syndrome.

Bilateral Neck Swelling

Bilateral parotid swelling suggests Mikulicz's syndrome, which is bilateral enlargement of the parotid, other salivary and lacrimal glands. (Sjögren's syndrome should be considered on the differential diagnosis of Mikulicz's syndrome.) Look for xerostomia. Another cause of bilateral parotid swelling is parotitis. Parotitis can be caused by dehydration, drug effect (sulfonamides, iodides, PTU and many others), infections (choriomeningitis or mumps), malignancy (consider leukemia, lymphoma, and Waldenström's macroglobulinemia), metabolic diseases (alcoholism, malnutrition, Vitamin A deficiency, diabetes mellitus, refeeding syndrome, and pellagra), and autoimmune disease

such as SLE or sarcoidosis. Uveitis or facial nerve involvement in the setting of parotid enlargement due to sarcoidosis is Heerfordt's syndrome. *Beware; facial nerve paralysis in the setting of a parotid tumor suggests malignancy until proven otherwise.*

Cysts are another kind of mass in the neck. A dermoid cyst is usually felt as a mass in the sternal notch. Thyroglossal duct cyst presents as a mass in the midline just above the thyroid. Pinch the mass and have the patient stick out the tongue; movement of the mass with tongue extension confirms a thyroglossal duct cyst. Brachial cleft cysts generally present as a single nodule anterior to the sternocleidomastoid muscle. Cystic hygroma feels like a lipoma. (Sometimes a lipoma will firm up if you put ice on it — like butter in the refrigerator.) The ice test works well for lipomas on the extremities or the back. Exercise caution about putting ice on the neck of an elderly person. (When in doubt, don't.)

Tracheal Deviation

Sometimes tracheal deviation will be visible. (We will palpate the trachea later.) Tracheal deviation suggests pleural effusion, pneumothorax, substernal goiter, aortic aneurysm, or old scarring from tuberculosis.

Limited Range of Motion

Have the patient look as far to each side as possible (without turning the shoulders) and gently flex and extend the neck. Limited range of motion is caused by muscle spasm or vertebral abnormalities. Muscle spasm can be produced by muscle strain (consider compensation for other spinal or visual problems), neck inflammation from infection or mass (think about mastoiditis or meningitis), Parkinsonism, or torticollis (vide supra). Vertebral abnormalities can result from trauma, infection, neoplasm, arthritis or dislocation.

PALPATION

Basic Structures

Palpate along the submental area, noting any masses or areas of tenderness. Next, move down to the thyroid cartilage (the larynx) and then to the cricoid cartilage just above the sternal notch. Inability to palpate the cricoid cartilage suggests a substernal goiter (check for superficial venous distension and Pemberton's sign, vide infra) or kyphosis. Fixation of the lower larynx with swallowing suggests peritracheal adhesions due to surgery or syphilis (Demarquay's sign).

Thyroid Gland

Palpate the spongy isthmus of the thyroid by gently pressing in an area of the firm cricoid cartilage at the sternal notch to calibrate your fingertips to the quality of the thyroid tissue. Normally the isthmus of an old person's thyroid gland feels like a piece of chicken skin. (Endocrinologists call this feeling bosselated). Once you have that awareness, gently move the overlying skin lateral and upward, and then gently push down and medially to feel the gland squirt underneath the fingertips. Masses will feel like lumps passing under the fingers. Move to the opposite side and use your left hand to recalibrate your left fingertips and examine the right lobe of the thyroid. If abnormalities in the thyroid gland are noted, then define the structures and have the patient look up, to extend the neck, and swallow. A mass in the thyroid gland will elevate with swallowing. A systolic thrill may be felt in some patients with Grave's disease. Lack of a carotid pulsation on one side of the thyroid suggests malignancy (Berry's sign).

Trachea

Have the patient close mouth, then gently grasp the cricoid cartilage with the fore-finger and middle finger of your right hand. Inability to grasp the cricoid cartilage because of a caudally displaced larynx suggests chronic lung disease. (Normally there are three finger breadths between the thyroid cartilage and the sternal notch.) Feeling the trachea in midline is normal. Now note the tracheal movement with inspiration. A slight downward movement in the midline is normal. This downward pull with inspiration may be accentuated in chronic pulmonary disease and correlates inversely with the FEV1. If you cannot detect tracheal mobility, then consider pulmonary emphysema, mediastinal malignancy, or aortic aneurysm. If the trachea pulls to one side, this suggests an unequal transmission of pressure in the chest. Possible causes include a pneumothorax on the ipsilateral side, a tension pneumothorax on the contralateral side, or upper lobe scarring and traction from a mass or old fibrosis.

Feeling a downward tracheal pulsation coincident with the pulse and not associated with inspiration (tracheal tug or Oliver's sign) suggests thoracic aortic aneurysm. (An up-and-down movement is significant but an in-and-out movement is not.) A palpable tracheal diastolic pulse suggests aortic aneurysm (Hall's sign).

William Silver Oliver (1836–1908) was a British military surgeon who served mainly in India. In a letter to the editor in Lancet in 1878 he described his sign: "Place the patient in the erect position, and direct him to close his mouth, and elevate his chin to the fullest extent, then grasp the cricoid cartilage between the finger and thumb, and use gentle upward pressure on it ... if dilatation or aneurysm exist, the pulsation of the aorta will be distinctly felt, transmitted through the trachea to the hand. This act of examination will increase laryngeal distress should this accompany the disease."

Neck Masses

Abnormal structures palpated in the neck include lymph nodes and soft tissue masses. Lymph nodes will be covered in more detail in

Chapter 11. Feeling lymph nodes suggests infection, lymphoma or metastatic cancer. To feel for masses, use your fingertips and have a delicate, gentle sliding or rotational movement. Have your fingertips slide along and between muscle boundaries.

Midline neck masses. Masses felt in the midline are either thyroglossal duct remnants (cysts), Delphian lymph nodes located along the thyrohyoid membrane (think thyroid cancer or Hashimoto's thyroiditis) or, if lower in the neck, a pyramidal lobe of the thyroid gland. A thyroglossal duct cyst felt below the submental area and above the thyroid cartilage may vanish when the patient swallows, because it moves below the hyoid. Having the patient open his or her mouth and look up will cause the mass to reappear. A mass at the cricoid level just above the sternal notch is probably a pyramidal lobe of the thyroid gland. Careful palpation can confirm the attachment to the thyroid isthmus. A mass at the sternal notch suggests a tuberculous abscess, dermoid cyst or a fatty tumor associated with Cushing's syndrome, similar to the Dowager's hump. Fullness of the sternal notch in leukemia is Jaccoud's sign.

Sigismond Jaccoud *(1830–1913) was a Swiss physician who became a renowned lecturer and teacher. He published his lectures as books and published a 3000-page, three-volume work on pathology. In addition to his famous sign in leukemia, he is recognized for his observations on the arthropathy of rheumatic fever and systemic lupus erythematosis.*

Lateral neck masses. Brachial cysts and carotid body tumors can cause swelling in the lateral neck. A brachial cyst feels soft and spongy, and is located just in front of the upper third of the sternocleidomastoid muscle. Seeing cholesterol crystals in the aspirated cyst fluid confirms the diagnosis. Carotid body tumors occur at the carotid bifurcation. The mass does not move up or down but may slide from side to side. Other soft tissue masses in the neck include lipomas, neuromas, sarcomas, and hemangiomas. Feeling crepitus in

the neck suggests pneumothorax or esophageal rupture.

AUSCULTATION

When listening over the trachea or the base of the neck in a patient with stridor, hearing harsh, high-pitched, prolonged airway sounds suggests tracheal obstruction. Diminished breath sounds in the sternal notch suggest tracheal stenosis (Aufrecht's sign). The patient is usually in respiratory distress with stridor but there are relatively decreased breath sounds in the lung bases. Some patients with sleep apnea will develop a sonorous expiratory wheeze at the base of the neck (Shephard's sign). Listen with the patient supine and breathing through nose.

Emanuel Aufrecht *(1844–1933) was a German physician who trained under Ludwig Traube (1818–1876) and Rudolf Virchow (1821–1902).*

Hearing a gurgling sound in the lateral neck with hand compression on the back of the neck suggests an esophageal diverticulum (Boyce's sign). Hearing a thyroid bruit suggests hyperthyroidism, but beware of transmitted cardiac murmurs. A buzzing sound over the thyroid in Grave's disease is Guttmann's sign. Also remember that a multinodular goiter usually does not produce a bruit. Carotid bruits are covered in Chapter 16.

SPECIAL TESTS

Pemberton's Maneuver to Detect a Substernal Goiter

Have the patient raise arms straight up over the head (as if being held up by a thief). This closes the thoracic outlet. If within one minute the patient's head turns red or the patient feels dizzy or congested, that is a positive Pemberton's sign (see Figure 70).

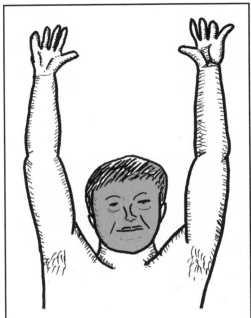

Figure 70. Pemberton's Sign.

Have the patient raise arms straight up over the head (as if being held up by a thief), to close the thoracic outlet. If within one minute the patient's head turns red or the patient feels dizzy or congested, that is a positive Pemberton's sign. The symptoms are caused by a large substernal goiter compressing the great vessels.

Kocher's Thyroid Maneuver

Push gently on each lobe of the thyroid with your thumbs. If the patient develops stridor then the test is positive and suggests thyroid cancer, thyroiditis, or significant goiter.

Emil Theodor Kocher (1841–1917) won the 1909 Nobel Prize in Physiology and Medicine for his work on the physiology, pathology and surgery of the thyroid gland. Kocher did much experimental work on the thyroid gland and was the first to excise the thyroid goiter in 1876. By 1912 Kocher had performed 2,000 thyroid excisions. When he died in 1917, more than 7,000 thyroid operations had been done in his clinic. The mortality decreased steadily from 14% in 1884 to 2.4% in 1889 and 0.18% in 1898, truly remarkable when the era in which he was undertaking the operation is considered. He described myxedema following thyroid surgery.

Kocher was a precise and masterful surgeon who relied on accuracy and scrupulous aseptic technique. Kocher's other surgical contributions include a method for reducing dislocations of the shoulder and improvements in operations on the stomach, the lungs, the tongue, and cranial nerves, and for hernia. He also devised many new surgical techniques, instruments, and appliances. The forceps and incision for gallbladder surgery that bear his name remain in general use.

The Lymph Nodes

"The great difficulty in education is to get experience out of ideas."
— **George Santayana**

"I have three treasures. Guard and keep them:
The first is deep love,
The second is frugality,
And the third is not to dare to be ahead of the world.
Because of deep love, one is courageous.
Because of frugality, one is generous.
Because of not daring to be ahead of the world, one becomes the leader of the world."
— **Lao-tzu**

Searching for occult lymphadenopathy is an important aspect of the physical examination. If potentially pathological lymph nodes are discovered, then one's diagnosis must explain the lymphadenopathy. A key consideration is if the lymph nodes are regional or generalized (more than two chains involved). Tender lymph nodes are usually significant because tenderness implies inflammation.

Lymph nodes larger than a centimeter are generally significant. Rubbery-feeling lymph nodes suggest lymphoma, while rock-hard lymph nodes suggest malignancy (metastatic disease). Matted lymph nodes (clusters) suggest chronic inflammation, sarcoidosis, or malignancy. In an elderly person most causes of lymphadenopathy are malignant disease.

SEQUENCE OF THE EXAMINATION

As a general rule, lymph nodes are searched for while examining a body part.

Generally the order is epitrochlear, cervical, supraclavicular, axillary, periumbilical, inguinal and femoral.

Epitrochlear Lymph Nodes

Epitrochlear lymph nodes are always abnormal if palpable. Consider infection in the forearm or hand, syphilis, drug abuse, dermatitis, or systemic disease such as SLE, or sarcoidosis. Shake hands with the patient and with your other hand support the elbow with your palm as your fingers feel along the brachialis border. This is easily accomplished when checking for forearm muscle tone (see Chapter 6).

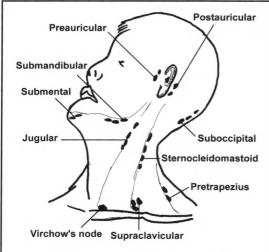

Figure 71. Cervical Lymphadenopathy.
The general order of palpating the cervical lymph nodes is submental, submandibular, preauricular, posterior auricular, occipital, anterior cervical (jugular), posterior cervical (sternocleidomastoid and pretrapezius), and supraclavicular. The text discusses possible conditions causing lymph node enlargement in these chains.

Cervical Lymph Nodes

The general order of palpating the cervical lymph nodes is submental, submandibular, preauricular, posterior auricular, occipital, anterior cervical or jugular, posterior cervical (sternocleidomastoid and pretraezius) and supraclavicular (see Figure 71). Submental and submandibular lymph nodes suggest oral or dental infection. Preauricular lymph nodes are seen in viral illness, lymphoma, Romana syndrome (trypanosomiasis), and cat-scratch fever. Posterior auricular lymph nodes are sometimes seen in toxoplasmosis or measles. Occipital lymph nodes suggest HIV infection. Anterior cervical lymph nodes are located along the me-

dial border of the sternocleidomastoid muscle and can be seen in upper respiratory infection. While erythema nodosa produces tender nodules in the legs, cervical lymphadenopathy is a common finding. Chronic cervical lymph nodes raise the possibility of lymphoma, metastatic cancer, tuberculosis, or actinomycosis. Posterior cervical lymph nodes can be seen in HIV infection, scalp infections and seborrheic dermatitis. Winterbottom's sign is swelling of the posterior cervical lymph nodes in African trypanosomiasis.

Supraclavicular Lymph Nodes

Supraclavicular lymph nodes are always abnormal and concerning. The sentinel nodes of internal malignancy (usually of GI origin) are on the left side. Virchow's node of internal malignancy is medial and deep, while Troisier's nodes are large and visible. Lung and breast cancer may metastasize to the supraclavicular fossa.

Rudolf Ludwig Karl Virchow (1821–1902) was the most distinguished German physician of the 19th Century. He emphasized that diseases arose, not in organs or tissues in general, but primarily in their individual cells. He was a tireless champion for social reforms and made the methods of natural science the basis of the medical sciences. He wrote a classic paper on thrombosis (describing his famous triad of changes in the vessel, changes in the blood flow, and changes in the blood), which included one of the earliest descriptions of leukemia. He coined the terms "thrombosis," "embolus," "amyloid" and many other commonly used terms.
Virchow introduced the standardized approach to the autopsy, improving the opportunity for more accurate clinical-pathological correlation. He researched the contamination of meat by parasites, leading to the development of public meat inspection. Virchow also was the father of German anthropology, participating in several archeological expeditions to Troy and Egypt.

To examine these nodes, have the patient relax with arms at sides. If you think you feel something, remember that aneurysms, the omohyoid muscle or cervical vertebra may be mistaken for lymph nodes. Feel along the supraclavicular and infraclavicular space. Focus on the medial portion of the clavicle and have the patient perform a Valsalva maneuver to bring up a suspected Virchow's node. If you feel a mass, stop and see if it pulses (subclavian artery aneurysm).

Charles Emile Troisier (1844–1919) was a French pathologist. In addition to describing his enlarged supraclavicular lymph nodes as a sign of internal gastrointestinal malignancy, Troisier was also the first to describe hepatomegaly and brownish skin pigmentation in diabetes mellitus as a result of hemochromatosis.

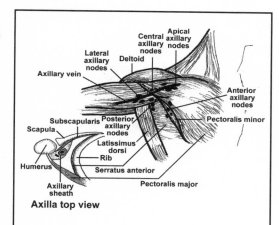

Figure 72. Axillary Lymphadenopathy.
The top view of the axilla in the lower left portion of the figure shows the four-walled structure; lymphatic drainage is different for each wall. The chest wall lymph nodes (central and apical axillary lymph nodes) drain the chest, breasts and arm. The medial arm (lateral axillary) nodes drain the arm. The anterior axillary nodes in the pectoral area drain the breast and chest wall, and the subscapular posterior axillary nodes drain the posterior arm and part of the posterior chest wall. Note the relationship of the axillary vein to the lateral, central, posterior and apical chains.

Axillary Lymph Nodes

Consider the axilla as a four-walled structure since lymphatic drainage is different for each wall. *The chest wall* lymph nodes (central and apical axillary lymph nodes) drain the chest, breasts and arm. *The medial arm* (lateral axillary) nodes drain the arm. *The anterior axillary* nodes in the pectoral area drain the breast and chest wall, and *the subscapular* posterior axillary nodes drain the posterior arm and part of the posterior chest wall.

◆ AXILLARY INSPECTION

Look carefully for skin lesions (rash or infection), pigmentation, edema, masses, or asymmetry.

◆ AXILLARY PALPATION

Support the patient's arm at the elbow with your same arm (left arm supporting left arm) to relax and abduct the arm. With your free hand, feel along the inner edge of the pectoral muscles and feel the length of the muscle from the apex of the axilla to the chest wall. Feel along the ribs with the patient's arm relaxed at the side. Next, feel along the medial aspect of the arm, starting in the apex of the axilla. Finally, feel along the posterior axillary wall.

Posterior Mediastinal Lymph Nodes

Posterior mediastinal lymph nodes may be appreciated by checking d'Espine's sign by listening over the spinous process of the upper thoracic vertebral bodies (T4–T5) and hearing loud tubular breath sounds (see Chapter 14).

Periumbilical Lymph Nodes

These key sentinel lymph nodes suggest abdominal (usually GI) or pelvic malignancy. Palpating these nodes is also called Sister Mary Joseph's sign.

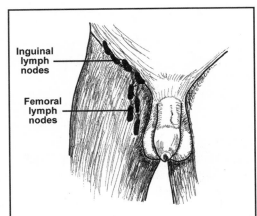

Figure 73. Inguinal and Femoral Lymph Nodes.

Inguinal nodes lie along the inguinal ligament and drain the genital and pelvic area. Feeling a furrow (Bailey's groove) between significant inguinal nodes suggests lymphogranuloma venereum. Femoral nodes course vertically down the leg. These lymph nodes tend to react to nonspecific conditions and may be present in dermatophyte lesions of the feet.

Inguinal and Femoral Lymph Nodes

Inguinal nodes lie along the inguinal ligament and drain the genital and pelvic area. They do not drain the feet, so they are not enlarged in dermatophyte lesions of the feet. Inguinal nodes are useful for biopsy because they tend to show pathology. Feeling a furrow (Bailey's groove) between significant inguinal nodes suggests lymphogranuloma venereum. Femoral nodes course vertically down the leg. These lymph nodes tend to react to nonspecific conditions and may be present in dermatophyte lesions of the feet.

CHAPTER 12

The Back

"Young men, be not proud in the presence of a decaying old man; he was once that which you are, he is now that which you will be."

— **Pope Clement III**

"Perhaps the most valuable result of all education is the ability to make yourself do the thing you have to do, when it ought to be done, whether you like it or not; it is the first lesson that ought to be learned; and however early a man's training begins, it is probably the last lesson that he learns thoroughly."

— **Thomas H. Huxley**

"There are few people who at the first sign of age do not show in what respects their body and mind will eventually fail."

— **François, 6th Duc de La Rochefoucauld**

The back examination is useful because it is a large expanse with clues to many organ system abnormalities. Because of the large surface area, skin conditions are frequently seen here. Musculoskeletal disorders also show signs of illness, from the kyphosis produced by vertebral compression fractures, to the muscle spasm of disc disease or muscle strain and the nerve root compression of degenerative or neoplastic disease. In addition, low back pain is such a common complaint in elderly people that familiarity with the back examination is essential.

RELEVANT ANATOMY

The spinal column is composed of 24 mobile vertebrae, stacked on top of each other like blocks (see Figure 74). Between them are the intervertebral discs which act like cushions. Each vertebra is linked to its adjacent neighbors (above it and below it) by the facet joints. The spinal cord is enclosed within the spinal canal, and spinal nerves branch off from the spinal cord at each vertebral level. The human spine is so flexible that it can bend to almost 270 degrees. It carries a heavy head and can support over 300 pounds per square inch.

135

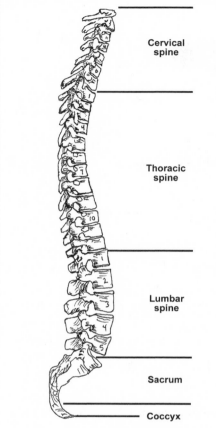

Figure 74. Normal Spine.

The spinal column is composed of 24 mobile vertebrae (seven cervical vertebrae, twelve thoracic vertebrae, and five lumbar vertebrae), stacked on top of each other like blocks. Between them are the intervertebral discs which act like cushions. Each vertebra is linked to its adjacent neighbors (above it and below it) by the facet joints. Note the subtle "S" curvature.

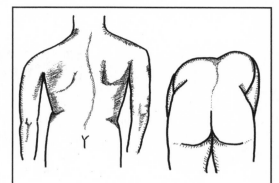

Figure 75. Scoliosis.

Curvature of the thoracic spine in the lateral dimension is scoliosis. Scoliosis looks like an "S" from the back. The spinous processes rotate in the direction of the concavity, and the convex shoulder is often elevated, the scapula more prominent, and the pelvis tilted.

INSPECTION

The first part of the back examination is to inspect the skin and the spinal contour. A soft, pillow-like, triangular swelling that outlines the scapula suggests scapular fracture (Comolli's sign). Curvature of the thoracic spine in the lateral dimension is scoliosis. Scoliosis looks like an "S" from the back (see Figure 75). The spinous processes rotate in the direction of the concavity, and the convex shoulder is often elevated, the scapula more prominent, and the pelvis tilted.

An increase in kyphosis suggests possible thoracic compression fractures of osteoporosis. A transverse abdominal crease may be evident on abdominal examination. If the angle of the spinal curvature is sharp, the kyphosis is called a gibbus deformity. Weak back muscles or hip disorders can produce lordosis of the lower thoracic spine.

Loss of lumbar lordosis suggests lumbar compression fractures. Stiff lumbar lordosis that does not straighten with forward flexion suggests musculoskeletal low back pain. Limited spinal range of motion in early tuberculosis is Lorenz's sign. Painful spine extension suggests tuberculosis of the spine (Anghelescu's sign). Seeing a decrease in flank swelling after relieving a hydronephrosis is the flush tank sign. The pelvis is tilted in lumbosacral disease and horizontal in sciatica (Vanzetti's sign).

PALPATION

After inspecting the spinal contour, palpate the spinous processes from the cervical

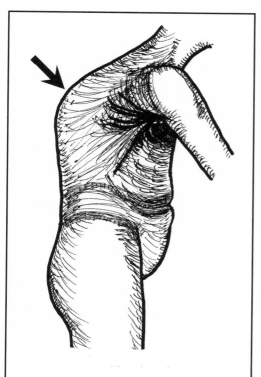

Figure 76. Kyphosis.

An increase in the forward curve of the upper back (as shown by the arrow) is kyphosis and suggests possible thoracic compression fractures. A transverse abdominal crease may be evident on abdominal examination. If the angle of the spinal curvature is sharp, the kyphosis is called a gibbus deformity.

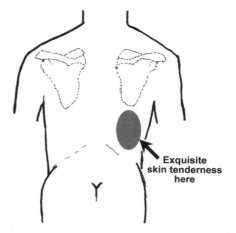

Figure 77. Boas' sign.

Exquisite hypesthesia of the skin along the right flank to light touch is Boas' sign. The sign reflects possible acute cholecystitis.

region to the lumbar area. Tenderness over any spinous process suggests compression fracture, epidural abscess, septic discitis, or metastatic cancer. Skin tenderness over the right flank suggests acute cholecystitis (Boas' sign). Skin tenderness over one side along a dermatome suggests herpes zoster or diabetic thoraco-abdominal syndrome. Tenderness over the greater trochanter suggests trochanteric bursitis. Tenderness over the ischial tuberosity suggests ischiogluteal bursitis.

Ismar Isidor Boas (1858–1938) was a German physician who is considered to be one of the fathers of gastroenterology. Shortly after Kuss-maul's introduction of the gastric tube, Boas and Anton Ewald (1845–1915) introduced the test

meal to measure gastric secretion. He was the first to recognize occult blood in the gastrointestinal tract and developed an approach for its use in the care of patients.

Boas' point is a tender area to the left of the spinous process of the twelfth thoracic vertebra as a sign of gastric ulcer. Boas' sign is hypesthesia along the right flank as a sign of acute cholecystitis.

PERCUSSION

Make a fist and gently thump down the spinous processes and over each flank. Tenderness over the flank suggests pyelonephritis. Tenderness over (or localized to) a spinous process suggests compression fracture, epidural abscess, septic discitis, or metastatic cancer. The appearance of red spots over the spinous processes of T1–T5 after percussing them suggests bronchial lymphadenopathy (Cattaneo's sign).

AUSCULTATION

While listening over the back is generally not performed except as a key part of the respiratory examination, posterior mediastinal lymph nodes may be appreciated by checking d'Espine's sign by listening over the vertebral bodies (T4-T5) and hearing loud tubular breath sounds (see Chapter 14).

SPECIAL CIRCUMSTANCES

The Elderly Person with Low Back Pain

Low back pain can be a crucial clue to significant systemic illness (vide infra). While there is considerable variation, the following rules of thumb are useful to organize your thinking. Osteoarthritis produces pain at the extreme ranges of motion, and with vibration. A strain and/or sprain usually produce reduced mobility. Disc problems often cause pain that increases with bending forward. Spinal stenosis causes an aching pain relieved by sitting and aggravated by arching backward. Prolonged extension and rotation tend to increase facet joint pain. Severe flank pain with a kidney stone is Thorton's sign. A patient who arises from a chair with one hand on his back above a bent leg suggests sciatica (Minor's sign).

◆ REVIEW HISTORICAL FEATURES FOR SYSTEMIC ILLNESS

The first step is to review any red flags in the patient's history for systemic illness. These red flags are low back pain and fever, weight loss, pain that causes pacing at night, or pain where the patient cannot find a comfortable position in bed for sleep. Severe back and neck pain on leg extension while the supine patient's knee is flexed to ninety degrees suggests meningitis (Kernig's sign).

◆ CHECK FOR LOWER SPINAL CORD DYSFUNCTION

Next, check the anal sphincter tone and look for a sensory defect in a saddle distribution. *Noting a perianal sensory defect or a lack of anal sphincter tone is a medical emergency* and suggests a cauda equina lesion or lower spinal cord compression.

◆ CHECK LOUVEL'S SIGN

The next step in the evaluation of low back pain is to check Louvel's sign. Have the patient cough or perform Valsalva's maneuver. An increase in the back pain implies radiculopathy.

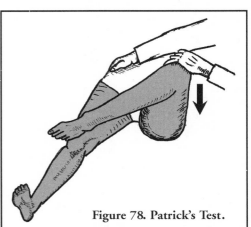

Figure 78. Patrick's Test.

This useful test tends to localize the discomfort to the site of pathology. Place the patient's ankle on the contralateral knee and then gently press down on the flexed knee. If this maneuver produces pain in hip, this suggests articular disease of the hip. If the test causes pain radiating from the back down the leg, this implies radiculopathy. Pain felt in the lower spine suggests a possible vertebral compression fracture.

◆ PERFORM PATRICK'S TEST

If Louvel's sign is not present, then check Patrick's test. Place the patient's ankle on the contralateral knee and then gently press down on the flexed knee. This useful test tends to localize the discomfort to the site of pathology. If this maneuver produces pain in hip, this suggests DJD of the hip. Consider radiculopathy if the test causes pain radiating from the low back down the leg. Pain felt in the lower spine suggests a vertebral compression fracture.

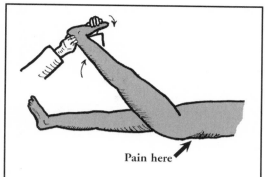

Figure 79. Straight Leg Raise.

Gently raise the leg to approximately 90° with the foot passively dorsiflexed. No pain to 90° of hip flexion is the norm. Early pain (within 10°) in the low back on straight leg raise suggests strain of the low back muscles (Demianoff's sign). Pain at less than 40° suggests sciatica or radicular low back pain. Pain at greater than 40° is seen in musculoskeletal low back pain or radicular low back pain (Goldthwait's sign).

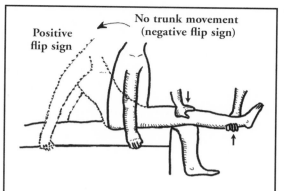

Figure 80. Flip Sign.

The flip sign is a useful confirmatory test if the straight leg test is positive for nerve root irritation. With the patient seated, gently raise the leg by extending the knee, performing, in essence, a seated straight leg raise. A positive flip test is having the patient shift the trunk backward to increase the angle at the hip. A negative flip sign (no trunk movement with knee extension) raises doubt regarding a positive straight leg raise test.

♦ CHECK STRAIGHT LEG RAISES

The next part of the examination of low back pain is to perform a straight leg raise. Early pain (within 10°) in the low back on straight leg raise suggests strain of the low back muscles (Demianoff's sign). Pain at less than 40° suggests sciatica or radicular low back pain. Pain at greater than 40° is seen in musculoskeletal low back pain or radicular low back pain (Goldthwait's sign). No pain to 90° is the norm. Repeat the test with the foot passively dorsiflexed (see Figure 79). The interpretation is the same.

Check the straight leg raise on opposite (non-painful) side. Pain in the other leg suggests sciatica. If the straight leg test is positive for nerve root irritation, then check the flip sign (see Figure 80). A negative flip sign raises doubt regarding a positive straight leg raise test.

♦ TEST FOR L4 RADICULOPATHY

Stretch the femoral nerve by having the patient lie on his or her side with the painful leg in the air. Hold the knee in extension and hyperextend the hip by 15°. Passively flex the knee. If this produces pain in the anterior thigh, this suggests L4 radiculopathy.

Now check active knee extension. Weakness suggests L4 radiculopathy. If weakness is present, then check for a sensory defect over medial malleolus.

♦ CHECK FOR L5 RADICULOPATHY

Next, check ankle dorsiflexion by having the patient walk on his or her heels. Weakness suggests foot drop or an L5 radiculopathy. Check for sensory loss over the great toe and dorsal foot to confirm this.

♦ CHECK FOR S1 RADICULOPATHY

Finally check plantar flexion by having the patient rise up on toes. Weakness or inability suggests a S1 radiculopathy. Check for sensory loss over the lateral malleolus and the plantar aspect of the foot. Confirm by seeing if there is a diminished ankle jerk. If the ankle jerk is increased, then this suggests a contralateral upper motor neuron lesion.

Table 12.1. Neurological findings in lumbosacral disc disease

Spinal Level	Pain	Numbness	Weakness	Reflexes
L4 root	L4 dermatome	Medial knee and calf	Knee extension, foot inversion	Reduced knee jerk
L5 root	L5 dermatome	Between great and first toe	Foot and big toe dorsiflexion	No change
S1 root	S1 dermatome	Lateral foot and sole	Foot eversion	Reduced ankle jerk
Midline disc herniation	Bilateral legs	Perineum	Bowel, bladder dysfunction	Reduced anal wink

Additional Back Pain Pearls

Back pain in the prone patient by pushing the foot to the buttocks and hyperextending the thigh suggests lumbosacral spine disease (Ely's sign). Back pain in a supine patient on flexing the good leg and thigh, and hyperextending the painful side by lowering it off the examination table, suggests lumbosacral disease (Gaenslen's sign). Pain along the sciatic or external cutaneous nerves of the thigh with the patient lying supine when the painful knee is passively flexed suggests lumbosacral disease (Nachlas's sign). If trunk flexion while standing causes knee flexion and contralateral leg extension, then that suggests lumbosacral disease (Neri's leg sign).

Pain when sliding the thumbs medially from the posterior superior iliac spines suggests probable muscle strain; pain on moving laterally from the midline suggests inflammation such as abscess (Mennell's sign). Pain in the sacroiliac joint on sitting suggests sacroiliac disease (Larrey's sign). Pain on moving or tilting the pelvis suggests a pelvic fracture (Larrey's fracture sign). Pain on compressing the pelvis suggests sacroiliac disease, not hip disease (Erichsen's sign).

CHAPTER 13

The Breasts

"By three methods we may learn wisdom: First, by reflection, which is noblest; second, by imitation, which is easiest; and third, by experience, which is the bitterest."
— **Confucius**

"Humility is the foundation of all the other virtues; hence, in the soul in which this virtue does not exist there cannot be any other virtue except in mere appearance."
— **Saint Augustine**

The main point of the breast examination is to search for breast cancer. It is important to be thorough and consistent.

RELEVANT ANATOMY

The breasts lie on the anterior chests between the sternal border and the lateral chest wall approximately from the third to the sixth intercostal spaces (see Figure 81). Cooper's ligaments that radiate in a circular, star-like fashion support the glandular tissue. The upper outer quadrant contains the most tissue and is the most likely site of breast cancer. A portion of tissue may extend to the axilla (the tail of Spence).

Sir Astley Paston Cooper (1768–1841) was an English surgeon who improved surgical technique and became an expert in vascular surgery.

He was knighted for removing a sebaceous cyst from the scalp of King George IV. He was the premier surgical instructor and educated John Keats (1795–1821). Cooper did not write much, but his works were of highest quality. He described multiple breast cysts, Cooper's fascia of the spermatic cord, and Cooper's ligament. He showed that perforation of the tympanic membrane did not result in deafness, and that deafness caused by Eustachian tube obstruction could be relieved by myringotomy. Cooper was one of the founders of the Royal Medical and Chirurgical Society.

PREPARING FOR THE EXAMINATION

Have the patient draped in a gown and be sure to respect the patient's privacy and modesty. Male examiners may benefit from the

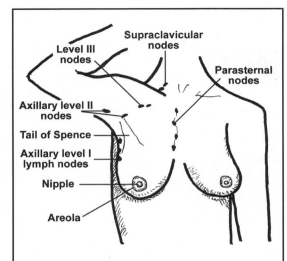

Figure 81. Breast Anatomy.

The breasts lie on the anterior chests between the sternal border and the lateral chest wall approximately from the third to the sixth intercostal spaces. Cooper's ligaments that radiate in a circular, star-like fashion support the glandular tissue. The upper outer quadrant contains the most tissue and is the most likely site of breast cancer. A portion of tissue may extend to the axilla (the tail of Spence). The lymph node drainage is also shown.

presence of a female chaperone. Take your time and be systematic. The primary intent is to find a possible mass. The care, attentiveness, and thoroughness of the examiner are more important than the geometry of the examination.

INSPECTION

Note the size and basic symmetry of the breasts. Retractions are abnormal and suggest malignancy. Have the patient perform actions that stretch Cooper's ligaments to expose a subtle retraction. These maneuvers can reveal changes even if a mass is not palpable. Have the undraped patient place her hands on her head and then place her hands pushing on her hips to contract the pectoralis muscles. Finally have the patient lean forward so the breasts

swing away from the chest wall. Also look for depressions, bulges or skin changes. The vascularity should be symmetric. Pay careful attention to any rashes or ulcerations. It is not uncommon for elderly women to have seborrheic keratoses under their breasts.

Nipples

Pink nipples rule out Addison's disease and previous pregnancy.

Supernumerary nipples are more common in men. They are associated with reduplication of renal arteries and renal cell cancer. An absent nipple with absent pectoralis muscle and mitral valve prolapse is Poland's syndrome.

Nipple retraction suggests breast cancer (Benzadon's sign). The nipple may point to the mass.

Nipple inversion may be congenital. Ulceration and scaling around the nipple suggests Paget's disease of the breasts or malignant melanoma.

PALPATION

Use a circular motion with the pads of the fingers (see Figure 82), pressing very gently, since a firm motion may mask subtle changes. Using a satin cloth may bring out masses by reducing the friction of palpation. Start at the nipple and move outward, including the tail of Spence.

Gently compress the nipple and note any discharge. A serous or bloody discharge suggests malignancy. Hypothalamic or pituitary dysfunction, as well as drugs such as phenothiazines, can cause a milky discharge.

Continue your examination and note any areas of tenderness. Check the consistency for symmetry and feel carefully for any nodules. A hard consistency suggests cancer while a squishy mass (Halsted's sign) suggests muci-

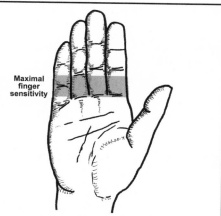

Maximal finger sensitivity

Figure 82. Finger Sensitivity for the Breast Exam.

This illustration shows the location of maximal finger sensitivity to feel breast masses. The area along the base of the fingers seems most sensitive when using light palpation.

nous carcinoma. In a male, consider a breast mass that is evident to the flat portion of the fingers (not just the finger tips) malignant until proven otherwise.

If nodules are present, then check for retractions, edema or redness. Note the exact location of the lesion and measure the size in all dimensions. Pay careful attention to the margin. Is it well-defined or diffuse? Is the shape round, irregular or flat and coin-like? Is it mobile or fixed? Also search for axillary, supraclavicular, and parasternal lymphadenopathy (see Figure 81).

CHAPTER 14

The Respiratory System

"The natural sound of the chest, on percussion, fails over the whole space occupied by the fluid. From this result simply, we could not indeed be certain whether the disease is pleurisy or pneumonia.... But mediate auscultation ... enables us to ascertain with precision, not merely the existence of the effusion, but its quantity. The signs by which the stethoscope effects this are, 1st, the total absence, or great diminution, of the respiratory sound; and, 2nd, the appearance, disappearance, and return of egophony."
— René-Théophile-Hyacinthe Laennec

"That the lungs partially deprived of air, should yield a tympanitic sound, and when the quantity of air in them is increased, a non-tympanitic sound appears opposed to the laws of physics. The fact ... is corroborated both by experiments on the dead body ... and also by this constant phenomenon, viz.: that when the lower portion of a lung is entirely compressed by any pleuritic effusion, and its upper portion reduced in volume, the percussion-sound at the upper part of the thorax is distinctly tympanitic."
— Josef Skoda

The goal of the pulmonary examination is to appreciate the quality of respiratory efficiency, gas exchange, and to note the presence of disease. Complete evaluation of the bedfast patient is often less than optimal because chest expansion is not always symmetrical and percussion notes may be less resonant.

INSPECTION

The Respiratory Rate

First determine the respiratory rate. (See Chapter 4 for more details regarding respiration as a vital sign.) While this vital sign is often recorded in the chart (most often as 20 breaths per minute) it is instructive to cultivate the discipline to obtain it yourself. An increased rate is an important clue to infection (frequently pneumonia), reactive airways disease, congestive heart failure, pulmonary embolus, and metabolic acidosis. A decreased respiratory rate (less than 10 breaths per minute) is seen in severe myxedema, CNS depressants (narcotics and benzodiazepines), and CNS disease (pontine hemorrhage, hypoglycemia, meningitis).

Respiratory Effort

Respiratory effort is noted by becoming aware of labored breathing. Normally the breathing is quiet and unlabored, and the examiner tends to proceed without paying much attention to the nature of the respiratory effort. Patients with air hunger will often breathe with an open mouth. Seeing pursed lips (mainly in expiration) suggests small airways disease with terminal bronchiole collapse. The terminal bronchioles do not collapse during inspiration so this is usually seen during expiration. Expiring with pursed lips increases the end expiratory pressure, keeping the airways open. It takes more work to put the first breath into a balloon than to add a breath to an already half-filled balloon.

Audible Breath Sounds

Also pay attention to whether the breathing is audible. Wheezing is a musical sound that is an important clue to reactive airways or local obstruction. Coughing indicates lower airway irritation, and stridor (a high-pitched shrieking sound) implies airway obstruction. *Inspiratory stridor is a medical emergency and suggests obstruction in the oral airway or epiglottis.* Expiratory stridor without inspiratory stridor suggests lower airway obstruction.

Patterns of Respiration

The respiratory pattern is another very important initial observation (see Figure 8). Normally the pattern is slow and regular. Deep rapid respirations suggest metabolic acidosis (Kussmaul's sign if the patient is in diabetic ketoacidosis). Also see if the patient has the cyclical pattern of Cheyne-Stokes' respiration. The pattern of Cheyne-Stokes' respiration is one of increasingly deep respirations followed by a steady diminution of breathing until an apneic episode occurs. The significance of Cheyne-Stokes' respiration is prolonged circulatory time or primary neurological disease.

Some patients will show pupillary dilation with rapid breathing and pupillary contraction with apnea. The differential diagnosis of Cheyne-Stokes' respiration is primary CNS disease, CHF, meningitis, pneumonia, medications, and obesity.

Irregular respiration, with periods of deep and shallow breathing and frequent sighs, suggests increased intracranial pressure (Biot's sign). Inspiration interrupted by cough suggests pleuritic pain.

Demeanor and Skin Color

Pay careful attention to the patient's demeanor and skin color. Patients in respiratory distress may appear restless, agitated, or drowsy. The patient's eyes may be prominent. Obviously the patient's skin color gives important clues to the level of oxygen saturation. Cyanosis suggests at least five grams of deoxyhemoglobin. If it just involves the nail beds then the peripheral circulation is clamped down or slowed.

Posture

The patient's posture and position are important to observe. Patients with respiratory failure will often sit leaning forward using their accessory muscles. Hypertrophy of the sternocleidomastoid may be present and the patient may have calluses on the extensor surface of their forearm or on their distal thigh (Dahl's sign) as evidence of the chronicity of their lung disease. Patients who sit leaning forward with their legs dependent (Fowler's position) may have severe heart failure. Patients leaning forward, with their head protruding as if sniffing flowers, may have epiglottitis.

George Ryerson Fowler (1848–1906) was a tireless American surgeon who completed the first thoracoplasty. He practiced in Brooklyn, New York, and was one of the first to adopt Joseph Lister's (1827–1912) antiseptic technique. Fowler's sitting position, with the body at a 45° angle, was for postoperative patients to help

*improve their breathing. The English physician
Charles Powell White (1728–1813) first used this
posture in women after delivery to facilitate
uterine drainage. Fowler founded the Brooklyn
Red Cross (1884) and introduced first aid instruction to the New York National Guard.*

Breathing difficulty when sitting up and
relieved when supine is platypnea and implies
severe upper lobe disease. Patients lying on
one side (lateral decubitus position) tend to
place the good lung in the dependent position
to maximize ventilation-perfusion matching.
However, if a pleural effusion is present, it will
tend to be on the dependent side.

Clubbing of the Fingernails

See if the fingers are clubbed by looking
for Schamroth's sign (see Figure 16). Have the
patient place both forefinger nails together and
look between them. If you can see a small diamond space between them, then the nails are
not clubbed. If the diamond is not visible,
Schamroth's sign is positive and clubbing is
present. Pulmonary causes of clubbing include
bronchogenic carcinoma, alveolar cell carcinoma, pulmonic abscess, interstitial pulmonary fibrosis, sarcoidosis, beryllium poisoning
and pulmonary arteriovenous fistula (not an
exhaustive list). There are also cardiac and GI
causes of clubbing (see Chapter 5).

Chest Shape and Symmetry

Note the patient's chest shape and symmetry. A barrel-shaped chest (increased AP diameter) suggests air trapping due to chronic
lung disease. The AP diameter may not really
be increased but an optical illusion due to decreased abdominal diameter in people with
emphysema. A thin, wiry habitus with distended arm veins suggests emphysema.

Venous Patterns

Note the venous pattern over the chest.
Unilateral venous distension suggests an under-

lying pulmonary neoplasm. Juicy collaterals
can be seen in superior vena cava syndrome.
Fine telangiectasias along the border of the
costal margin are commonly seen in elderly
men.

Chest Wall Deformities

Chest wall deformities can have a significant impact on respiratory dynamics. Abnormalities commonly seen in elderly people are
scoliosis and kyphosis (see Figures 75 and 76).
Less commonly you may see an older person
with pectus excavatum (funnel chest). The
sternum is depressed creating a funnel-like
shape. Pectus excavatum is associated with
congenital abnormalities in the respiratory
tract and heart, as well as Marfan's syndrome.
Another sternal abnormality is pectus carina-
tum (pigeon chest). In this condition the sternum sticks out like a ridge on the chest. It is
associated with acromegaly, Marfan's syndrome,
and congenital problems of the diaphragm.

Tracheal Location

Next, look at the tracheal position. (You
may have already performed this during the
neck examination.) Normally the trachea is
slightly to the right of the midline. Atelectasis and consolidation shifts the trachea toward
the involved side. Pleural scarring will cause
the trachea to deviate to the involved side during inspiration. Pneumothorax will pull the
trachea to the opposite side, while massive
pleural effusion and goiter will push the trachea
to the opposite side.

Chest Movement
During Respiration

The next part of the chest inspection is to
observe the chest movement during respiration. If the patient is using accessory muscles,
this implies the FEV1 is decreased to 30% of
normal (generally FEV1 between 1.0 and 1.5).

This patient often is sitting up, leaning forward, with hands propped on knees. There is sternocleidomastoid tension, with the muscle being thicker than the patient's thumb.

Look for diaphragm movement, which will sometimes be seen as a flickering along lateral chest with inspiration. A loss of this movement on one side, indicating a paralyzed hemidiaphragm, is Litten's sign. In overweight people the diaphragmatic movement may not be visible.

Watch the sides of the chest from the back to see if the chest moves symmetrically. Symmetric decreased expansion suggests extreme old age, emphysema, and ankylosing spondylitis (which usually presents in young men with back pain). Symmetric increased expansion suggests paralysis of the diaphragm with compensatory intercostal contractions. Decreased chest expansion due to substernal goiter is Bryson's sign.

Asymmetric expansion suggests pneumonia, a large pleural effusion, rib fracture, or pneumothorax. With hemiplegia, the affected side moves more than the unaffected side during quiet respiration, but is more sluggish with forced respiration (Jackson's breathing sign).

Paradoxical Chest Movements

Look carefully to see if there are any paradoxical movements. Paradoxical sternal movement suggests trauma or multiple rib fractures. Paradoxical abdominal movement is where the abdomen moves out with expiration. It is a sign of a paralyzed diaphragm, respiratory failure, or fatigue during a COPD exacerbation. Intermittent paradoxical abdominal movement due to fatigue is called respiratory alternans. Epigastric depression with inspiration suggests large pericardial effusion or paralyzed diaphragms (Duchenne's sign).

Guillaume Benjamin Amand Duchenne *(1806–1875), the great and lonely French neurologist, had significant family troubles. His wife died of puerperal fever, and his mother-in-law spread rumors that the death could be attributed*

to Duchenne himself, since he was the only person present at the birth. By the latter part of his career, Duchenne became well established, earning the respect of Jean-Martin Charcot who called Duchenne "The Master." One of Duchenne's lasting imprints on the field of neurology was development of the meticulous techniques of neurological exam. His attention to observational detail extended beyond the standard exam. Apart from Duchenne's description of the disorders to which his name is attached, he was also the first to distinguish upper and lower motor neuron causes of 7th nerve paralysis, and he made several important contributions to our understanding of lead palsy. It was Duchenne who described the cogwheel rigidity of Parkinson's disease.

Duchenne was probably the first person to use biopsy procedures to obtain tissue from a living patient. He was also one of the first to use photography to illustrate disease processes, as well as the facial expression of emotion. Charles Darwin used Duchenne's photographs in his book, The Expression of Emotions in Man and Animals. In his later career, Duchenne deteriorated rapidly due to cerebral vascular disease. As the consummate observer, he documented his progressive hemiparesis during his final days, recording his decline using his remaining good hand.

Rib Retractions

Rib retractions are a sign of a flail chest if the ribs themselves show paradoxical movement. If the interspaces show retractions, there is an imbalance between the negative pressure generated and the ability of the lung to expand. Generalized retractions are a sign of significant inspiratory obstruction. Focal retractions suggests bronchial obstruction, flail chest, and constrictive pericarditis (Broadbent's sign), if over the heart. Unilateral loss of normal retractions suggests pleural effusion, pneumothorax, or consolidation.

Bulging Interspaces

Bulging interspaces on inspiration suggest a tension pneumothorax, a large pleural effusion, emphysema, or reactive airways disease.

Elevation of supraclavicular space in an asynchronous manner suggests pleural effusion, as the lung floats like a cork on the pleural fluid. The side with the fluid will elevate first.

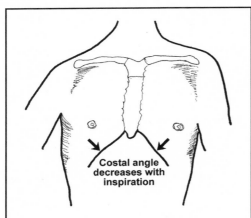

Figure 83. Hoover's Sign.

Normally the costal angle should increase as the intercostal muscles open the chest, as the diaphragm contracts. Hoover's sign is paradoxical closing of the costal angle with inspiration, due to loss of intercostals' contribution secondary to air trapping. This sign indicates chronic obstruction with an FEV1 less than one liter. Restrictive lung disease by itself does not produce Hoover's sign.

The Costal Angle (Hoover's Sign)

An especially useful observation is to watch the costal angle during respiration (Hoover's sign). Normally this angle should increase as the intercostal muscles open the chest, as the diaphragm contracts. Hoover's sign is paradoxical closing of the costal angle with inspiration, due to loss of intercostals' contribution secondary to air trapping (see Figure 83). This sign indicates chronic obstruction with an FEV1 less than one liter. Restrictive lung disease by itself does not produce Hoover's sign.

Unilateral Movements

If there are unilateral movements, consider the source of the inequality. If one side moves more laterally, this implies significant atelectasis (pulling up from above) or a subphrenic abscess (pushing up from below). If one side moves more medially, then consider intercostal paralysis, pleural effusion, or tension pneumothorax. Unilateral narrowing of the intercostal spaces suggests pneumothorax or inflammation (Przewalski's sign). If you see decreased medial movement with normal lateral movement, consider cardiac enlargement, severe right heart failure, and pericardial effusion.

PALPATION

Palpate the Lateral Chest Walls

Palpation over the lateral chest wall can provide helpful information on respiratory excursion. Feeling an area of localized warmth in a febrile patient could represent an empyema. Appreciating a mass in the chest wall could

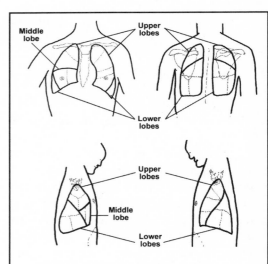

Figure 84. Lung Surface Anatomy.

This illustration shows the location of the upper, middle and lower lobes of the lungs (with the subsegmental lung areas) relative to landmarks on the chest and back. Note the anterior location of the right middle lobe and the posterior and lateral locations of the lower lobes.

represent a rib fracture (there may be an area of point tenderness and possibly ecchymosis), tuberculosis, nocardia, or actinomycosis. A mass felt in an interspace suggests abscess (possibly actinomycosis, tuberculosis or empyema necessitans) or lymphadenopathy from lymphoma. Feeling crepitus suggests subcutaneous emphysema from a rib fracture, ruptured bleb with pneumothorax, esophageal rupture, or abdominal perforated viscus with retroperitoneal air tracking.

Pain on Palpation

Localized pain on palpation suggests early herpes zoster, rib fracture, or costochondritis (Tietze's syndrome, named for the German surgeon Alexander Tietze [1864–1927]). Sternal tenderness can be a sign of fracture, leukemia (classically the lower third of the sternum), other blood marrow abnormalities, metastatic prostate cancer, or xiphoidalgia. Pneumonia can produce tenderness and spasm of the insertion of the sternocleidomastoid muscle.

Palpate the Trachea

If you have not already done so, palpate the trachea. Check the lateral tracheal wall with the clavicular heads to determine whether it is midline. Deviation from the midline is significant. See Chapter 10 for more information on tracheal palpation.

Palpate Rib Expansion

Next, palpate the rib expansion segmentally. First, place your hands on each upper lobe with the thumbs under each clavicular head. Watch for symmetrical thumb expansion with each inspiration. To check the middle and lingular segments, place your hands across lower chest with each thumb at the fifth intercostal space on the sternum. Watch for symmetrical thumb expansion with each inspi-

ration. A lack of symmetrical movement suggests bronchial stenosis on the side with the reduced movement. To evaluate the lower lobes, place your hands across the lower chest anteriorly with each thumb at the costal margin. Watch for symmetrical thumb expansion with each inspiration. Paradoxical movement, with a decrease in the costal angle with inspiration, caused by severe air trapping in chronic lung disease (FEV1 less than one liter), is Hoover's sign. Repeat the lower lobe examination posteriorly at the level of the tenth rib. A normal movement is one to two centimeters.

René-Théophile-Hyacinthe Laënnec (1781–1826) was the French physician who introduced the stethoscope into the physical examination, after he obtained the idea from children he saw playing in the streets of Paris. By placing to their ears one end of a long piece of wood, the children were able to listen to the transmission of sounds made by the scratching of a pin at the other end. He described and named the physical signs of rales, rhonchi, crepitation, and egophony, and compared his physical findings to observations he made during autopsy. Among many others, he also described pectoriloquy, bronchial and vesicular breathing sounds, and bronchiectasis. He called this method of examination the "mediate" method and told of it in his book, De l'auscultation mediate, published in 1819.

Laënnec also contributed significant work in the study of tuberculosis, a disease that likely claimed his mother. Although the infectious nature of the disease eluded him, Laënnec was first to understand that tuberculous lesions could occur anywhere in the body, and therefore was not confined to lungs as was previously believed. He was also first to describe and name melanoma, as well as understand that the black spots it might produce in the lungs were not soot or tuberculosis, but metastatic melanotic disease.

Tactile Fremitus

Have the patient say "toy coin" each time you touch the chest with the ulnar side of your hand (see Figure 85). The "oy" sound is the key to producing the vibration. Feeling increased vibration (fremitus) over an area of dullness to percussion suggests consolidation

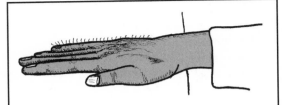

Figure 85. Tactile Fremitus.

Have the patient say "toy coin" each time you touch the chest with the ulnar side of your hand. Use both hands to compare sides simultaneously. Begin at the apices posteriorly and work down the back, then go anteriorly to the apices. Normally the right apex will have slightly more fremitus than the left because of the aortic position. Feeling increased vibration (fremitus) over an area of dullness to percussion suggests consolidation or direct communication between the bronchus and the chest wall. Appreciating decreased fremitus over an area of dullness suggests pleural effusion or pneumonectomy.

or direct communication between the bronchus and the chest wall. Appreciating decreased fremitus over an area of dullness suggests pleural effusion or pneumonectomy. Use both hands to compare each side simultaneously. Begin at the apices posteriorly and work down the back, then go anteriorly to the apices. Normally the right apex will have slightly more fremitus than the left because of the aortic position. Note the level of the diaphragm.

PERCUSSION

Make sure your hands are warm before you begin. (This is important before performing palpation, as well.) The feel of the resonance is more useful to me than the sound of the percussion note. It is especially helpful in a noisy setting such as a crowded emergency room where subtleties of sound are more difficult to appreciate.

Start at the back and check each side to compare the quality of the sensation. Having

a loose wrist and a floppy hand is a key. As you percuss, consider the characteristic of the structure you are percussing. One trick is to practice over a table, going from the center toward the legs. Close your eyes and practice until you can stop over the leg.

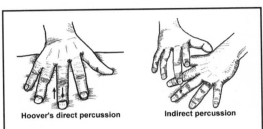

Hoover's direct percussion   Indirect percussion

Figure 86. Two Percussion Techniques.

Hoover's direct percussion is particularly useful in percussing the cardiac border. Place your dominant hand on the skin, raise your middle finger or forefinger, and tap on the skin directly. The indirect percussion technique is what students are generally taught as percussion. Place your non-dominant hand on the skin, and with your dominant middle finger tap the middle finger of your non-dominant hand at the DIP joint. The significance of dullness to percussion is that it implies consolidation, pleural fluid or pleural scarring. The percussion note is more resonate in pneumothorax (Biermer's sign).

Percussion Techniques

There are three basic techniques to percussion. The first is the light pat. Gently pat the back on each side, starting at the apices and moving down to the diaphragm. The second technique is direct percussion (see Figure 86). Place your dominant hand on the skin, raise your forefinger and tap on the skin directly. The third percussion technique is indirect percussion (which students are generally taught as percussion). Place your non-dominant hand on the skin, and with your dominant middle finger tap the middle finger of your non-dominant hand at the DIP joint.

The significance of dullness to percussion is that it implies consolidation, pleural fluid or pleural scarring. Parenchymal consolidation suggests pneumonia or cancer. Dullness to percussion and absent breath sounds due to hydatid disease in the lungs is Bird's sign. If you suspect pleural fluid, recheck your percussion with the patient in the lateral decubitus position with the dull side up. Look for any change in dullness due to fluid shift. No change in dullness with a change in position implies either consolidation or loculated fluid. The percussion note is more resonate in pneumothorax (Biermer's sign).

Michael Anton Biermer (1827–1892) was a German physician who trained under Rudolph Virchow. He carefully described and named pernicious anemia (first described by Sir Thomas Addison in 1849) and was the first to describe retinal hemorrhages. He also described the change in resonance over a pneumothorax and a change in the percussion note when a patient with a pleural effusion changes position.

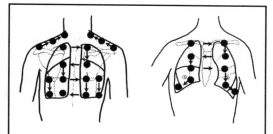

Figure 87. Patterns of Percussion.

It is important for the patient to be upright if at all possible. Percuss down the posterior mid-clavicular line, comparing each side. Note the diaphragmatic excursion by checking level of diaphragm in expiration and then deep inspiration. Normally this excursion is about 4cm. After percussing the diaphragms, percuss down the mid-axillary line on each side. Next, percuss across the trapezius from the shoulder to the base of the neck, to check Kronig's isthmus. Percuss the clavicles. Dullness on one side suggests upper lobe disease. Finally, percuss over the right middle lobe in the right mid-chest and along the left anterior chest.

The Sequence of Percussion

It is important for the patient to be upright if at all possible. Percuss down the posterior mid-clavicular line on each side. Note

the diaphragmatic excursion by checking level of diaphragm in expiration and then deep inspiration. Normally this excursion is about 4cm. Compare each side. After percussing the diaphragms, percuss down the mid-axillary line on each side. Finding an elevated left hemidiaphragm is clearly abnormal and implies volume loss, paralysis of the left hemidiaphragm or a left upper quadrant abdominal mass. Finding an elevated right hemidiaphragm is normal but can suggest volume loss, a right upper quadrant mass, or a paralyzed right hemidiaphragm.

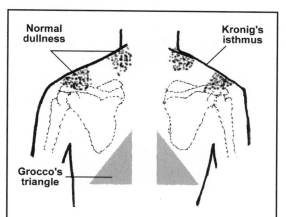

Figure 88. Kronig's Isthmus and Grocco's Triangle.

Kronig's isthmus (of resonance) is appreciated by percussing across the trapezius from the shoulder to the base of the neck, checking on each side. This area, in a bathing suit strap distribution, is significantly more resonant than the shoulder or the base of the neck. Loss of this normal resonance suggests upper lobe disease. The medial base of the lung is called Grocco's triangle. Dullness in the triangle near the spinous process is sometimes noted contralateral to a pleural effusion (or significant pneumonia) and ipsilateral to a massive left-sided pleural effusion or pericardial effusion.

Next, percuss across the trapezius from the shoulder to the base of the neck, to check Kronig's isthmus (of resonance) on each side. This area, in a bathing suit strap distribution, is significantly more resonant than the shoulder or the base of the neck. Loss of this area of normal resonance suggests upper lobe disease.

Percuss the clavicles. Dullness on one side suggests upper lobe disease. Finally, percuss over the right middle lobe in the right mid-chest and along the left anterior chest.

Special Circumstances to Interpret Percussion Findings

Dullness in the medial base of the lung (Grocco's triangle) near the spinous process can sometimes be appreciated contralateral to a pleural effusion (or significant pneumonia) and ipsilateral to a massive left pleural effusion or pericardial effusion. Dullness below the left scapula (Ewart's sign) suggests a large pericardial effusion. Dullness to percussion below the right scapula (Conner's sign) suggests a large pericardial effusion. Feeling increased rib vibration in the anterior chest to percussion posteriorly suggests a pleural effusion (Kellock's sign). Change in the percussible dullness with change in position suggests pleural effusion (D'Amato's sign). With small pleural effusion there is dullness in the T9 to T11 interspaces.

Hyperresonance just above an area of dullness (Skodaic hyperresonance) is a useful sign of a pleural effusion. Noting hyperresonance over the mid-clavicle suggests pneu-

mothorax. Confirm by appreciating decreased breath sounds over the hyperresonant side. Noting a band of hyperresonance near the diaphragm suggests subphrenic abscess or lower lobe pneumonia.

Joseph Skoda (1805–1881) was an Austrian physician who was an expert at auscultation and percussion of the chest. He described over one hundred separate pulmonary noises, validating his finding by autopsy.

His famous courses on diseases of the chest began in 1834 and soon attracted young colleagues from the Austrian monarchy as well as from other European countries. Skoda ended his life as a famous and wealthy physician but used the greater part of his possessions for charity and also for financial support of his cousin in Plzen, the founder of the Skoda automobile factory.

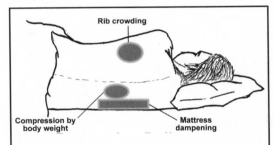

Figure 90. Percussion Dullness in a Bedfast Patient.

Sometimes an elderly patient is too ill to sit up and percussion must be accomplished with the patient in the lateral decubitus position. This position can add some artifacts of lung compression, producing dullness in the mid lung fields of both the dependent and upward lungs.

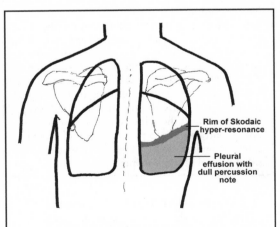

Figure 89. Skodaic Hyperresonance.

Hyperresonance just above an area of dullness (Skodaic hyperresonance) is a useful sign of a pleural effusion. The mechanism is compressed lung just above the level of pleural fluid.

Sometimes an elderly patient is too ill to sit up and percussion must be accomplished with the patient in the lateral decubitus position. This position can add some artifacts of lung compression, producing dullness in the mid-lung fields of both the dependent and upward lungs (see Figure 90).

AUSCULTATION

Make sure that the listening area is quiet. *Do not listen through the patient's clothing.* Warm your stethoscope, either by carrying it in your pants pocket or by vigorously rubbing it. Another strategy is to place a rubber membrane on the bell. Have the patient breath deeply through his or her open mouth. Listen to at least two respiratory cycles at each location. If patient has been intubated, listen for bilateral breath sounds and over the epigastric area to help determine the tube placement. All breath sounds should increase in pitch with inspiration and decrease with expiration.

Begin at the bases and work up the back. The reason to start here is to be able to appreciate any basilar crackles secondary to atelectasis or early congestive heart failure. These crackles might disappear by the time you get to the bases if you had started at the apices and worked down.

If you hear additional noises, make sure they are coming from the patient's chest and not from the skin, muscles or other extraneous source. Make sure that your stethoscope bell is securely placed flat on the chest and that you are not breathing on your stethoscope tubing. Try breathing on the tubing to appreciate the low-pitched rustling sound your breath produces. Also make sure that your earpieces are securely in your ears to exclude environmental noise. Body hair can produce a crackling sound that resembles dry cellophane crackles.

d'Éspine's Sign

When you reach the level of the mid-scapula (about T5), listen over the vertebral spinous process for d'Éspine's sign (see Figure 91). This is an important sign of a posterior mediastinal mass. Listen on either side of the vertebral column and compare the quality and intensity of the sounds with the sounds over the spinous process. Normally the lateral sounds are louder and more distinct. D'Éspine's sign is positive when the vertebral breath sounds are loud, and upper airway sounds are of greater intensity than the corresponding lateral lung sounds. It implies continuity between a main stem bronchus and the vertebrae, and

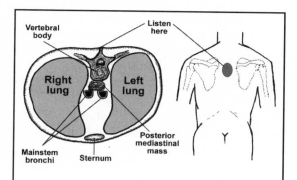

Figure 91. D'Éspine's Sign.
D'Éspine's sign is an important sign of a posterior mediastinal mass. When you reach the level of the mid-scapula (about T5), listen over the vertebral spinous process and on either side of the vertebral column. Compare the quality and intensity of the sounds in the lung fields with the sounds over the spinous process. Normally the lateral sounds are louder and more distinct. D'Éspine's sign is positive when the vertebral breath sounds are loud, and upper airway sounds are of greater intensity than the corresponding lateral lung sounds. It implies continuity (a mass) between a main stem bronchus and the vertebra.

suggests malignancy, lymphoma, metastatic cancer, tuberculosis, sarcoidosis, and other causes of mediastinal lymphadenopathy. Listen for egophony, bronchophony, and whisper pectoriloquy. These may be more sensitive than the change in breath sounds for posterior mediastinal lymphadenopathy. If d'Éspine's sign is present, try percussing over the spinous processes of T1–T5. The appearance of red spots over the spinous processes of T1–T5 after percussing them suggests bronchial lymphadenopathy (Cattaneo's sign). False positives of d'Éspine's sign can occur in severe kyphosis, which should be obvious.

The Quality of Breath Sounds

Next, appreciate the quality of the breath sounds. Alveolar (vesicular) breath sounds are normal but pathological processes cause these sounds to disappear. Upper airway or bronchial (tubular) breath sounds are normal over an airway, but hearing these sounds in the peripheral lung fields suggests consolidation, lymphadenopathy, or a pleural effusion. Also pay attention to the inspiratory-to-expiratory ratio of breath sounds. Chronic obstructive lung disease increases the expiratory phase of respiration. Hearing equal inspiratory and expiratory sounds suggests respiratory obstruction (Grancher's sign). Localized prolongation of expiratory sounds is Jackson's sign.

The Loudness of Breath Sounds

Loudness of the breath sounds can be quantitated by the breath intensity index. Zero equals no breath sounds. One is barely-heard breath sounds. Two is faint but definite breath sounds. Three is normal breath sounds. Four is augmented breath sounds.

Increased breath sounds over an area of dullness suggest consolidation. If there is upper lobe consolidation, consider tuberculosis, Pancoast's tumor, or aspiration pneumonia. Signs of middle lobe consolidation suggest pneumonia, malignancy, or conditions producing lymphadenopathy (middle lobe syndrome). Lower lobe consolidation suggests pneumonia, aspiration or pulmonary infarct.

Decreased breath sounds over an area of consolidation suggest pleural effusion or pneumonectomy.

Adventitious Breath Sounds

Next, listen carefully for any adventitious sounds. If there is stridor, then listen over the trachea or at the base of the neck to see if loudness is greatest there. If it is heard on inspiration (*a red flag of a medical emergency*), then consider epiglottic obstruction, epiglottitis, vocal cord dysfunction, tracheal obstruction, whopping cough, neoplasm, foreign body, tracheal stenosis, or palatal obstruction. If the stridor is only in expiration, this suggests lower airway obstruction such as foreign body.

Wheezes

Wheezes are musical sounds that indicate obstruction of airways. Obstruction during expiration suggests a source within the chest. Obstruction in the trachea (outside the chest) can be heard during inspiration. Hearing both inspiratory and expiratory wheezes is more concerning than hearing either alone. Focal wheezes help to localize the site of obstruction. End-expiratory wheezes suggest reactive airways (asthma) and imply bronchiolar disease. Peak flow is reduced significantly. Hearing wheezes throughout expiration suggests asynchrony of one lung area with another, such as in organophosphate poisoning.

Hearing end-inspiratory wheezes implies small airway opening in deflated section of lung. This finding suggests chronic bronchitis, bronchiectasis, or organophosphate poisoning. Hearing wheezes throughout inspiration implies a fixed stenosis or obstruction of the upper tracheal bronchial tree, such as in interstitial fibrosis or hypersensitivity pneumonitis.

Crackles (Rales)

Inspiratory crackles are commonly heard in elderly people. Early inspiratory crackles imply significantly decreased FEV1/FVC due to broncho-obstructive disease, chronic bronchitis, emphysema, or reactive airways disease.

Dry crackles suggest interstitial lung disease. Moist crackles suggest congestive heart failure. Localized mid-expiratory crackles can be a sign of bronchiectasis or pneumonia.

Mid-inspiratory crackles suggest bronchiectasis, while late-inspiratory crackles suggest restrictive (alveolar) disease caused by congestive heart failure, idiopathic pulmonary fibrosis, sarcoidosis, or drug toxicity.

For expiratory crackles, note the location of the crackles. Changing location of crackles with changes in the patient's position suggests congestive heart failure. This implies an increased pulmonary capillary wedge pressure (above 25mmHg). Fixed crackles suggest fibrosis or pneumonia.

Also note the quality of the crackles. Peripheral lesions tend to increase the pitch (fineness) of the crackles. Fine crackles (like crackling cellophane) suggest interstitial fibrosis, sarcoidosis, or asbestosis. Coarse crackles suggest chronic pulmonary fibrosis. Post-tussive rales (crackles) suggest parenchymal disease or lung abscess.

Rhonchi

Rhonchi are coarse, flapping sounds, that suggest fluid or mucus in an airway.

Amphoric Breathing

A low-pitched sound resembling blowing over a soft-drink bottle (an amphora) is amphoric breathing. One trick is to listen over the occiput while the patient whispers "Wahoo," to appreciate the nature of the sound. Amphoric breathing is never heard in the presence of alveoli, so this finding suggests alveolar destruction. It signifies a large bullae or lung abscess, with air going into and out of a cavity. Disappearance of amphoric breathing suggests that something has occupied the void (aspergillus fungus ball or fluid).

Pleural Friction Rubs

Pleural friction rubs are leathery, creaky sounds, usually in inspiration and expiration, but sometimes only in inspiration. They tend to be localized. They do not have a musical quality like a wheeze, and suggest two inflamed pleural surfaces (the parietal and visceral pleura) rubbing together. Hearing a pleural friction rub implies neoplasm, pulmonary infarction, pneumonia, tuberculosis, or systemic lupus erythematosus. A sternal friction rub, heard when the patient raises and lowers arms, suggests aortic arch aneurysm or fibrotic mediastinal tumor (Perez's sign).

SPECIAL TESTS

Post-tussive Rales

Listen for rales after a cough (post-tussive rales), as they may signify a lung abscess.

Egophony (Goat Sound)

This "E" to "A" change is considered the most sensitive sign of pulmonary consolidation. Have the patient say "E." Compressed lung will bleat like a goat changing it to an "A" sound. For practice, listen over the skull or the base of the neck where this "E" to "A" change is normal. Egophony may be present along the top of a pleural effusion. It may also be present over a massive pleural effusion due to significant lung compression. Extensive pulmonary fibrosis can also produce egophony.

Whisper Pectoriloquy

Whisper pectoriloquy is the second best sign of consolidation. Have patient whisper, "Sixty-six whiskeys, please" (because of the sibilance). With abnormal bronchial breathing the sounds will be more distinct and you can easily appreciate the words whispered.

Bronchophony

In bronchophony, spoken sounds seem more distinct when listening over a consolidated or compressed lung. Have the patient say a sentence like "UNC is number one." With consolidation the sentence will be heard clearly over the involved area.

Expiratory Time

Have the patient take a deep breath and exhale as quickly as possible. Listen over the upper posterior chest. Hearing expiratory sounds for over three seconds suggests airway obstruction. A more accurate method is to listen over the trachea and use a six-second threshold.

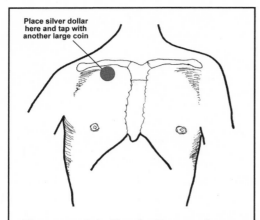

Figure 92. Coin Test for Pneumothorax.
Have the upright patient hold a large silver coin such as a pre–1964 silver dollar (Susan B. Anthony dollars are too small) flat against the chest, just below the mid-clavicle. Smaller coins such as quarters or nickels will not work. Tap the coin with another silver dollar while you listen to the chest with your stethoscope. A pneumothorax or a large bulla will produce a loud bell-like sound rather than the usual metallic tap.

The Coin Test for Pneumothorax

Have the patient, sitting upright, hold a large silver coin such as a silver dollar (Susan B. Anthony dollars are too small) flat against the chest, just below the mid-clavicle. Tap the coin with another coin while you listen to the chest with your stethoscope. A pneumothorax or a large bulla will produce a loud bell-like sound rather than the usual metallic tap.

Smaller coins such as quarters or nickels will not work. Supine patient positioning will not work. Tuning forks sometimes work.

Shephard's Sign of Sleep Apnea

Some patients with sleep apnea will develop a sonorous expiratory wheeze at the base of the neck. Listen with the patient supine and breathing through the nose.

Guarino's Auscultatory Percussion

This is a very sensitive method to detect pulmonary masses greater than one-and-one-half centimeters in size. With your non-dominant hand percuss the manubrium. As you percuss, listen to the percussion note, beginning at the bases and moving upward. A lesion will produce audible dullness. Remember that the sound transmissions are linear, so the lesion is located along the line connecting the manubrium and the auscultatory finding.

SPECIAL CIRCUMSTANCES

Discriminating a Pleural Effusion from Consolidation

Both conditions produce dullness to percussion, so percuss above the dullness. In pa-

Table 14.1. Physical findings in various lung conditions					
Condition	*Tracheal Shift*	*Chest Expansion*	*Fremitus*	*Percussion*	*Breath Sounds*
Pneumothorax	away	unclear	decreased	increased	reduced
Pleural effusion	away	decreased	decreased	dull	reduced
Consolidation	no shift	decreased	increased	dull	tubular
Consolidation with atelectasis	toward	decreased	decreased	dull	reduced
Pleural thickening	toward	decreased	decreased	dull	reduced

tients with large effusions there is a decrease in the lower extremity blood pressure on the affected side when compared to the upper extremity (Williamson's sign). Hearing a rim of hyperresonance just above the dullness (Skodaic hyperresonance) suggests pleural effusion. The tympanitic note above a pleural effusion changes when the patient opens and closes the mouth (Williams' sign). Increased resonance of the thoracic spinous processes suggests pleural effusion (Korányi's sign). Percussing an S-shaped line of dullness on the chest suggests a pleural effusion (Damoiseau-Ellis sign) (see Figure 93).

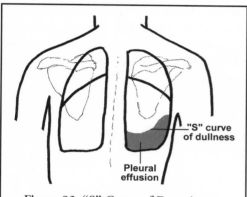

Figure 93. "S" Curve of Damoiseau.
Percussing an S-shaped line of dullness on the posterior chest suggests a pleural effusion (Damoiseau-Ellis sign).

Listen to the quality of breath sounds in the area of dullness. Hearing an increased intensity of sounds suggests consolidation. Hearing a decreased intensity suggests pleural effusion.

Listen for egophony by having the patient say "E." Compressed lung will bleat like a goat, changing it to an "A" sound. If egophony is present in an area of dullness, this suggests consolidation (Shilbey's sign). Egophony just above an area of dullness suggests pleural effusion. "U" to "A" egophony over a pleural effusion is Karplus' sign. Hearing no sound at all over an area of dullness implies resection.

Listen for whisper pectoriloquy by having the patient whisper, "Sixty-six whiskeys, please." Clearly hearing the phrase in an area of dullness suggests consolidation. Hearing no sound suggests pleural effusion.

If the signs suggest a pleural effusion, then gently move patient while listening over the effusion. Hearing a sloshing sound suggests hydropneumothorax. Also note the location of the effusion. A right-sided pleural effusion suggests congestive heart failure. A left-sided effusion suggests pancreatitis, pulmonary infarct, pericarditis, ascites, or a ruptured thoracic duct.

Signs of Cavitary Lung Disease

In pulmonary cavities the percussion note may change when the patient opens and closes the mouth (Wintrich's sign). Listening over a pulmonary cavity sometimes discloses harsh inspiratory sounds that quickly diminish in intensity (Seitz's sign). Forced inspiration can lower the pitch of the sound over a cavity (Friedreich's lung sign). Cough following apical percussion producing an area of apical tympany suggests cavitary disease (Erni's sign). Aphonia can be due to lung abscess (Behier-Hardy sign).

Signs of Pleural Inflammation

Decreased rib expansion can be due to an inflammatory process in the lungs (Bethea's sign). Pain from pleural irritation referred to the shoulder is Capp's sign. Chest pain that increases with bending toward the pain suggests intercostal neuralgia. Increase in pain with bending away from the pain suggests pleuritic pain (Schepelmann's sign). With pleuritic inflammation the patient will lie with the good side down (Andral's decubitus sign).

Gabriel Andral (1797–1876) was a French physician who was the founder of the science of hematology and is credited with the integration of that science into clinical and investigative medicine. He is known for having cataloged the most important diseases of the bladder and is

Table 14.2. Soft signs of tuberculosis

Sign	Physical Description
Abraham's	Dullness under the acromial process
Burghart's	Fine rales under the clavicles
De la Camp's	Dullness lateral to T5 and T6
Jurgensen's	Fine crepitant rales in the lung fields
Lombardi's	Varicosities over C7-T3 spinous processes
Murat's	Tactile fremitus over painful hemithorax
Riviere's	Dullness across back at T6
Rothshchild's	Flattening of sternal angle
Roussel's	Pain on percussion between clavicle and fourth rib

said to be the originator of the word "anemia" and "hyperemia." He was also the first physician to see the potential of the chemical analysis of the blood.

Palpable intercostal muscle rigidity suggests pleural inflammation (Pottenger's sign). Disappearance of this sign can indicate empyema (Ramond's sign). Pain on palpation on the left upper abdominal quadrant (the mirror image of Murphy's point) suggests lower lung pleural inflammation (de Mussey's sign). Pleural inflammation can produce sensitivity of the upper back and shoulder muscles to palpation (Sternberg's sign).

CHAPTER 15

The Cardiovascular System

"The teacher who is indeed wise does not bid you to enter the house of his wisdom but rather leads you to the threshold of your mind."

— **Kahlil Gibran**

"Physical examination must be carried out with a watchful eye, a sensitive touch, discerning ears, and an alert sense of smell. Above all, what is needed is an alert mind, free of dogma and routine. Each clinical problem, no matter how routine it may appear to be on the surface, calls for an unprejudiced approach. Each possible clue must be pursued; nothing can be taken for granted."

— **Maxwell M. Wintrobe**

The primary purpose of the cardiac examination is to assess the structure and function of the heart as a muscular pump and to evaluate it for possible malfunctions. Since heart disease is so common in elderly people, this examination often provides significant information. Proficiency in cardiac examination is also important because settings such as nursing homes and residences may not have ready access to high technology.

INSPECTION

Maculo-papular skin lesions on the upper extremities can be seen in end-stage heart failure (Robertson's sign).

Examining the Neck Veins

The first step of the cardiac examination is to examine the neck veins. Have the patient begin supine, then elevate the examining table until the top of the venous pulse wave is visible. Always examine the patient from the right side, looking at the right side of the neck. This approach provides a more accurate determination of venous waves since it is a straight shot from the right jugular veins to the superior vena cava and right atrium.

Have the patient turn the head slightly to the left, then look just lateral to the lateral head of the sternocleidomastoid to see if the internal jugular pulsation is visible. (If so use it.) Sometimes the pulsation will be just inferior to the lateral head and occasionally it will be

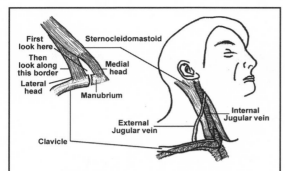

Figure 94. Examining the Jugular Veins.
Turn the patient's head slightly to the left and look between the two heads of the sternocleidomastoid; if the internal jugular pulsation is visible, use it. Sometimes the pulsation will be just inferior to the lateral head. Also look along the right supraclavicular fossa for the external jugular vein. Confirm the vein, by gently compressing it at the base of the neck and watching it distend, and then release it. The text shows you how to interpret the findings.

between the two heads of the sternocleidomastoid.

Look along the right supraclavicular fossa for the external jugular vein. Confirm the vein, by gently compressing it at the base of the neck and watching it distend, and then release it.

◆ ESTIMATE THE CENTRAL VENOUS PRESSURE

Note the height of the column of blood in each of the veins and use whichever vein is most distended. Note the highest level of the pulsation. More than three centimeters above the clavicle with the patient at forty-five degrees is abnormal. The level of the clavicle is ten centimeters of water when the patient is sitting upright (at 90°). You can estimate the central venous pressure by standing back and determining the relative position of the right atrium (about midway down the sternum and in the mid-axillary line) and the height of the column of blood. From this estimation up to sixteen centimeters of water is normal.

◆ NOTE THE VARIATION IN JUGULAR VENOUS PRESSURE WITH RESPIRATION

Next, pay attention to the variations in

the JVP with respiration. You should see them collapse with inspiration, which is normal. An increase in JVP with inspiration (Kussmaul's sign) suggests a problem with right atrial filling, usually caused by constrictive pericarditis or right ventricular failure. (Consider right ventricular infarction.)

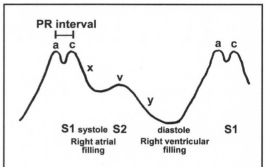

Figure 95. Jugular Venous Waveforms.
The "a" wave represents the right atrial contraction while the "c" wave is the cusp of the tricuspid valve pushing back into the right atrium at the beginning of systole. The a–c interval mirrors the pr interval on the electrocardiogram. The "x" descent occurs with right atrial filling. The "v" wave represents the volume of blood filling the atrium and the "y" descent indicates right ventricular filling after the opening of the tricuspid valve.

◆ LOOK FOR THE "X" AND "Y" DESCENTS

Now carefully study the venous waveforms. Look particularly for two downward motions for each upward motion. (Sometimes the second descent will look like a little bounce at the end of systole.) The downward motions are the "x" and "y" descents. Each descent is normally seen for each cardiac cycle.

If only one descent is seen, then determine which descent is missing by feeling the pulse. Seeing the descent coincident with the pulse means the "x" descent is visible and the "y" descent is missing, implying a problem with right ventricular filling, such as cardiac tamponade or tricuspid stenosis. (TS has giant "a" waves.) Seeing the descent discordant with the pulse means the "y" descent is visible and the "x" descent is missing, implying a problem with right atrial filling, such as pericardial constriction or tricuspid regurgitation. (TR has giant "v" waves.) If the pulsation is synchronous with the pulse, palpate the vein. (A bounding pulse is probably the carotid artery.)

♦ LOOK FOR THE "A" WAVE

Note the "a" (atrial contraction) wave at the top of the venous pulse. Bounding giant "a" waves are seen in tricuspid stenosis (along with the loss of the "y" descent). Intermittent large "a" waves are canon "a" waves, seen in third degree AV block (when right atrium contracts while the tricuspid valve is closed). Seeing two pulsations suggests visible "a" and "c" waves, implying first degree AV block since the interval between the "a" wave (atrial contraction) and the "c" wave (cusp of the tricuspid valve at the beginning of right ventricular systole) reflects the PR interval on the electrocardiogram. Sometimes the two waves are the "a" and the "v" waves.

♦ LOOK FOR THE "V" WAVE

Note the "v" wave (volume of blood entering the right atrium), which is usually the little bounce you see after the "x" descent. Large "v" waves suggest tricuspid insufficiency (Lancisi's sign).

Giovanni Maria Lancisi (1654–1720) was from a wealthy bourgeois family. His mother died in childbirth, and an aunt who was a nun reared Lancisi initially. When the nun died, Lancisi returned to his father's home in Rome. Lancisi obtained his MD in 1672 when he was still a month shy of 18. In 1684 he was appointed professor of anatomy in Rome, where he taught for 13 years.

In 1688 Pope Innocent XI made Lancisi pontifical doctor. He filled the post under succeeding popes. In return for curing the pope of a renal calculus, Lancisi was named canon of the church of St. Lorenzo. Clement conferred Roman nobility on Lancisi. The highest families in Rome also consulted Lancisi.

Apical Impulse

After examining neck veins, the next step is to see if the apical impulse is visible in the vicinity of the fifth intercostal space. Not seeing the apical impulse is usually a normal finding. You can check to see it in forced expiration or in the left lateral decubitus position. You can also check after palpation. The location can be a clue to pericardial effusion if there is a fullness in the epigastric area (Auenbrugger's sign).

Josef Leopold Auenbrugger (1722–1809) was the Austrian physician who introduced percussion to modern medicine. As a child he learned to tap with his fingers on the wine barrels in his father's cellar to determine how full they were based on the sound. He tapped directly on the chest wall, not with the intermediation of a finger of the opposite hand, as is currently common. He refined this technique and tested his theories at autopsy and by filling barrels and cadavers with fluids. His discovery was published in Vienna in 1861 in a book entitled "A New Discovery that Enables the Physician from the Percussion of the Human Thorax to Detect the Diseases Hidden Within the Chest." Jean-Nicolas Corvisart, Napoleon's favorite physician, happened upon a description of Auenbrugger's work and tested it for several years. Auenbrugger also wrote the libretto for the comic opera Der Rauchfangkehrer by Salieri (a contemporary of Mozart).

♦ LOCATION OF THE APICAL IMPULSE

Obviously the location of the apical impulse depends on intrathoracic pressures, so first check the trachea to see if it is midline. Finding a laterally displaced apical impulse with left tracheal displacement suggests mediastinal shift to the left. Normally the PMI is just medial to the midclavicular line at the fifth intercostal space. The nipple is almost never in the midclavicular line and should not be used as a constant landmark. For variations in the PMI see Table 15.1.

♦ TIMING AND RHYTHM OF
   THE APICAL IMPULSE

Regular rate and rhythm suggests sinus rhythm. An irregular rhythm suggests atrial fibrillation, or bigeminy if regularly irregular.

Table 15.1. Observations of the point of maximal impulse	
PMI Characteristic	*Implication*
• Lateral to the midclavicular line or below the 6th intercostal space	• Left ventricular enlargement
• Right-sided apical impulse	• Dextrocardia
• Subxiphoid impulse	• Right ventricular enlargement
• Right upper sternal pulsation	• Ascending aortic aneurysm
• Greater than 2 centimeters in size	• Left ventricular hypertrophy or dilation
• Systolic retraction (Broadbent's sign)	• Pericardial constriction or right ventricular hypertrophy
• Double impulse	• Asymmetric septal hypertrophy, right bundle branch block, left ventricular dyskinesia or an early diastolic filling wave (visible S3), aortic stenosis (uncommon)
• Diastolic impulse	• Pericardial constriction

PALPATION

Use your fingertips or the area between the MCP and PIP joints. Practice and attention will determine which area is most sensitive for you. Acute tenderness to palpation of the lower third of the sternum suggests leukemia or metastatic cancer (Mosler's sign).

Point of Maximal Impulse

♦ LOCATION

The PMI is normally at the fifth intercostal space in the midclavicular line. Feeling a PMI displaced lateral to midclavicular line or below fifth intercostal space is abnormal. Generally a displaced PMI suggests left ventricular hypertrophy or dilated cardiomyopathy. Feeling an apical systolic retraction suggests constrictive pericarditis, tricuspid insufficiency, or restrictive cardiomyopathy.

♦ SIZE

The PMI is normally the size of a penny. A quarter-sized PMI is abnormal and suggests left ventricular hypertrophy.

TIMING

Normally the systolic impulse is one-half to two-thirds of systole. Feeling a sustained PMI suggests left ventricular hypertrophy. You can verify this by listening to P2 at the left upper sternal border. The PMI is sustained if P2 is coincident with or later than the palpable PMI.

CHARACTERISTICS OF THE PMI

Feeling a double impulse suggests a palpable S3 (it is only significant if you hear an S3), a palpable S4 (more significant than an audible S4 and suggesting ischemic heart disease and increased afterload) or ventricular aneurysm. Lateral pulsation of the left hemithorax suggests left ventricular aneurysm.

Left Lower Sternal Border

After palpating the PMI, move your hand slightly medial to palpate along the lower left sternal border. Systolic movement here (feeling a right ventricular lift) is never normal. Presence of a right ventricular lift suggests severe right ventricular hypertrophy. You can accentuate the lift by passively elevating the legs to increase venous return. Occasionally a pericardial friction rub is palpable here.

Left Second Intercostal Space

When you have felt along the left lower sternal border, move your hand up to feel the second left intercostal space. Your middle finger should sink into the interspace. Feeling a pulsation here is always abnormal and suggests pulmonary hypertension. Consider primary pulmonary hypertension, atrial septal defect, pulmonic stenosis, dissecting aortic aneurysm (sometimes with a diastolic thrill) or pulmonary embolus.

Sternal Notch Palpation

From the left upper sternal border move your fingers to the sternal notch. Feeling a pulsation here suggests ascending aortic aneurysm.

Right Upper Sternal Border

Now move from the sternal notch to the right upper sternal border. Feeling a pulsation here suggests a tortuous brachiocephalic artery, ascending aortic aneurysm, or aortic regurgitation.

Precordial Thrills

Palpable turbulence over the precordium is called a precordial thrill. Feeling this turbulence defines grade 4 and higher murmurs. Generally precordial thrills are located along the valvular outflow tract. You will appreciate a thrill if it is present when palpating the locations suggested above.

Carotid Artery Pulses

Next, palpate between the sternocleidomastoid and the trachea to feel the carotid artery pulse (see also Chapter 18). Have the patient turn slightly toward you to relax the neck muscles. Do not go above the thyroid cartilage so that you avoid inadvertently massaging the carotid sinus. Check the pulse rate and note the regularity of the pulse. An irregularly irregular rate suggests atrial fibrillation. In atrial fibrillation there is a difference between the apical pulse and the brachial pulse (Jackson's pulse deficit).

Feeling a regular pulse with alternating strength (pulsus alternans) is an important sign of heart failure from any cause.

Note whether the carotid upstroke is rapid or delayed (compare it with the PMI). Feeling a delayed upstroke (pulsus parvus et tardus) suggests aortic stenosis, any left ventricular outflow obstruction, or any significant decrease in stroke volume. Remember that vascular stiffness due to aging can reduce the delay, causing a more normal feeling upstroke.

Note whether the impulse is vigorous or not. A vigorous upstroke with a rapid collapse (Corrigan's water hammer pulse) suggests increased pulse pressure due to aortic insufficiency. Very rarely mitral insufficiency can give a vigorous upstroke. Also note whether the peak of the upstroke is single, double or multiple. A single peak is normal. Feeling a double peak (bisferiens pulse) suggests asymmetric septal hypertrophy or combined aortic stenosis and insufficiency. A confirmatory trick is to listen over the brachial artery while slowly increasing the pressure on the artery. With enough pressure you will hear a systolic bruit that splits into two distinct bruits.

Feeling multiple peaks (carotid shudder) suggests combined aortic stenosis and insufficiency. A carotid shudder can also be felt in isolated aortic valve lesions, including calcification of the aortic ring.

Note the collapse of the arterial pulse. A rapid collapse suggests aortic insufficiency. Also note the presence of a thrill. Feeling unequal carotid pulses suggests carotid stenosis. (Check for asymmetric arcus senilis, with the side without the arcus being the side with the stenosis).

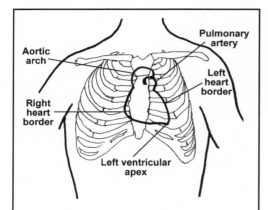

Figure 96. Cardiac Silhouette.

The determination of the silhouette is usually straightforward since the densities of the heart and lungs are so dissimilar. The first percussive note that changes in resonance represents the border of the heart, not the percussion note of maximal dullness. Direct percussion is often better than the traditional indirect percussion. If the palpable point of maximal impulse is more than a centimeter medial to the percussed dullness, consider a pericardial effusion to account for the dullness rather than the cardiac border.

PERCUSSING THE CARDIAC SILHOUETTE

Once the cardiac palpation is complete you should percuss the cardiac silhouette (see Figure 96). This is useful to locate the cardiac apex and especially useful to determine the cardiac border in cases of suspected pericardial effusion when the apical impulse cannot be palpated.

The determination of the silhouette is usually straightforward since the densities of the heart and lungs are so different. *The first percussive note that changes in resonance represents the border of the heart, not the percussion note of maximal dullness.* Direct percussion (see Figure 86) is often better than the traditional indirect percussion, but use what works best for you after trying both techniques with con-

firmation by chest x-ray or echocardiogram. To perform direct percussion tap the chest with the pad of the middle finger in a slapping motion, letting the fingertip slide or stroke along the chest wall after the contact. Some experts percuss the gastric air bubble and Traube's semi-lunar space first to rule out situs inversus.

Ludwig Traube (1818–1876) was a German internist who learned physical diagnosis under Josef Skoka (1805–1881). Traube was an important scientist and one of the most popular teachers of his time.

Traube introduced measurement of temperature as a routine clinical observation. In 1852 Traube produced the first graphic presentation of a fever course with simultaneous recording of pulse and respiratory frequency. Clinical signs described by Traube include the summation gallop, the pistol shot pulse of aortic insufficiency, pulsus alternans, and Traube's semi-lunar space, a crescent-shaped space about 12mm wide, just above the costal margin due to gas in the stomach.

Start at the left mid-axillary line at the fifth intercostal space and slowly move toward the sternum. Note the point where the percussion notes changes slightly, then move up to the fourth intercostal space and repeat the process.

Check the relationship between the cardiac border and the PMI. A displaced PMI just inside the percussed cardiac border suggests left ventricular enlargement. Finding the PMI more than a centimeter inside the cardiac border suggests a large pericardial effusion. Cardiac enlargement in the setting of thyrotoxicosis is Grocco's cardiac sign.

Now percuss along the upper left sternal border to check for pulmonary hypertension. This is most useful if palpation reveals a pulsation in this area, but get into the habit of routinely checking this area for practice and to appreciate the range of normal.

Finally, percuss along the right sternal border. This helps to determine overall heart size. Dullness along the right sternal border suggests right ventricular enlargement or a pericardial effusion (Moschcowitz's sign). The higher the level of dullness, the more likely it is due to effusion. Sometimes percussing the upper right sternal border is useful in cases of suspected ascending aortic aneurysm. Finding dullness at the right upper sternal border is Potain's sign of aortic aneurysm.

Eli Moschcowitz (1879–1964) was two years old when his family emigrated from Russia to America. He studied medicine at the Mount Sinai Hospital, graduating in 1903. Moschcowitz began working as a pathologist at the Beth Israel Hospital, where he described "his" disease (TTP) and remained for some twenty years. He distinguished himself both as a pathologist and as a clinician, and was an invaluable asset to his colleagues. "In hospitals, people should be treated and not diseases."

CARDIAC AUSCULTATION

As with most clinical procedures, preparation, orientation, and self-discipline is key. Use a good stethoscope. (This can be challenging in isolation suites equipped with toy-like disposable stethoscopes.) Make sure the patient is comfortable and let the patient know that you are going to listen carefully to his or her heart. Have the examining room as quiet as possible. Turn off any electrical devices, ask people to stop talking, and close the door. The better you get at cardiac auscultation, the more important these simple points become.

Begin with the diaphragm, take your time, and perform the examination correctly and carefully. Orient yourself to the cardiac cycle by feeling the carotid pulse. In each location, listen carefully to S1, then to S2, systole (the space between S1 and S2), early diastole (just after S2) and late diastole (just prior to S1). Focus all your awareness on each specific item until you are sure of what you are hearing.

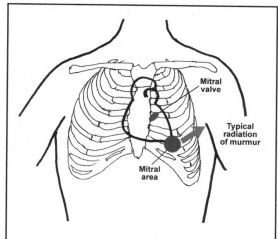

Figure 97. Mitral Area.
The mitral area is located at the apex. Take a moment to focus on the heart sounds and to orient yourself to the cardiac cycle. This is the best place to hear S1, S3 and S4 gallops and mitral valve murmurs.

Start at the Apex (Mitral Area)

Take a moment to focus on the heart sounds and to orient yourself to the cardiac cycle. This is the best place to hear S1, S3 and S4 gallops and mitral valve murmurs. It is also useful to compare the quality of the sounds with the PMI you palpated.

♦ DETERMINE THE HEART RATE AND RHYTHM

Appreciate the heart rate. A fast rate (tachycardia) is greater than 100 beats per minute. A slow rate (bradycardia) is less than 60 beats per minute. A normal heart rate is between 60 and 100 beats per minute.

Note the heart rhythm. A steady, predictable rhythm is regular and normal. An occasionally irregular rhythm suggests premature ventricular contractions, premature atrial contractions, or atrial fibrillation with second-degree AV block. (Think possible digitalis toxicity if the patient is on digitalis.) A predictably irregular rhythm suggests bigeminy, trigeminy, respiratory variations, and second-degree AV block. (Go back and check the neck veins.) Finding an irregularly irregular rhythm suggests atrial fibrillation or atrial flutter with variable AV block. Check the pulse deficit by subtracting the peripheral (radial) pulse rate from the auscultated pulse rate.

◆ LISTEN TO S1

Note especially the intensity of S1 relative to S2. Normally S1 is louder than S2 at the apex. The loudness of the mitral valve closure depends upon three things: the degree of valve opening (whether it has had time to passively swing shut because of heart block), the force of ventricular contraction shutting the valve, and the integrity of the valve. Think of slamming a door. The amount of noise you make will depend on how far open the door is, how hard you slam it, and the integrity of the door.

◆ HEARING A SOFT S1

S1 equal to or softer than S2 in the mitral area implies first-degree AV block, left ventricular failure, left ventricular hypertrophy, left bundle branch block or significant mitral insufficiency. Sometimes obesity and emphysema will also reduce the intensity of S1. You can often determine the likely mechanism. In first-degree AV block you may recheck the neck veins for "a" and "c" waves since these waves reflect the "pr interval" on the EKG. Left ventricular failure will show jugular venous distension, bibasilar rales, an S3 gallop, hepatomegaly, and pedal edema. (Consider myocardial infarction, ischemia or ventricular aneurysm.) Left ventricular hypertrophy, usually from chronic hypertension, characteristically produces an enlarged, displaced PMI. Left bundle branch block produces a paradoxically split S2.

◆ HEARING A LOUD S1

Hearing a very loud S1 suggests mitral stenosis, a hyperdynamic state (from fever, hyperthyroidism, or anemia) or an atrial myxoma (very rare).

◆ HEARING A VARIABLE S1

Once you have appreciated the loudness of S1 compared to S2, note any beat-to-beat variation in the intensity of S1. Appreciating an irregularly irregular rhythm and a variable intensity of S1 suggests atrial fibrillation. Decreasing intensity of S1 until a dropped beat suggests second degree AV block Mobitz type I (Wenckebach). You may first appreciate a sense of hearing grouped beats. Hearing a regular bradycardia with a variable S1 suggests third degree AV block. Another cause of a variable S1 is ventricular tachycardia.

◆ HEARING A SPLIT S1

Next, pay attention to whether S1 is single or double. Hearing a single sound is nor-

Table 15.2. Differentiating the causes of a split first-heard sound	
Reason for Split	**Differentiating Clues**
Split S1 from right bundle branch block	• Wide split S2
S4 and S1	• S4 gallop is not as crisp as an ejection click, may be palpable, disappears when the bell of your stethoscope is pushed, disappears during extrasystole, cannot be heard away from the ventricular outflow tract
S1 and ejection click	• Ejection clicks are usually crisp and high pitched, move closer to S1 when the patient stands, may be heard with other clicks or mitral valve prolapse murmur

mal. Reduplication of S1 suggests a split S1, hearing an S4 gallop and S1, or hearing S1 and an early ejection click. A split S1 suggests right bundle branch block, which produces delayed closure of tricuspid valve. Listen for wide split S2 as well.

There are a few tricks to tell if the reduplicated first heart sound is really an S4 gallop and S1. An S4 is not as crisp and high-pitched as an ejection click. Also, you may have been able to palpate the S4 during your cardiac palpation of the PMI. Listen through your bell with the patient in the left lateral decubitus position. An S4 should disappear when the bell is pushed. An S4 will disappear during an extra systole. Having the patient perform three sit-ups may accentuate an S4.

S1 and an early ejection click can also cause a split-sounding S1. An ejection click is usually crisp and high-pitched. It will move closer to S1 when the patient is standing. You may hear a mitral valve prolapse murmur or other clicks as well.

♦ LISTEN TO S2

Hearing a split S2 here suggests an S3 gallop or a wide split S2 with loud P2 or S2 and an opening snap (vide infra). An S3 gallop is caused by impaired ventricular compliance in early diastole. It suggests congestive heart failure until proven otherwise and can be accentuated with mild exercise such as having the patient perform two or three sit-ups.

♦ LISTEN TO SYSTOLE (THE TIME INTERVAL COINCIDENT WITH THE PULSE)

Hearing a murmur best here suggests mitral regurgitation, mitral prolapse, tricuspid regurgitation, or ventricular septal defect (radiates to back, to left paravertebral area). Hearing an extra sound during systole at this location suggests an ejection click, the click of mitral valve prolapse, or a pericardial friction rub. (It sounds like the heart is beating inside a paper sack.)

♦ LISTEN TO EARLY DIASTOLE

Hearing an extra sound most commonly suggests an S3 gallop. The gallop is produced by decreased ventricular compliance and is a key finding of congestive heart failure. It implies a low ejection fraction. Other conditions that can produce an S3 gallop include mitral regurgitation, tricuspid regurgitation, cardiomyopathy and right ventricular myocardial infarction. Less common sounds in early diastole are the opening snap of mitral stenosis, a pericardial knock, an atrial myxoma tumor plop, and the beginning of a mitral stenosis murmur.

♦ LISTEN TO LATE DIASTOLE

An extra sound in late diastole suggests an S4 gallop. The S4 is produced by decreased ventricular compliance when ventricle is full. It is probably normal in elderly people. If the S4 is palpable as well as audible, then consider hypertension, pulmonary hypertension, and cardiac ischemia.

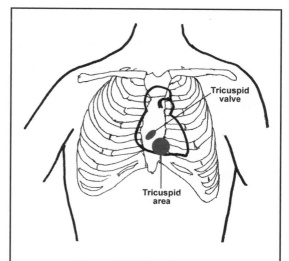

Figure 98. Tricuspid Area.
The tricuspid area is located at the left lower sternal border. Tricuspid murmurs and some asymmetric septal hypertrophy murmurs are heard best here.

Move to the Left Lower Sternal Border (Tricuspid Area)

When you have completed your examination of the apex, move to the left lower sternal border. Tricuspid murmurs and some asymmetric septal hypertrophy murmurs are heard best here.

♦ LISTEN TO S1

Hearing a split S1 here suggests a bundle branch block or a right-sided S4-S1.

♦ LISTEN TO S2

Hearing a split S2 here but not at the apex suggests that either P2 is too loud or there is a right ventricular S3 gallop. You may hear the S3 increase in inspiration, by pushing on the liver or passively elevating the legs to increase venous return. Loss of the second heart sound after swallowing suggests obstruction of the lower esophagus (Meltzer's sign). Appendicitis can increase the intensity of the second heart sound (Mannaberg's sign).

♦ LISTEN TO SYSTOLE

A murmur heard best here suggests tricuspid regurgitation, mitral regurgitation, mitral valve prolapse, or aortic stenosis. Hearing an extra sound here suggests an ejection click, a click of mitral valve prolapse or a pericardial friction rub.

♦ LISTEN TO EARLY DIASTOLE

Hearing an extra sound suggests an S3 gallop (possibly right ventricular), an opening snap, the beginning of mitral stenosis murmur, or an aortic regurgitation murmur.

♦ LISTEN TO LATE DIASTOLE

An extra sound in late diastole suggests an S4 gallop (possibly right ventricular).

Left Upper Sternal Border (Pulmonic Area)

Once your examination of the left lower sternal border is completed, move up to the

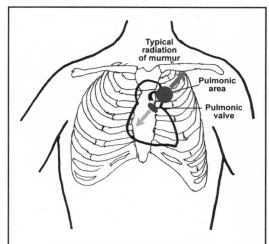

Figure 99. Pulmonic Area.
The pulmonic area is located at the left upper sternal border. Pulmonic valve murmurs and patent ductus arteriosus are loudest here and it is the best place to hear split of S2. Having the patient sit upright (or examining a patient in a wheelchair) will increase the respiratory changes and bring out the P2 in this location.

left upper sternal border. Pulmonic valve murmurs and patent ductus arteriosus are loudest here and it is the best place to hear split of S2. Having the patient sit upright (or examining a patient in a wheelchair) will increase the respiratory changes and bring out the S2 in this location.

♦ LISTEN TO S1

S1 will sound softer than S2 at this location.

♦ LISTEN CAREFULLY TO S2

Normally S2 is louder than S1 at this location. Hearing P2 louder than A2 suggests pulmonary hypertension or aortic stenosis.

♦ FOCUS ON THE SPLIT IN S2

Focus on the nature of the split (hearing a muffling or two distinct sounds) in the S2. Hearing a split in inspiration and no split in expiration is normal. Appreciating a narrow fixed split suggests pulmonary hypertension. The split is narrow because of reduced compli-

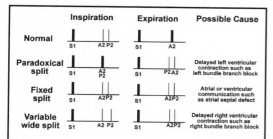

Figure 100. Splitting of S2.

Hearing a split in inspiration and no split in expiration is normal. Appreciating a narrow fixed split suggests pulmonary hypertension. A wide split where the two sounds never come back together suggests right bundle branch block (check for a split first heart sound). Hearing a paradoxical split where you hear no split in inspiration but a split in expiration (A2 after P2) suggests left bundle branch block, aortic stenosis, tricuspid regurgitation, or patent ductus arteriosis with left to right shunt.

ance in the pulmonary vascular bed. A wide split where the two sounds never come back together suggests right bundle branch block (check for a split first heart sound), left ventricular PVC, mitral regurgitation, massive pulmonary embolus, severe right heart failure, pulmonic stenosis, ventricular septal defect with left to right shunt or atrial septal defect (including post-operative).

Other causes of an apparent split S2 are hearing an S2 and S3 (the split will be louder over the ventricle than the base), S2 and an opening snap, S2 and a pericardial knock, and S2 and an atrial myxoma tumor plop.

Hearing a paradoxical split where you hear no split in inspiration but a split in expiration (A2 after P2) suggests left bundle branch block, aortic stenosis, tricuspid regurgitation, or patent ductus arteriosis with left to right shunt.

♦ LISTEN TO SYSTOLE

A murmur heard best here in systole suggests pulmonic stenosis. A pulmonary systolic murmur radiating to the left clavicle is Petteruti's sign.

♦ LISTEN TO EARLY DIASTOLE

Murmur heard best here in diastole suggests pulmonic regurgitation.

♦ LISTEN TO LATE DIASTOLE

An extra sound heard just before systole is likely a right-sided S4.

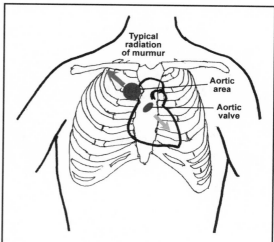

Figure 101. Aortic Area.

The aortic area is located at the right upper sternal border. Aortic valve murmurs are often heard best here, although they can radiate along the entire aortic outflow tract from the left lower sternal border to the right subclavicular area.

Right Upper Sternal Border (Aortic Area)

When your examination of the pulmonic area is finished, move over to the right upper sternal border.

♦ LISTEN TO S1

S1 should be softer than S2 here.

♦ LISTEN TO S2

Hearing a muffled A2 or not hearing A2 at all suggests aortic stenosis.

♦ LISTEN TO SYSTOLE

A murmur heard best here suggests aortic stenosis, aortic sclerosis, or asymmetric septal hypertrophy.

◆ LISTEN TO EARLY DIASTOLE

A murmur heard best here suggests aortic regurgitation.

◆ LISTEN TO LATE DIASTOLE

A late diastolic rumble (Austin Flint murmur) suggests aortic insufficiency.

CHARACTERIZING CARDIAC MURMURS

Murmurs are characterized by their grade, pitch, timing in the cardiac cycle, change in intensity, quality, location heard best, and radiation.

Grade

The grade of a murmur is a basic measure of its loudness (see Table 15.3).

Pitch

A low-pressure gradient, a large opening, or both, cause low-pitched murmurs. A high-pressure gradient, a small opening, or both, cause high-pitched murmurs.

Timing

◆ SYSTOLIC MURMURS

Almost all systolic murmurs begin in early systole. If the murmur lasts throughout systole (holosystolic), think of mitral insufficiency or tricuspid insufficiency.

◆ DIASTOLIC MURMURS

Almost all diastolic murmurs begin in early diastole. Consider aortic insufficiency and pulmonic insufficiency if the murmur ends before mid diastole. Late diastolic low-pitched murmurs include mitral stenosis and tricuspid stenosis. A high-pitched late diastolic murmur suggests coronary artery stenosis. A holodiastolic murmur suggests atrial septal defect or acute rheumatic fever (Carey Coombs' murmur).

◆ CONTINUOUS SOUNDS

A sound heard continuously throughout the cardiac cycle suggests a pericardial friction rub, a venous hum, or an AV fistula. A pericardial friction rub is a leathery sound like a heart beating inside a paper sack. It is heard best at the left lower sternal border and is more of a scratchy, swishing sound than a continuous sound. Hearing a three-component friction rub implies acute pericarditis until proven otherwise.

A hepatic venous hum is a continuous low-pitched sound. It is usually associated

Table 15.3. Grading criteria for cardiac murmurs	
Grade	Criterion
1	• Faint murmur, softer than S1 and S2
2	• Faint murmur, about the same intensity as S1 and S2
3	• Murmur louder than S1 and S2, without a thrill
4	• Loud murmur with a palpable thrill
5	• Loud murmur with a palpable thrill heard with the lightest touch of the stethoscope to the skin
6	• Murmur that can be heard without the stethoscope

with severe liver disease. It should disappear with pressure over the liver (Rusconi's sign). Another hum is a cervical venous hum. This sound resembles the sound heard when a seashell is placed against the ear to "hear the ocean." Cervical hums should disappear with Valsalva's maneuver or compressing the ipsilateral jugular vein.

Arteriovenous fistulas can also produce continuous or swishing sounds. A patent ductus arteriosis is heard best at left upper sternal border. A ruptured aneurysm of the sinus of Valsalva is heard best at the right upper sternal border. A coronary AV fistula is heard best at left lower sternal border, and a pulmonary AV fistula is usually heard best outside the cardiac area.

Change in Intensity

Hearing a crescendo (going from soft to loud) systolic murmur should make you think of aortic stenosis. Decrescendo murmur starts loud and diminishes in loudness. A diamond-shaped murmur is caused by turbulence during systole and either increased flow across a normal valve or normal flow across an abnormal valve. Note when the murmur ends. A diamond-shaped murmur ending before S2 is aortic stenosis, while a diamond-shaped murmur ending after S2 is pulmonic stenosis.

Quality

The quality of a murmur describes its musical or mechanical characteristics. Descriptive terms are harsh, musical, blowing, rumbling or grinding.

Loudest Location

The loudest location is the site where the murmur is heard best. Aortic valve murmurs tend to be heard in the right second intercostal space. Pulmonic valve murmurs are best heard in the left second intercostal space. Mitral valve murmurs are loudest at the apex, and tricuspid valve murmurs are heard best at the left lower sternal border.

Radiation

As the term implies, the radiation of a murmur is the track the sound tends to travel or radiate. Aortic murmurs radiate along the aortic outflow, from the left lower sternal border to the right second intercostal space to the right infraclavicular area. Pulmonic murmurs radiate along the pulmonary outflow tract. Mitral insufficiency murmurs radiate to the axilla or the subscapular portion of the back (especially rupture of the chordae tendinea with anterior leaflet dysfunction). Tricuspid insufficiency radiates to the venous system. Septal rupture from a myocardial infarction radiates to the paravertebral area.

SPECIFIC MURMURS CHARACTERISTICS

Tricuspid Stenosis

Tricuspid stenosis is a diastolic, soft, rumbling murmur heard best at the left lower sternal border. This murmur will increase in intensity with inspiration. Other clinical signs include giant "a" waves on the jugular venous pulse, loss of the "y" descent on jugular venous pulse, an increase in jugular venous pressure on inspiration (Kussmaul's sign) and a jugular presystolic click. Otherwise this clinically resembles mitral stenosis.

Tricuspid Insufficiency

Tricuspid insufficiency is a harsh, holosystolic murmur heard best at the left lower sternal border. This murmur can radiate to the axilla in severe pulmonary hypertension. Maneuvers that change the quality of the murmur

Table 15.4. Typical characteristics of common murmurs

Murmur	Timing	Characteristic Sound	Radiation
Tricuspid stenosis	Diastolic	Soft rumbling, increases with inspiration	None
Tricuspid insufficiency	Systolic	Holosystolic, fine to coarse; increases with inspiration	No pattern
Pulmonic stenosis	Systolic	Diamond-shaped, coarse; increases with inspiration	Left upper sternal border, under left clavicle
Pulmonic insufficiency	Early diastolic	Soft, high-pitched, short decrescendo increases with inspiration	Left sternal border
Mitral stenosis	Diastolic	Rumbling, low-pitched crescendo	None
Mitral insufficiency	Systolic	Blowing or coarse, holosystolic	Left axilla
Aortic stenosis	Systolic	Mid-to high-pitched, coarse, diamond-shaped	Under right clavicle and carotids
Aortic insufficiency	Early diastolic	Soft, high-pitched, early diastolic decrescendo	Left lower sternal border, right upper sternal border

include an increase in intensity with inspiration (Carvallo's sign), an increase with increased venous return, and an increase with pushing on the liver (Vitmus' sign).

Primary causes of tricuspid insufficiency include endocarditis and rheumatic disease. A secondary cause is right ventricular dilation. Other clinical signs of tricuspid insufficiency include seeing prominent "v" waves in the jugular venous pulse, seeing winking ear lobes (White's sign), hearing a murmur over peripheral veins, and feeling liver pulsations.

Pulmonic Stenosis

Pulmonic stenosis is a diamond-shaped systolic murmur heard best at the left upper sternal border. Primary causes include congenital abnormality and rheumatic disease. Secondary causes are atrial septal defect and

ventricular septal defect. Other clinical signs of pulmonic stenosis are a right ventricular heave and hearing a wide split S2 with soft P2. The murmur may radiate to the left carotid artery.

Pulmonic Insufficiency

Pulmonic insufficiency is an early diastolic decrescendo murmur heard best at the left upper sternal border. Syphilis and SBE tend to spare the pulmonic valve, and endocarditis is very rare. Rheumatic heart disease involving this valve is even more rare.

A secondary cause of pulmonic insufficiency is pulmonary hypertension. (In this case the pulmonic insufficiency murmur due to pulmonary hypertension is called a Graham Steell murmur). Other clinical signs include a palpable pulmonary artery and finding dullness to percussion to the left of the sternum.

Mitral Stenosis

Mitral stenosis is a low-pitched diastolic rumble with presystolic accentuation. The loudness of the rumble may correlate with the degree of stenosis. Beware if patient has aortic insufficiency, as this could be an Austin Flint murmur producing relative mitral stenosis. A mitral stenosis murmur is heard best at the apex with the patient in left lateral decubitus position.

Causes of mitral stenosis include rheumatic fever, calcified mitral annulus, carcinoid syndrome, SLE, and rheumatoid arthritis. Other clinical signs of mitral stenosis include hearing a loud S1, a loud P2, and an opening snap. The S2–OS interval may help in estimating severity. (The shorter the interval, the greater the gradient across the valve.) Patients with mitral stenosis may have flushed cheeks.

Mitral Insufficiency

Mitral insufficiency is a harsh, whooping, or honking holosystolic murmur heard best at the apex. Mitral insufficiency murmurs radiate to the axilla. Primary causes include mitral valve prolapse, bacterial endocarditis, or rheumatic conditions. Secondary causes include cardiac enlargement, papillary muscle dysfunction, mitral annular calcification or Gallavardin's phenomenon of aortic stenosis (vide infra). Other clinical signs of mitral insufficiency include systolic clicks. (Check for these with the patient standing or in patients with pectus excavatum.)

Aortic Stenosis

The aortic stenosis murmur is a harsh, diamond-shaped, systolic murmur that radiates along the aortic outflow tract. The peaking of the murmur moves toward S2 as the valve area narrows. Gallavardin's phenomenon is when the aortic stenosis murmur becomes more pure and musical as one listens toward the apex. It is important to know about this so you do not mistakenly diagnose a nonexistent mitral murmur. Classically the aortic stenosis murmur is heard best at the right upper sternal border. It radiates to the right supraclavicular area. Lack of radiation to this area should raise the question of another cause for the murmur. The aortic stenosis murmur increases after a premature ventricular contraction, due to the increased gradient across the valve produced by the enhanced diastolic filling with the compensatory pause.

Louis Gallavardin (1875–1957) was one of the premier French cardiologists of the twentieth century. He made important early contributions to our understanding of fatty degeneration and diastolic hypertension. He was also the first to report coronary artery spasm as a cause of myocardial infarction, and one of the first to describe the mid-systolic click of mitral valve prolapse. He described pulmonary edema as a result of mitral stenosis and the phenomenon in aortic stenosis that bears his name. Gallavardin had a prodigious memory and was the consummate physical diagnostician when physical diagnosis was at its peak. He had an impressive knowledge of art objects and rare books. As an octogenarian, Gallavardin was still able to point out from memory and with precision the subtle nuances of an El Greco painting at the Seville museum.

The causes of aortic stenosis include calcific degeneration or a bicuspid valve. Other clinical signs of aortic stenosis are paradoxical split of S2 and pulsus parvus et tardus. You can estimate the degree of stenosis by feeling the delay between the PMI and the carotid pulse. (The greater the delay, the greater the stenosis.) Some clinicians are remarkably adept and consistent at estimating the valve area using combinations of these techniques.

Subaortic Stenosis (IHSS)

Subaortic stenosis is a harsh, diamond-shaped, mid-systolic murmur heard best at the left sternal border. The murmur becomes louder during a PVC, softer on the beat following PVC, softer with squatting, and louder with standing. IHSS is caused by a subvalvular muscular ring or obstructive cardiomyopathy. Other clinical signs include feeling a diminished pulse after a PVC or appreciating a bisferiens pulse.

Aortic Insufficiency

Aortic insufficiency is an early diastolic decrescendo murmur heard best at the right upper sternal border. It is useful to have the patient sitting upright, leaning forward, and exhaling. The patient should be holding breath (in expiration) since the quality and acoustic frequency of the murmur is similar to the breath sounds and can be completely obscured by them. Sometimes there is a late diastolic rumble (Austin Flint murmur).

Austin Flint (1812–1886) was one of the most eminent nineteenth century physicians. Flint made several important contributions to the knowledge of diseases of the heart and the respiratory system. He coined the term "bronchiovesicular breathing." He also introduced the binaural stethoscope. His murmur is a presystolic or late diastolic (mitral) heart murmur, best heard at the apex of the heart. It is present in some cases of aortic insufficiency and is thought to be due to the vibration of the mitral valve caused by regurgitation of blood from the aorta into the heart before contraction of the ventricles. Flint's law pertains to the relationship of elevated audible pitch and diminished percussion resonance in pulmonary consolidation.

If the murmur radiates to the left lower sternal border, consider rheumatic valve disease or syphilitic aortitis. Radiation to the right lower sternal border suggests aortic dissection, bacterial endocarditis or aneurysm of the sinus of Valsalva. Radiation to the left axilla (called a Cole-Cecil murmur) is a useful way, when present, to differentiate aortic insufficiency from pulmonic insufficiency. Maneuvers to increase intensity of the aortic insufficiency murmur include arterial occlusion, squatting or sitting up.

Other clinical signs of aortic insufficiency include Duroziez's sign, Hill's sign or Corrigan's pulse.

Paul Louis Duroziez (1826–1897) studied in Paris, and as a student he won the Corvisart Prize for his discussion on digitalis. In 1856 he became chef de clinique with Jean-Martin Charcot and in 1870 served as a surgeon in the Franco-Prussian War. He was in general practice and held no official hospital appointment, but was widely acclaimed because of his articles on mitral stenosis as well as other cardiac disorders. Highly respected by his physician colleagues, he was elected president of the Société de Médecine in 1882.

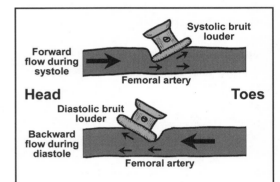

Figure 102. Duroziez's Sign.

Gently place the diaphragm of the stethoscope over the femoral artery and push down to produce a bruit (a universal finding with enough compression), with the end of the stethoscope facing the head. (The stethoscope will be tilted about 30° with the caudal end above the skin.) Continue to push and an early diastolic sound will be heard in aortic insufficiency that creates a to-and-fro swishing sound. Tilt the stethoscope so that the caudal portion is compressing the artery and the other end is up (a 30° angle in the other direction). An increase in the diastolic sound with this maneuver is Duroziez's sign.

♦ DUROZIEZ'S SIGN

To check Duroziez's sign, gently place the diaphragm of the stethoscope over the femoral artery (see Figure 102). Gently push down to produce a bruit (a universal finding with enough compression), with the end of the stethoscope facing the head. (The stethoscope will be tilted about 30° with the caudal end above the skin.) Hearing two systolic sounds suggests a high output condition such as hyperthyroidism, anemia, blood loss, or AV fistula in the leg.

(Consider previous cardiac catheterization.) Continue to push and an early diastolic sound will be heard in aortic insufficiency that creates a to-and-fro swishing sound. Tilt the stethoscope so that the caudle portion is compressing the artery and the other end is up (a 30° angle in the other direction). An increase in the diastolic sound with this maneuver is Duroziez's sign. Hearing Duroziez's sign but not finding Hill's sign (below) suggests atherosclerotic disease in the leg or a low output cardiac state. The time for surgical repair may have passed.

◆ Hill's Sign

Hill's sign is helpful in determining the severity of the aortic incompetence and the amount of increased stroke volume. It cannot be obtained in atrial fibrillation because the systolic blood pressure varies so much with the variable R-R interval. With the patient supine, measure the brachial and dorsalis pedis blood pressures. Normally the blood pressure in the legs will be up to 20 millimeters of mercury higher than the arms. An apparent increase in leg blood pressure of more than 20 millimeters of mercury correlates with the degree of aortic insufficiency or the increase in stroke volume. Takayasu's disease can give a false positive result by reducing the upper extremity blood pressure.

◆ Corrigan's Pulse

Corrigan's pulse is a bounding pulse with wide pulse pressure and quick relaxation. It resembles an old water hammer.

OTHER CARDIAC SOUNDS

Means-Lerman Scratch

A Means-Lerman scratch is a mid-systolic sound over the upper sternum. It occurs in end expiration and is associated with hyper-thyroidism. It is caused by a pulmonary ejection murmur in the setting of a hyperdynamic heart.

Clicks

Systolic ejection clicks suggest mitral valve prolapse. The click moves earlier in systole with standing. Additional causes are tricuspid valve prolapse, a bicuspid aortic valve, or a prosthetic valve. Hypertension and tortuous aortic root can produce an early systolic click with no change with position. This is usually in the setting of a hyperdynamic state such as anemia, hyperthyroidism or medication effect. Rarely in mitral valve prolapse will there be an early diastolic click.

Mechanical heart valves produce characteristic mechanical clicks. One trick to tell if click is from a mechanical valve is to listen over the shoulder near the AC joint. The high-pitched click will be transmitted to bone while the native clicks will not.

Mediastinal Crunch

Mediastinal crunch (Hamman's sign) is a characteristic crunching sound coexistent with heartbeat. It implies mediastinal emphysema or pneumopericardium. There is loss of cardiac dullness to percussion. The crunch usually extends into the neck.

Splash of Air Embolism

Roll patient immediately onto left side to decrease risk of cerebral air embolism.

SPECIAL TESTS

Hepatojugular Reflux to Check for Right Ventricular Failure

Note the initial jugular venous pulse level. Put your right palm and fingers just below the right costal margin and gently push down for about thirty seconds while noting the jugular venous pressure during several respirations. Note the increase in jugular venous pressure. Seeing more than a centimeter increase is abnormal, denoting positive hepatojugular reflux (Pasteur's sign).

Clinical Maneuvers That Affect Murmurs

◆ RESPIRATORY EFFECTS

All right-sided murmurs increase with inspiration. Many left-sided murmurs decrease with inspiration but this may be difficult to hear. Therefore, respiratory variation can help differentiate corresponding right-sided from left-sided murmurs, for example, tricuspid regurgitation from mitral regurgitation.

◆ CHANGES IN POSITION

Standing decreases venous return and decreases ventricular filling. Therefore, standing decreases the intensity of all murmurs *except* IHSS murmur and mitral valve prolapse. In end-stage cardiac disease there is no decrease in the pulse with lying supine (Schapiro's sign).

Squatting increases peripheral resistance and increases ventricular filling. It brings out the murmurs of ventricular septal defect, aortic insufficiency and mitral insufficiency.

Sitting up and leaning forward accentuates the second heart sound and increases the aortic insufficiency murmur. The left lateral decubitus position increases murmur of mitral stenosis. Some people feel that the exercise component of moving accounts for the increase in the murmur.

◆ INCREASING PERIPHERAL RESISTANCE

This maneuver is most helpful in excluding murmurs than ruling in a murmur. Ways to increase the peripheral resistance include squatting and isometric handgrip. Have the patient squeeze (hard) a rolled-up blood pressure cuff or towel. Hearing an increase in systolic murmur with an increase in peripheral resistance excludes aortic stenosis and IHSS. Hearing a decrease in the systolic murmur excludes mitral regurgitation and ventricular septal defect. Hearing a decrease in a diastolic murmur excludes aortic insufficiency and mitral stenosis.

◆ ARTERIAL COMPRESSION

Use a blood pressure cuff on each arm and inflate them above systolic pressure and hold there. This will increase left-sided regurgitant murmurs such as aortic regurgitation (an excellent maneuver), mitral regurgitation or ventricular septal defect.

SPECIAL CIRCUMSTANCES

Differentiating Various Murmurs

Changes in a murmur with inhalation can help distinguish a right-sided murmur from its corresponding left-sided murmur. All right-sided murmurs increase with inspiration (Carvallo's sign). Increased volume either increases the gradient across a stenotic valve or the amount of regurgitation in a regurgitant murmur. All left-sided murmurs do not increase with inspiration. Increasing the afterload by isometric handgrip can differentiate systolic murmurs at the apex from murmurs at the base. An increase in a systolic murmur with handgrip excludes an aortic or pulmonic murmur. A decrease in a systolic murmur with handgrip excludes mitral or tricuspid murmur.

José Manuel Rivero Carvallo (1905–1993) was a Mexican cardiologist who in 1946 described the increase in the intensity of the pansystolic murmur of tricuspid regurgitation during inspiration to distinguish it from mitral regurgitation.

How to Differentiate Systolic Murmurs at the Base
(Aortic Stenosis from Pulmonic Stenosis)

First, note the carotid upstroke compared to the PMI. A delayed carotid upstroke suggests aortic stenosis. Listen carefully to S2. Hearing a diminished S2 suggests aortic stenosis. Hearing a paradoxically split S2 suggests aortic stenosis.

Listen in the second intercostal space on each side of the sternum. A murmur heard best in the left second intercostal space suggests pulmonic stenosis. An increase in the murmur with inspiration suggests pulmonic stenosis.

A murmur heard best in the right second intercostal space suggests aortic stenosis, as does radiation of the murmur to under the right clavicle.

How to Tell Aortic Stenosis from Aortic Sclerosis

First, note the blood pressure. Aortic stenosis may reduce the pulse pressure to less than 40mmHg, while aortic sclerosis does not affect the pulse pressure. Next, check the carotid upstroke compared to the PMI. Appreciating a delayed upstroke suggests aortic stenosis (pulsus parvus et tardus). Listen carefully to S2. Hearing a diminished S2 suggests aortic stenosis, as does hearing a paradoxically split S2. Check to see if the murmur radiates to the right clavicle. Aortic stenosis radiates to the right clavicle and aortic sclerosis does not. Also check for radiation to the right carotid artery. Aortic stenosis radiates to the right carotid artery and aortic sclerosis does not.

How to Tell Aortic Stenosis from IHSS

First, check the carotid upstroke compared to PMI. Feeling a delayed upstroke suggests aortic stenosis (pulsus parvus et tardus), feeling two short pulses (pulsus bisferiens) suggests IHSS. You can confirm it: listen over brachial artery and gently push down on the proximal portion with your stethoscope until you heard a soft compression bruit. In bisferiens pulse you will hear two soft bruits for each cardiac cycle.

Listen carefully to S2. Hearing a diminished S2 suggests aortic stenosis. Hearing a louder, clearer S2 suggests IHSS. Listen during an extrasystole. IHSS gets louder during an extrasystole. Aortic stenosis gets softer during the extrasystole but then the following beat has a louder AS murmur, due to the increased gradient caused by the increased filling. Listen to the patient as the patient stands. An IHSS murmur increases with standing while the aortic stenosis decreases with standing. Listen to the patient as the patient squats. IHSS murmurs decrease with squatting while aortic stenosis murmurs do not decrease with squatting.

How to Identify Aortic Insufficiency

Aortic insufficiency is an early decrescendo murmur that is loudest at base or left lower sternal border. Pulses may be bounding (Corrigan's water hammer pulse) and the pulse pressure will be over 40mmHg. Pedal pulses are often surprisingly easy to palpate. Head bobbing may be present, coincident with each heartbeat (de Musset's sign). Pupillary contractions coincident with the pulse suggest aortic insufficiency (Landolfi's sign). Retinal arteries may pulsate (Becker's sign). The uvula may pulsate (Mueller's sign). The fingertips may flush with transillumination coincident with the pulse. Downward pulling of the trachea coincident with the pulse, the tracheal tug, is Cardarelli's sign. The murmur increases in intensity with patient exhaling and leaning forward. Severe regurgitation will increase in intensity when blood pressure cuff on arm is inflated to over systolic pressure.

Hearing an additional late diastolic mur-

Table 15.5. Signs of aortic aneurysm	
Name	*Manifestation*
Chalier's sign	Double click over the anterior chest
Dorendorf's sign	Supraclavicular fullness due to an aortic arch aneurysm
Glasgow's sign	Soft bruit over the brachial artery
Hope's sign	Double heart beat at the apex
Potain's sign	Dullness to percussion along the right upper sternal border
Sansom's sign	Soft murmur heard over the patient's closed lips

mur loudest at the apex (Austin Flint murmur) suggests aortic regurgitation. A swishing sound can be heard over the femoral artery in aortic insufficiency (Duroziez's sign). A faint double sound over the femoral arteries suggests aortic insufficiency (Traube's sign).

Hill's sign can determine the severity of the regurgitant volume sign, provided the patient has a regular cardiac rhythm. With patient supine, measure the brachial systolic blood pressure with the popliteal systolic blood pressure. The measured systolic pressure in the leg is usually no more than 20mmHg higher than the arm systolic pressure. The higher the systolic pressure in the leg (over the 20mmHg difference) the greater the degree of aortic regurgitation (Hill's sign).

How to Differentiate Systolic Murmurs at the Apex or Left Sternal Border
(Tricuspid Regurgitation from Mitral Regurgitation)

Tricuspid regurgitation will increase with inspiration (Carvallo's sign) while mitral stenosis will not. Tricuspid regurgitation may increase with liver compression (Vitum's sign). Tricuspid regurgitation may cause the right earlobe to pulse. Tricuspid regurgitation will produce a large "v" wave in the jugular veins. Mitral regurgitation will radiate the left axilla. Hearing a click suggests mitral regurgitation.

How to Differentiate Diastolic Murmurs Heard Best at the Apex or Left Lower Sternal Border
(Mitral Stenosis from Tricuspid Stenosis)

Seeing a soft malar flush suggests tight mitral stenosis (mitral facies). Hearing an early diastolic opening snap suggests mitral stenosis. Appreciating an increase in the murmur in left lateral decubitus position suggests mitral stenosis. Hearing an increase in the murmur with inspiration suggests tricuspid stenosis.

Evaluation of the Elderly Patient with Suspected Pericardial Effusion

♦ CHECK FOR PULSUS PARADOXUS

First, check for pulsus paradoxus. Determining less than 10mmHg of pulsus rules out pericardial tamponade. More than 10mmHg of pulsus paradoxus suggests large pericardial effusion or severe right ventricular failure. Next, check the neck veins. Seeing an increase in the venous column with inspiration (Kussmaul's sign) suggests pericardial constriction, severe tricuspid stenosis (giant "a" waves) or right ventricular failure.

♦ CHECK FOR LOSS OF THE "X" OR "Y" DESCENTS

Loss of the "x" descent suggests a problem with right atrial filling, including pericardial constriction. The descent may reappear with patient sitting upright. Loss of the "y" descent implies a problem with right ventricular filling, such as pericardial tamponade.

♦ CHECK FOR LOSS OF A VISIBLE PMI

Look for epicardial bulging (Auenbrugger's sign) and palpate for the PMI. It may be inside the area of cardiac dullness on percussion (below). Percuss the cardiac silhouette. Lateral displacement of the right heart border is Rotch's sign and blunting of the right cardiohepatic angle is Ebstein's sign. A large pericardial effusion makes the first rib seem more prominent along the sternal border (Ewart's second sign).

♦ CHECK FOR MOSCHCOWITZ TRIAD

Check for Moschcowitz triad of pericardial effusion, which is widening of the cardiac silhouette, an increase in cardiac dullness in the second intercostal space, and an abrupt transition of pulmonary resonance to cardiac dullness.

♦ LOOK FOR DRESSLER'S SIGN

Check for Dressler's sign which is flatness of the lower one-half of the sternum to percussion.

♦ CHECK FOR DULLNESS IN THE LUNG BASES

Check for signs of dullness in the posterior lung fields. Dullness at the left lower lung field is Ewart's sign of pericardial effusion, while right-sided dullness is Conner's sign. Disappearance of Ewart's or Conner's signs when the patient sits up and leans forward is Bamberger's sign of pericardial effusion.

♦ ADDITIONAL SIGNS OF PERICARDIAL EFFUSION

Sudden collapse in the distended neck veins with diastole suggests pericardial tamponade (Friedreich's sign). Anterior bulging of the lower sternum suggests pericardial effusion (Pitre's sign). Protuberance of the epigastrium suggests massive pericardial effusion (Auenbrugger's sign). Dullness at the angle of the scapula that disappears when the patient leans forward is Bamberger's sign of pericardial effusion. Percussible dullness in the left third intercostal space suggests large pericardial effusion (Sansom's sign). Lateral displacement of the percussed cardiac border with expiration suggests a large pericardial effusion (Greene's sign). A large pericardial effusion can blunt the percussible right cardio-hepatic angle, producing

Table 15.6. Signs of pericarditis	
Name	*Manifestation*
Bouillaud's sign	Systolic retractions along the anterior axillary line
Broadbent's sign	Precordial retractions coincident with the heart beat
Cegka's sign	No change in the area of cardiac dullness with inspiration
Fisher's sign	A late diastolic murmur in constrictive pericarditis
Gorham's sign	Pericardial friction rub in the setting of a myocardial infarction
Heim-Kreysig's sign	Systolic cardiac retractions
Pin's sign	Patient with chest pain who prefers to sit leaning forward with knees drawn up
Wynter's sign	Lack of abdominal respiratory movements in the setting of pericarditis

dullness along the lower right sternal border (Ebstein's sign). Dullness at the right lower sternal border suggests large pericardial effusion (Rotch's sign). In pericardial effusion the transition on percussion from the lungs to the right heart border is abrupt (Moschcowitz's sign). A large pericardial effusion produces egophony and bronchial breathing at the lower border of the left scapula (Ewart's sign).

CHAPTER 16

The Abdomen

"I do not know how dosages of H2-blockers were calculated in this country, but I imagine that the objective was to eradicate every trace of acid — an approach entirely in keeping with the long Calvinist tradition of U.S. gastroenterology."

— **Howard Spiro**

"L'Homme pense; donc je suis," dit l'Univers.

— **Paul Valery**

The abdominal examination is one where the skill and attentiveness of the examiner is directly transmitted to the patient. We instinctively shield the abdomen when we are physically threatened and feel vulnerable when someone puts his or her hand on our bare abdomen.

POSITIONING THE PATIENT

Have the patient supine in a warm room with a good light. Support the head so that the abdomen is relaxed. The patient's arms should be at the sides or over the chest, but not behind the head since this will tense the abdominal muscles (see Figure 103).

Use extra pillows to support the head if

the patient has kyphosis. Drape the groin with a simple sheet. Modify the position as needed if the patient has dyspnea from congestive heart

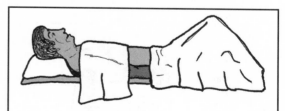

Figure 103. Positioning and Draping for the Abdominal Examination.

The patient should be supine in a warm room with a good light. Support the head so that the abdomen is relaxed. The patient's arms should be at the sides or over the chest, but not behind the head since this will tense the abdominal muscles. Use extra pillows to support the head if the patient has kyphosis. Drape the groin with a simple sheet. Modify the position as needed if the patient has dyspnea from congestive heart failure.

failure. Once the position is established, explain what you are going to do at each step of the examination.

Special circumstances that may require modification include a wheelchair-using patient, a patient with severe congestive heart failure who cannot lie flat, or a patient with back injury. In these circumstances you may have to examine the patient upright, paying careful attention to the effects of gravity on organ position such as the liver. The main point is to be thorough and not to use the patient's disability as an excuse to cut corners.

ABDOMINAL INSPECTION

General Appearance

The first consideration is the patient's overall demeanor and whether there is a primary gastrointestinal complaint. The patient writhing in pain suggests obstruction while the patient lying quiet and still may have peritoneal inflammation. The evaluation of the patient with acute abdominal pain is discussed

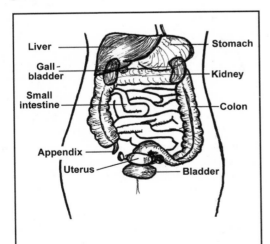

Figure 104. Abdominal Anatomy.
This figure shows the relative positions of the major abdominal organs.

later in this chapter. A scaphoid or boat-like abdomen suggests weight loss or malnutrition. Search for visible masses including the left supraclavicular fossa as signs of possible malignancy (Troisier's sign). The umbilicus often deviates to the side of intra-abdominal inflammation (Schlesinger's sign).

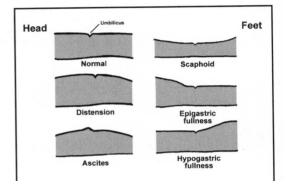

Figure 105. Abdominal Contours.
The abdominal contour can provide useful information. General distension with a normal umbilicus is caused by fat, peritoneal fluid or gaseous distension. Seeing a distended abdomen with an umbilicus that is everted suggests fluid (ascites). A scaphoid or boat-like abdomen suggests weight loss or malnutrition. Localized distension usually results from obstruction or enlargement of an individual organ or structure. Epigastric enlargement suggests enlarged stomach or gastric outlet obstruction. The hypogastric distension of an enlarged bladder tips the umbilicus up toward the head. Periumbilical swelling suggests early small bowel obstruction (Leudet's sign).

Check for Abdominal Distension

The next general observation is whether the abdomen is distended and, if so, whether the distension is general or localized. General distension is caused by fat, peritoneal fluid or gaseous distension. Often the nature of the umbilicus can help suggest an etiology of the distension. Abdominal fat can sometimes be differentiated from other causes in that the umbilicus is depressed. Seeing bulging flanks and an umbilicus that is flat or everted suggests fluid (ascites). In small or large bowel obstruction due to pancreatitis, the umbilicus may be sunken like a Cupid's bow and you may see peristaltic activity. Observing a ladder-like appearance of the lower abdomen suggests small bowel obstruction, while seeing a large inverted "U" appearance suggests large bowel obstruction.

Localized distension usually results from obstruction or enlargement of an individual organ or structure. Periumbilical swelling suggests early small bowel obstruction (Leudet's sign). The hypogastric distension of an enlarged bladder tips the umbilicus up toward the head. Ascites may cause the umbilicus to point toward the feet (Tanyol's sign). An enlarged right upper quadrant suggests hepatobiliary enlargement or mass, while a distended left upper quadrant suggests an enlarged spleen. A deep crease on inspiration along the right costal margin suggests echinococcal cyst of the liver (Lennhoff's sign). Epigastric enlargement suggests enlarged stomach or gastric outlet obstruction. Local abdominal distension proximal to obstruction is Wahl's sign. Intestinal dilation above an obstruction and no peristalsis below the obstruction suggests fecal impaction (Schlange's sign).

Look for Hernias

Next, look for hernias by having the patient raise the head off the pillow to accentuate the abdominal pressure. Hernias are named by their location. Common sites for hernias are midline (umbilical, epigastric), incisional, and in the groin (inguinal and femoral).

Check the Venous Pattern

The venous pattern over the abdomen is usually not apparent unless there is obstruction or malnutrition. Note the direction of blood flow. Normally blood flows away from umbilicus (veins above umbilicus drain toward the head, and veins below drain toward the groin). Blood flow toward the umbilicus suggests inferior vena cava obstruction. Superficial

venous distension, but with normal flow, suggests portal vein obstruction.

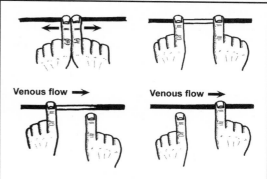

Figure 106. Determining the Direction of Venous Flow.

If distended veins are seen over the abdomen, determine the direction of flow by placing your index fingers together on the enlarged vein as shown in the upper left drawing. Move your index fingers apart along the vein about 5 to 6 centimeters to milk out the blood (upper right figure). Now lift up your right index finger and note the speed of filling. Repeat the venous stripping procedure and lift your left index finger. The direction of flow is the more rapid direction of filling.

Determine the direction of flow (not technically inspection, but it fits here) by placing your index fingers together on the enlarged vein. Move your left index finger along the vein about 5 to 6 centimeters to milk out the blood. Now lift up your right index finger and note the speed of filling. Repeat the venous stripping procedure and lift your left index finger. The direction of flow is the more rapid direction of filling.

Skin Findings

The abdomen has a generous expanse of skin, so a number of generalized skin lesions may appear here, including seborrheic keratoses, early scurvy (corkscrew hairs) and malignant melanoma. Jaundice may be more apparent over the abdomen. Also look for a transverse abdominal crease that suggests previous vertebral compression fractures. Prominent flaccidity of the skin suggests recent significant weight loss. A tense shiny quality to the skin suggests distension due to ascites. Fine telangiectasias from arterial obstruction may be seen.

Also pay attention to any surgical scars. The location may be useful to infer the procedure. (A few patients may not remember previous surgeries.) Check for possible scar-related malignancy. Hyperpigmented scars suggest excess ACTH, possibly from Addison's disease or an endocrine tumor.

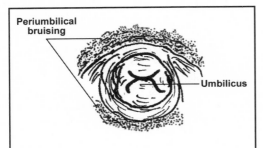

Figure 107. Cullen's Sign.
Periumbilical cyanosis or ecchymoses is called Cullen's sign and signifies retroperitoneal hemorrhage. Periumbilical jaundice is Ransohoff's sign of a ruptured common bile duct.

Look for the bruises of needle sticks, especially in recently hospitalized patients. Especially examine the course of the inferior hypogastric vessels. Injections of heparin or insulin into these vessels can cause significant effects. A bruise around the umbilicus is Cullen's sign of retroperitoneal bleeding (see Figure 107). Seeing jaundice around the umbilicus is Ransohoff's sign of common bile duct rupture. A bruise around the flank is Grey Turner's sign of retroperitoneal bleeding (see Figure 108).

Striae are usually in the lower quadrants and rarely around the shoulders. Old striae are silver and pale, while new striae are pink or purple.

Thomas Stephen Cullen (1868–1953) was the son of a minister. He graduated near the top of his class in medicine from the University of Toronto in 1890. His career was strongly influenced by the American surgeon Howard Kelly. Kelly, having been on a fishing holiday in

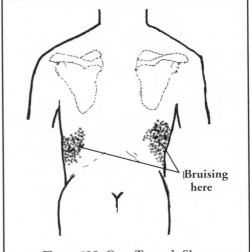

Figure 108. Grey Turner's Sign.
A bruise around either or both flanks is Grey Turner's sign of retroperitoneal bleeding.

Canada, performed an operation in Toronto at which Cullen was his assistant. Cullen was so impressed with Kelly's skills that in 1891 he became junior intern at Kelly's service at Johns Hopkins. He went into practice as a gynecologist in 1897, retaining his association with the medical school at Johns Hopkins where he became professor of gynecology in 1900.

Cullen's sign is periumbilical cyanosis, reticular cyanosis or ecchymosis due to subcutaneous intraperitoneal hemorrhage.

Movements with Respiration

Abrupt stop (or catch) with deep inspiration suggests pleuritic chest pain, a process involving the diaphragm, acute cholecystitis, or peritoneal inflammation. Seeing an area of reduced respiratory movement suggests underlying inflammation. For example, sigmoid diverticulitis may reduce respiratory movement in the left lower quadrant. Abdominal distension with expiration (respiratory paradox) suggests a paralyzed diaphragm.

Pulsatile Movements

Pulsatile movements across the abdomen suggest vascular aneurysm or wide arterial pulse pressure.

ABDOMINAL PERCUSSION

Technique

Make sure your hands are warm. Generally indirect percussion is used in the abdominal examination. See Chapter 14 (Figure 86) for more information on percussion technique.

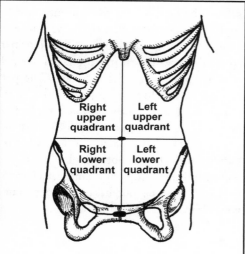

Figure 109. Four Quadrants.
The expanse of the abdomen is conveniently divided into four quadrants, as shown in this figure.

Percussing all Four Quadrants

Begin by gently percussing in all four quadrants, starting at the right upper quadrant and moving counterclockwise. Note any areas of tightening of the rectus muscle indicating underlying peritoneal inflammation. Skin sensitivity over inflamed internal viscera is Livingston's sign. Resonance in the medial right upper quadrant with borborygmi suggests duodenal ulcer (Günzberg's sign). Flank percussion producing inguinal pain suggests a kidney stone (Lloyd's sign). Left-sided abdominal dullness and right-sided abdominal resonance suggests chronic peritonitis (Thomayer's sign).

Percuss any Observable Areas of Distension

Tympany suggests gaseous distension while dullness suggests a mass. With distension and bulging flanks, check for a fluid wave. Briskly tap on one side just above and lateral to the iliac crest, with the other palm on the contralateral side above the other iliac crest. Seeing a rapid wave across the skin is a skin wave. Sensing a palpable percussion wave just following the skin wave suggests ascites. Producing vasoconstriction by tapping in the midline between the xiphoid and the umbilicus is Livierato's sign.

Percuss the Liver Span

Percuss the lower border of the liver, beginning in the right lower quadrant and moving upward toward the right costal margin. Percuss the upper border of the liver, beginning in the mid-thorax in the mid-clavicular line and moving down. Note the difference in the liver borders to determine the liver span in the mid-clavicular line. Ten to twelve centimeters of liver span is normal; more than twelve is hepatomegaly. A liver span less than nine centimeters suggests cirrhosis. Be aware that a pleural effusion and right lower lobe pneumonia can give a false sense of the upper liver margin. Hepatomegaly percussed to the left of the midline is Grocco's abdominal sign.

Williamson and Sapira's method of liver percussion: have the patient inhale deeply and hold it to flatten the diaphragm. Lightly percuss the upper and lower liver borders.

Check for Liver Displacement

Check for liver displacement where the size is normal but the position is abnormal. Upward displacement suggests a paralyzed right hemidiaphragm, massive ascites or malignancy. Downward displacement suggests a flattened diaphragm due to emphysema.

Resonance in the right upper quadrant at the mid-axillary line suggests free air under right diaphragm or gas in the hepatic flexure of the colon.

Check for Splenomegaly

♦ METHOD 1: CHECKING FOR AN INCREASE IN THE AREA OF SPLENIC DULLNESS

Start in the area of expected splenic dullness in the tenth interspace just above the left flank and below the mid-axillary line. Percuss toward the midline, noting the point where the dullness shifts. Dullness extending into the mid-axillary line or dullness extending into Traube's semi-lunar space suggests splenomegaly.

♦ METHOD 2: NOTING MOVEMENT OF THE INFERIOR BORDER OF THE SPLEEN

Percuss the lowest intercostal interspace in the anterior axillary line. Tympany is normal while dullness suggests splenomegaly. Have the patient inhale deeply. Dullness in an area of previous tympany suggests splenomegaly.

♦ METHOD 3: NIXON'S APPROACH

With patient in right lateral decubitus position (right side down), percuss from tenth interspace posteriorly toward the umbilicus. Less than eight centimeters of dullness is normal. More than eight centimeters of dullness suggests splenomegaly. False positives can be due to colonic mass or stool in the splenic flexure. False negatives can occur with colonic gas.

Any suggestion of splenic enlargement by any technique should be followed by careful palpation.

ABDOMINAL PALPATION

In most cases abdominal palpation will yield useful information. (In some cases the palpation will be a crucial examination.) Begin the examination by gently placing your warm hand on the epigastric area and letting your hand relax. Note any masses, pulsations, peristaltic activity, and areas of deformity or abnormality. This approach also subliminally reinforces the competence and thoughtfulness of the examiner. It also relaxes and reassures the patient.

It is sometimes helpful to have the patient flex knees and place the soles of the feet flat on the bed. Watch the patient's face for signs of discomfort. Gently palpate in each quadrant, being guided by your previous percussion for peritoneal irritation. Always palpate a suspected tender area last. The perception of a full feeling in the flanks by the examiner's hands gently compressing and relieving the area suggests ascites (Robertson's sign). A related approach is to lean over the patient and elevate both flanks about two inches and then drop your hands. Ascites will feel as if a water balloon has been dropped into your hand, while fat or gas will not have the same feeling of mass.

Palpate the Liver Edge

Hook your fingers along the right costal margin, with the PIP joints along the costal margin. Have the patient take a deep breath to cause the liver to descend. Difficulty of a patient to take a deep breath when the physician's fingers are pushing at the right costal margin suggests acute cholecystitis (Murphy's sign, also called Naunyn's sign).

John Benjamin Murphy (1857–1916), a tall surgeon with a colorful character and a parted red beard to match, was born in Appleton, Wisconsin. Best known for the two signs that bear his name, Dr. Murphy is also remembered for noting a pattern of symptoms that occur early in the process of appendicitis. He enthusiastically advised his contemporaries to remove the appendix of patients presenting with such symptoms and, like many an innovator, Murphy was roundly criticized by his peers for the surgical management he espoused. In the years that fol-

lowed, over 200 successful appendectomies proved the validity of his observations and popularized preemptive removal of the appendix in cases suspicious for appendicitis.

Two well-known clinical signs carry his eponym. The first, known simply as "Murphy's Sign," is a sign of gallbladder inflammation. The second sign, known as "Murphy's Sign II" or "Murphy's Punch," elicits pain in a patient with inflamed kidneys when the examiner gently but firmly punches along the costovertebral angle in the area of the patient's lower back. Murphy pioneered the anastomosis of the gallbladder and small intestine. He also broke new ground in the use of bone grafting. He was the first surgeon to successfully repair a traumatically severed femoral artery and was the first surgeon in the United States to artificially immobilize and collapse the lung of patients in the treatment of pulmonary tuberculosis.

A key issue is the texture of the liver and the nature of the liver edge. A soft, smooth edge is normal. A sharp well-defined edge suggests cirrhosis. A firm smoothness of the edge suggests congestion or infiltration. Feeling a hard nodular liver suggests malignancy. Liver pulsations suggest tricuspid regurgitation.

Palpate the Spleen

There are several methods to palpate a spleen, which probably contains a message in itself. If you feel a spleen tip, then check the consistency. A soft spleen that feels like a normal liver suggests acute enlargement. A hard spleen denotes a chronic process. In each palpation method, have the patient take a deep breath and then let it out. Gently advance your palpating hand during the exhalation and hold it in place. Have the patient take another deep breath and feel for the spleen tip.

◆ METHOD 1

With the patient supine, the examiner is on the patient's right side. Palpate with your right hand pushing gently under the left costal margin while pushing your left hand forward from the left flank to create a loose expanse of skin (see Figure 110).

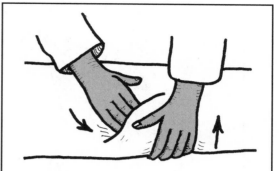

Figure 110. Palpating the Spleen.
With the patient supine, palpate with your right hand pushing gently under the left costal margin while pushing your left hand forward from the left flank to create a loose expanse of skin. Have the patient take a deep breath and then let it all out. Gently advance your palpating hand during the exhalation and hold it in place. Have the patient take another deep breath and feel for the spleen tip. The text describes other methods of palpation.

◆ METHOD 2

With the patient supine, the examiner stands on patient's left side and hooks fingers under the costal margin as the patient inhales deeply. This is a mirror image of the liver edge palpation strategy.

◆ METHOD 3

With the patient supine, the examiner is on the patient's right side. Place your right hand along the left costal margin and roll the patient toward you with your left hand (to the right lateral decubitus position) as you feel for the spleen tip.

◆ METHOD 4

With the patient supine and the examiner on the patient's right side, place your right hand along the left costal margin and roll the patient away from you (to the left lateral decubitus position) as you feel for the spleen tip.

There are other methods with the patient sitting and prone. Find a technique that works best for you and refine it. Method 1 is my personal choice.

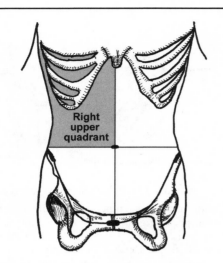

Figure 111. Right Upper Quadrant.
Structures in this location include the liver, gallbladder, large intestine, and the upper pole of the right kidney. Spasm of the rectus muscles in the right upper quadrant to percussion suggests hepatobiliary inflammation (D'Amato's abdominal sign). Masses in this area suggest hepatoma, hepatomegaly, or an enlarged gallbladder. Discomfort on palpation suggests cholecystitis, hepatitis, passive congestion and duodenal ulcer.

Right Upper Quadrant Palpation

Feeling a mass in this location suggests hepatoma, hepatomegaly, or an enlarged gallbladder. (If in the presence of jaundice, this is Courvoisier's sign of malignancy.) Discomfort on palpation suggests cholecystitis (with inspiration this is Murphy's sign), hepatitis, passive congestion and duodenal ulcer. Spasm of the rectus muscles in the right upper quadrant suggests hepatobiliary inflammation (D'Amato's abdominal sign). Large liver cysts can produce fremitus (Rovighi's sign). Right upper quadrant pain caused by a strike to the right lateral rectus, with the patient holding his or her breath, suggests cholecystitis (Riesman's abdominal sign).

Ludwig Georg Courvoisier (1843–1918) was raised in Basel, Switzerland, receiving his medical degree from the University of Basel in 1868.

One of his mentors at Basel was August Socin, one of the first surgeons in Europe to advocate for the antiseptic techniques of Joseph Lister. Courvoisier continued his studies in London, and spent an additional year in Vienna working with Theodor Billroth.

Courvoisier continued his association with Socin when he served in a German military hospital during the Franco-Prussian War. Following the war, he worked in a deaconess hospital in the small town of Riehen on the German-Swiss border for 30 years. He remained quite busy in practice by maintaining a private clinic in Basel as well. His primary achievements were in surgery of the biliary tract. His name is remembered by students of medicine today for his description of a painless, palpable gallbladder in association with pancreatic cancer. Despite his busy career, it is said that he still made time for his primary interest outside of medicine — collecting butterflies.

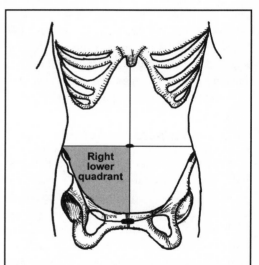

Figure 112. Right Lower Quadrant.
The right lower quadrant is the area of the cecum, appendix, ovary, and the lower pole of the right kidney. Feeling a mass in this location suggests inflammatory bowel disease, malignancy or vascular aneurysm. Discomfort on palpation suggests appendicitis or ischemia.

Right Lower Quadrant Palpation

Feeling a mass in this location suggests inflammatory bowel disease, malignancy or vascular aneurysm. Discomfort on palpation suggests appendicitis.

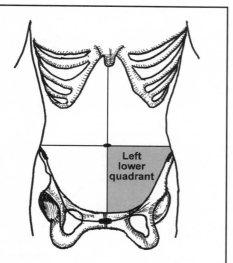

Figure 113. Left Lower Quadrant.

Left lower quadrant structures include the sigmoid colon, small bowel, and the ovary. Discomfort in this location suggests constipation, diverticulitis, bowel ischemia or vascular aneurysm. Pain on palpating midway between the umbilicus and the left inguinal ligament suggests acute ileal obstruction (Kink sign). Feeling a soft squishy mass suggests Crohn's disease (Lockwood's sign). Feeling a firm mass here suggests colon cancer or stool in the left colon.

Left Lower Quadrant Palpation

Feeling a mass here suggests colon cancer or stool in the left colon. Discomfort suggests constipation, diverticulitis or vascular aneurysm. Feeling a soft squishy mass with the sense of gas oozing through the bowel suggests Crohn's disease (Lockwood's sign). Pain on palpating midway between the umbilicus and the left inguinal ligament suggests acute ileal obstruction (Kink sign).

Left Upper Quadrant Palpation

Feeling a mass suggests splenomegaly. If the spleen is enlarged but not massive, consider

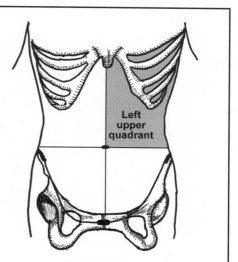

Figure 114. Left Upper Quadrant.

Structures in this area include the stomach, transverse colon, spleen, tail of the pancreas, and left kidney. Discomfort on palpation suggests abdominal aortic aneurysm and pancreatitis. Feeling a mass suggests splenomegaly, colon cancer or stool in the splenic flexure.

pernicious anemia, leukemia, lymphoma, hemolytic anemia, infections, and portal hypertension. If the splenomegaly is massive (felt below the umbilicus), consider chronic granulocytic leukemia, polycythemia rubra vera, Hodgkin's disease, and malaria. Splenomegaly with anemia suggests hypersplenism, leukemia and lymphoma. Splenomegaly with jaundice suggests portal hypertension or hemolytic anemia. An enlarged spleen with lymphadenopathy suggests lymphoma, chronic lymphocytic leukemia, and sarcoidosis. Splenomegaly with liver enlargement suggests portal hypertension, hemolytic anemia, leukemia, myeloid metaplasia, and polycythemia rubra vera.

Additional causes of a left upper quadrant mass are colon cancer and stool in the splenic flexure. Discomfort on palpation suggests abdominal aortic aneurysm and pancreatitis. Mallet-Guy's sign of pancreatitis is the presence of tenderness *only* on palpating the left upper quadrant while the patient rolls into the right lateral decubitus position.

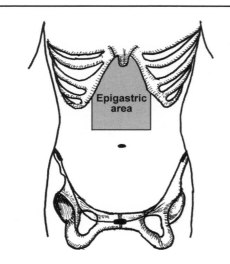

Figure 115. Epigastric Area.
The epigastric area is located in the mid-portion of the upper abdomen and is frequently described to supplement the four quadrant locations. Discomfort on palpation suggests peptic ulcer disease and pancreatitis. Feeling a mass in the epigastric area suggests gastric outlet obstruction or abdominal aortic aneurysm. The abdominal aortic aneurysm is a pulsatile mass greater than 3cm and usually extending to the right of the midline.

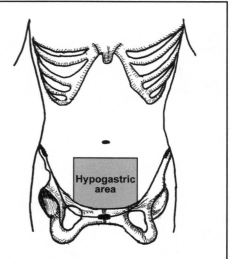

Figure 116. Hypogastric Area.
The hypogastric area contains the bladder, uterus, and bowel. Discomfort on palpation suggests cystitis. Feeling a mass here suggests urinary obstruction, uterine enlargement or femoral hernia. In rectus muscle hematoma the mass does not cross the midline and remains palpable when the muscle is relaxed (Fothergill's sign). Increased muscle tone along the lower rectus suggests peritoneal inflammation (Sumner's sign).

Epigastric Palpation

Feeling a mass in the epigastric area suggests gastric outlet obstruction or abdominal aortic aneurysm. The abdominal aortic aneurysm is a pulsatile mass greater than 3cm. It tends to make your fingers pulse out (laterally), not up. Confirm by listening for a bruit. Discomfort on palpation suggests peptic ulcer disease and pancreatitis.

Hypogastric Palpation

Feeling a mass here suggests urinary obstruction, uterine enlargement or femoral hernia. Discomfort on palpation suggests cystitis. In rectus muscle hematoma the mass does not cross the midline and remains palpable when the muscle is relaxed (Fothergill's sign). Increased muscle tone along the lower rectus

suggests peritoneal inflammation (Sumner's sign).

Check for Rebound Tenderness in All Quadrants

Be careful and considerate. You do not want to precipitate unnecessary discomfort. Gently push in the abdomen and then release by straightening your fingers. The presence of tenderness on the release suggests peritoneal irritation. Check for areas of hypesthesia over areas of rebound by stroking the skin very gently.

AUSCULTATION

In cases of suspected obstruction or in the case of a primary abdominal complaint, this part of the exam is always performed first.

Listen for Bowel Sounds

Listen to the abdomen with the diaphragm for at least thirty seconds. Absent bowel sounds suggest ileus while hearing high-pitched bowel sounds with tinkles and rushes suggests small bowel obstruction. Appreciating a leathery friction rub suggests localized peritonitis. If the friction rub is over the liver, it suggests primary hepatocellular carcinoma, metastatic cancer and liver abscess. If the friction rub is over the spleen, it suggests splenic infarction.

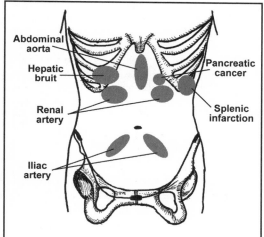

Figure 117. Location of Abdominal Vascular Bruits.

Hearing an epigastric bruit suggests an abdominal aortic aneurysm. Have the patient stand to see if the bruit shifts posteriorly, indicating an aneurysm of the gastroepiploic or other omental artery. A bruit over the liver suggests hepatoma. Subcostal bruits suggest renal artery stenosis. Hearing a bruit over the left upper quadrant suggests left renal artery stenosis, carcinoma of the body or tail of the pancreas, massive splenomegaly, and splenic artery stenosis or dissection.

Listen for Vascular Bruits

Hearing loud two-component (systolic and diastolic) bruits suggests the development of aorto-venous fistulae. Hearing an epigastric bruit suggests an abdominal aortic aneurysm. Have the patient stand to see if the bruit shifts

posteriorly, indicating an aneurysm of the gastroepiploic or other omental artery. Subcostal bruit suggests renal artery stenosis. Hearing a bruit over the left upper quadrant suggests left renal artery stenosis, carcinoma of the body or tail of the pancreas, massive splenomegaly, and splenic artery stenosis or dissection. A bruit over the liver suggests hepatoma. A caput medusa with a venous hum and a palpable thrill is Cruveilhier's sign.

Léon Jean Baptiste Cruveilhier (1791–1874), son of a French surgeon, began his medical studies under then-famous pathologist Guillaume Dupuytren. After several autopsies, however, he became disgusted with the study of medicine and joined a secret religious order. He later returned and cemented his relationship with Dupuytren.

Primarily a researcher, Cruveilhier was "a modest and honest physician," who built his reputation and vast practice via authorship. His testing of bone callus development elucidated the significance of the extraosseous periosteal tissue in normal bone fracture healing. By injecting mercury into the vasculature and bronchial system he was able to illustrate the ideas of infarction and embolism. His work prepared the way for the work of Virchow in the mid 1800's. Cruveilhier's sign, large veins radiating from the umbilicus secondary to portal hypertension, was based on his studies of human vasculature.

THE RECTAL EXAMINATION

"Bubo is an apostem breeding within the anus in the rectum with great hardness but little aching. This I say, before it ulcerates, is nothing else than a hidden cancer.... Out of bubo [cancer] goes hard excretions and sometimes they may not pass, because of the constriction caused by the bubo, and they are retained firmly within the rectum.... I never saw nor heard of any man that was cured ... but I have known many that died of the foresaid sickness." — John of Arderne

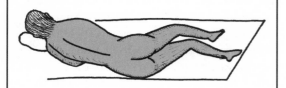

Figure 118. Positioning for the Rectal Examination.

The left lateral decubitus position with the patient's knees pulled up (right knee slightly higher than the right) is usually the most comfortable and modesty-preserving positioning for an elderly person. The left-handed examiner may prefer the right lateral decubitus position.

Inspect the Anal and Perineal Area

Generally the left lateral decubitus position with the patient's knees pulled up is the most comfortable and modesty-preserving positioning for an elderly person. Sometimes previous spinal injury will limit the degree of flexion but a satisfactory position can usually be found. Explain in detail why you are performing the examination and that you will first only look at the perineal tissue and that you explain each step of the internal examination before it occurs. Give the patient some tissue to hold for the completion of the examination to clean off any extra lubricant.

Pay particular attention to the border of the skin and the rectal mucosa. Flesh-colored tags suggests old fibrosed external hemorrhoids. Purple vascular structures distal to the pectinate line suggest external hemorrhoids. Tender, purple vascular structures proximal to the pectinate line suggest internal hemorrhoids. Seeing a dark red ring of tissue around the anus suggests rectal prolapse. Bryant's sign of intra-abdominal bleeding is seeing an ecchymotic ring around the rectum. Bruises can also be seen in sexual abuse. A tear in the distal anus is an anal fissure.

An opening in the perineal skin suggests an anal fistula. If the opening is less than 2cm from the anus and from nine to three on the "clock face," then consider anterior location

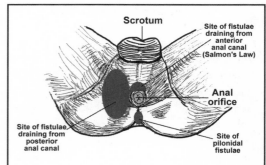

Figure 119. Perineal Inspection.

Carefully examine the border of the skin and the rectal mucosa. Flesh-colored tags suggests old fibrosed external hemorrhoids. Purple vascular structures distal to the pectinate line suggest external hemorrhoids. Seeing a dark red ring of tissue around the anus suggests rectal prolapse. Bryant's sign of intra-abdominal bleeding is seeing an ecchymotic ring around the rectum. Noting a tender tear in the distal anus is an anal fissure. An opening in the perineal skin suggests an anal fistula. The illustration shows the common sites for fistula drainage. If the opening is less than 2cm from the anus and from nine to three on the "clock face," then consider anterior location of a perirectal abscess (Salmon's Law). If the opening is more than 2cm from the anus, then consider a posterior location of a perirectal abscess (Salmon's Law). Seeing an opening near the coccyx suggests a pilonidal fistula.

of a perirectal abscess (Salmon's Law). If the opening is more than 2cm from the anus, then consider a posterior location of a perirectal abscess (Salmon's Law). Fluctuance between the anus and the ischial tuberosity suggests a posterior perirectal abscess.

Perform the Digital Rectal Exam

Arrange the guiac card in a convenient location and place some lubricant on your gloved forefinger. Explain to the patient that they will feel the sensation of pressure but that it should not be painful. Gently press against the anal opening and note the presence of the anal wink. Gently replace your finger against the anal opening *and wait*. With anal stimulation the first part of the anal reflex is con-traction. (This is not the time to vigorously try to advance.) After five to fifteen seconds you will sense a relaxation of the sphincter as the next part of the reflex occurs. Your finger may feel sucked into the opening. The reason to wait patiently is to minimize rectal spasm and discomfort, which will allow a more sensitive appreciation of any mucosal lesions. Note the anal sphincter tone. Test the lower spinal cord by having the patient try to contract around your finger and noting the difference in tone. Also have the patient bear down to push lower abdominal contents toward your finger.

Once your finger is completely inserted, slowly feel each quadrant by moving your slightly bent finger in a circle. Start at one o'clock and sweep around in a complete arc. Any areas of localized tenderness are abnor-mal and suggest a mucosal tear or perirectal abscess. Prostatitis can also produce exquisite anterior tenderness. The location of a posterior mass along the rectal shelf suggests malignancy. Stool in the rectal vault is not a rare finding and suggests compromise of the proximal muscular sling.

In men the prostate is easily felt anteriorly (see Figure 120). Note the size, symmetry, consistency and nodularity of the gland. Any nodules should be considered for biopsy.

Remove your finger and place any visible stool on the guiac card. Take some tissue and clean the lubricant off the anal opening.

SPECIAL TESTS

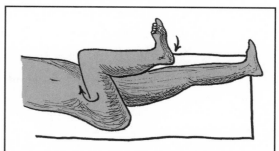

Figure 121. Obturator Muscle Test.
Flex the knee of the supine patient to 90°, then internally and externally rotate the hip. Pain in the corresponding lower quadrant suggests intra-peritoneal inflammation.

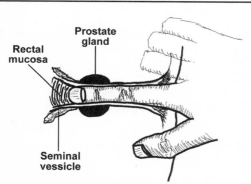

Figure 120. Rectal Examination.
Once your finger is completely inserted, slowly feel each quadrant by moving your slightly bent finger in a circle. Start at one o'clock and sweep around in a complete arc. Any areas of localized tenderness are abnormal and suggest a mucosal tear or perirectal abscess. Prostatitis can also produce exquisite anterior tenderness. The location of a posterior mass along the rectal shelf suggests malignancy. Stool in the rectal vault is not a rare finding and suggests compromise of the proximal muscular sling. In men the prostate is easily felt anteriorly. Note the size, symmetry, consistency and nodularity of the gland. Any nodules should be considered for biopsy. The Marfanoid finger in this illustration symbolizes how large it feels to the patient.

Obturator Muscle Test

Flex knee of the supine patient to 90°, then internally and externally rotate the hip. Pain in the corresponding lower quadrant suggests intraperitoneal inflammation.

Psoas Sign

Have the patient raise a leg while you push down on the knee. Pain in the lower quadrant is a positive sign. Repeat on the opposite side. Alternatively, have the patient lie

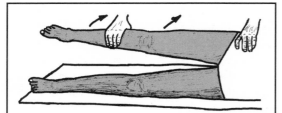

Figure 122. Psoas Muscle Test.
Have the patient lie on the left side and move the right knee back to extend the hip. Producing pain is a positive test. Another method (also with the patient lying with the left side down) is to have the patient raise the right leg while you push down on the knee. Pain in the lower quadrant is a positive sign.

on the left side and move the right knee back to extend the hip. Producing pain is a positive test.

Determining the Presence of Ascites

Look for a protuberant abdomen and bulging flanks. Palpate a fluid wave by having the patient supine. Lean over the patient and push up on the bulging flanks. Let your hands drop down to the bed and feel for the rebound of fluid back into your hand, as if a water balloon had been dropped into your hand.

SPECIAL CIRCUMSTANCES

The Elderly Patient with Abdominal Pain

Note the location, quality, radiation, severity, and timing, of the discomfort. Right upper quadrant discomfort suggests cholecystitis (check Murphy's sign), hepatitis, passive congestion, or duodenal ulcer. Right lower quadrant discomfort suggests appendicitis. Left lower quadrant discomfort suggests con-

stipation, diverticulitis or colon cancer. Left upper quadrant discomfort suggests pancreatitis or abdominal aortic aneurysm. Epigastric discomfort suggests peptic ulcer disease, pancreatitis and dissecting abdominal aortic aneurysm. Hypogastric discomfort suggests cystitis or diverticulitis. A patient with enterocolitis, hemorrhoids, and prostatitis may experience shooting pains to the rectum on sitting (Chair sign). Deep throbbing flank pain on deep flank palpation suggests a kidney stone (Signorelli's flank sign).

♦ BEGIN THE EXAM BY GENTLY PLACING YOUR HAND ON THE EPIGASTRIC AREA AND LET IT RELAX

Note any masses, pulsations, peristaltic activity, areas of deformity or abnormality. This approach also subliminally reinforces the competence and thoughtfulness of the examiner and relaxes and reassures the patient. Epigastric pulsation and expansion suggests abdominal aortic aneurysm (Corrigan's sign).

♦ AUSCULTATE THE ABDOMEN (AS DESCRIBED ABOVE) AND GENTLY PERCUSS IN ALL FOUR QUADRANTS

Note any areas of tightening of the rectus muscle indicating underlying peritoneal inflammation. Gently palpate in each quadrant, being guided by your previous percussion for peritoneal irritation. Always palpate a tender area last.

♦ HAVE PATIENT DO AN ABDOMINAL CRUNCH (HALF SIT-UP) WITH ARMS CROSSED OVER CHEST (CARNETT'S SIGN)

Do not perform this test if there is already abdominal rigidity, as this maneuver induces voluntary guarding. Palpate the abdominal wall when the patient is halfway up. A positive test is a *reduction* of abdominal wall discomfort due to protection by the tensed muscles. This suggests appendicitis, cholecystitis, renal colic, or ovarian cyst. A negative test is an increase in abdominal wall pain indicating an abdominal wall process rather than an intra-abdominal process. Abdominal pain on tensing the abdominal muscles suggests an abdominal wall problem, while pain on relaxing the abdominal muscles suggests a visceral cause (Carnett's sign). Loss of abdominal reflexes in the setting of peritonitis is Rosenbach's sign.

♦ CHECK FOR EXQUISITE SKIN TENDERNESS OVER THE RIGHT FLANK

Exquisite tenderness to light stroking of the flank is Boas' sign implying cholecystitis. This is not the jolting check for costovertebral angle tenderness. Also consider early herpes zoster.

♦ HAVE THE PATIENT COUGH TO SEE IF THAT LOCALIZES THE PAIN

♦ HAVE THE PATIENT PERFORM A VALSALVA MANEUVER FOR FIFTEEN TO TWENTY SECONDS, THEN ASK THE PATIENT TO LOCALIZE THE DISCOMFORT

♦ CHECK FOR REBOUND TENDERNESS

Be careful and considerate; you do not want to precipitate unnecessary discomfort. Gently push in the abdomen and then release by straightening your fingers. Presence of tenderness on the release suggests peritoneal irritation. Check for areas of hypesthesia over areas of rebound by stroking the skin very gently.

♦ PALPATE THE AREA OVER THE GALLBLADDER

Pain over the gallbladder is Murphy's sign. Pain in the right lower quadrant when palpating the right upper quadrant suggests acute appendicitis (Soresi's sign).

♦ PALPATE MCBURNEY'S POINT

Having this palpation produce sharp pain in right lower quadrant, right shoulder or subscapular area suggests acute appendicitis. Pain in left lower quadrant suggests diverticulitis. Pain in the epigastric or precordial area (Aaron's sign) suggests appendicitis.

Charles McBurney (1845–1913) was one of the surgeons pioneering the diagnostic and operative treatment of appendicitis. In 1888 he was appointed the surgeon-in-chief at Roosevelt Hospital, where most of his clinical work, including his famous studies on appendicitis, was completed. He rapidly made his hospital one of the international centers of surgical excellence.

McBurney's classic report on early operative interference in cases of appendicitis was presented before the New York Surgical Society in 1889. In it he described the area of greatest abdominal pain in this disease process, now known as McBurney's point. Five years later, he set forth in another paper the incision that he used in cases of appendicitis, now called McBurney's incision. He published numerous papers and was a keen hunter and fisher. He died of a coronary thrombosis while on a hunting trip.

♦ PALPATE LEFT ILIAC FOSSA (ROVSING'S SIGN)

Right lower quadrant tenderness suggests acute appendicitis.

Niels Thorkild Rovsing (1862–1927) was the most renowned Danish surgeon at the beginning of the twentieth century. An inspiring teacher, Rovsing was primarily recognized as a brilliant abdominal surgeon. He wrote extensively on diseases of the bladder and gallbladder. He became internationally recognized and his work on abdominal surgery was translated into German and English. In 1908, together with Eilert A. Tscherning (1851–1919), he founded the Danish Surgical Society.

The Elderly Person with an Abdominal Mass

Note the location, size, mobility, and quality of the mass. A right upper quadrant mass suggests hepatoma, hepatomegaly or an enlarged gallbladder (Courvoisier's sign). A right lower quadrant mass suggests inflammatory bowel disease or malignancy. A left lower quadrant mass suggests colon cancer or stool in the left colon. Feeling a left upper quadrant mass suggests splenomegaly, colon cancer, or stool in the splenic flexure. An epigastric mass suggests gastric outlet obstruction and abdom-

Table 16.1. Signs of appendicitis

Name	Clinical Feature
Bassler's sign	• Pain on pushing the palpating hand from the anterior iliac crest down and to the right
Brittain's sign	• Retraction of the right testicle with right lower quadrant palpation
Cope's sign	• Right lower quadrant pain on extending the thigh
Gray's sign	• Pain on palpation four centimeters below and to the left of the umbilicus
Mannaberg's sign	• Accentuation of the second heart sign in appendicitis
McBurney's sign	• Pain on palpation two-thirds of the distance between the anterior iliac spine to the umbilicus
Obturator sign	• Pain on pressing the obturator foramen suggests obturator nerve inflammation, such as appendicitis.
Roux's sign	• Soft cecal resistance to palpation suggests inflammatory bowel disease or appendicitis.
Rovsing's sign	• Producing pain in the right lower quadrant by pushing in the left lower quadrant
Sicard's sign	• A decreased right lower abdominal reflex in appendicitis
Ten Horn's sign	• Pain produced by gently stretching the right spermatic cord in the right scrotum
Williams' sign	• Inability of a supine patient to hold up the right leg due to pain and swelling of the inguinal ligament

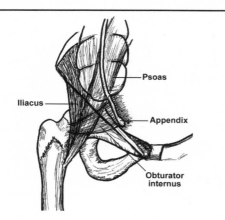

Figure 123. Muscles Near the Appendix.
This figure shows the relationship of the psoas, iliacus, and obturator internus muscles to the appendix. Note how an inflamed appendix might cause pain on contraction of these muscles. The obturator muscle test and psoas muscle test are based on this proximity.

inal aortic aneurysm (usually a pulsatile mass greater than three centimeters). Confirm by listening for a bruit. A mass in the hypogastric area suggests urinary obstruction, uterine enlargement, or femoral hernia.

Benign findings sometimes felt on the abdominal examination include the borders of the rectus muscle, stool in the colon, lipomas in the abdominal wall, bladder enlargement, the abdominal aorta, floating ribs and the sacral promontory.

The Elderly Person with Abdominal Distension

If the distension is generalized, note the umbilicus. If the distension is simply fat, the umbilicus is depressed. If there are bulging flanks and the umbilicus is flat or everted, con-

---

Table 16.2. Signs of possible malignancy

Name	*Clinical Feature*
Bouveret's sign	• Colonic obstruction with right lower fullness
Courvoisier's sign	• Jaundice and a palpable gallbladder suggests cancer of the head of the pancreas.
Strauss's sign	• Feeling a mass in the pouch of Douglas on rectal exam suggests metastatic gastric carcinoma.
Tansini's sign	• A scaphoid abdomen suggests primary gastric or pancreatic cancer, while protuberance suggests metastatic bowel disease.
Troisier's sign	• Visible enlargement of the left supraclavicular fossa

---

Table 16.3. Other signs of an acute abdomen

Name	*Clinical Feature*
Ballance's sign	• Persistent dullness on the left flank and shifting dullness on the right suggests splenic rupture.
Blumberg's sign	• Appearance of rebound tenderness is a poor prognostic sign while rebound tenderness that resolves is a favorable sign.
Chapman's sign	• Painful restriction of the upper body in a supine patient
Claybrook's sign/ Federici's sign	• Transmission of cardiac and respiratory sounds through the abdominal wall suggests a perforated viscus.
Dance's sign	• Retractions in the right lower quadrant suggest ileocecal intussusception.
Kehr's sign	• Severe pain in the left shoulder due to a ruptured spleen
Ransohoff's sign	• Periumbilical jaundice suggests rupture of the common bile duct.

sider ascites. In pancreatitis the umbilicus may be sunken like a Cupid's bow and you may see peristaltic activity. Seeing a ladder-like appearance of lower abdomen suggests small bowel obstruction. Seeing a large inverted "U" appearance suggests large bowel obstruction.

If the distension is localized again, note the umbilicus. An enlarged bladder tips the umbilicus up toward the head, while ascites may cause the umbilicus to point toward the feet (Tanyol's sign). An enlarged right upper quadrant suggests hepatobiliary enlargement or mass. An enlarged left upper quadrant suggests an enlarged spleen. An enlarged epigastrium suggests enlarged stomach or gastric outlet obstruction.

Hernias can be sought by having the patient raise the head off the pillow to accentuate abdominal pressure. The location of the hernia will define the type.

CHAPTER 17

The Lower Extremities

"Always look at the feet. Looking at a woman's legs has often saved her life."
— **William Osler**

"The human foot is a masterpiece of engineering and a work of art."
— **Leonardo da Vinci**

This chapter is primarily concerned with the orthopedic aspects of the lower extremity examination. The vascular assessment is contained in Chapter 18 and the neuromuscular evaluation is in Chapter 21. The assessment of balance and gait is reviewed in Chapter 23.

EVALUATION OF THE HIP

Observations of Standing Posture

The hip cannot be inspected or palpated directly, so most inferences derive from changes in movement. Observe the patient's standing posture, since hip problems will tend to cause the affected foot to advance slightly and rotate slightly inward. Also check Trendelenberg's sign (see Figure 125) by having the patient lift the right leg and seeing if the left hip

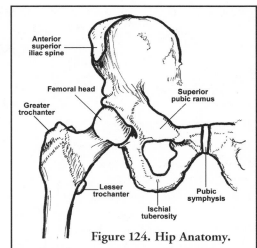

Figure 124. Hip Anatomy.

This illustration shows the skeletal anatomy of the hip. The labeled structures (with the notable exception of the femoral head) can be appreciated on careful physical examination.

elevates (normal) or does not (a positive test). Repeat on the other side. A positive test suggests degenerative joint disease, weakness of

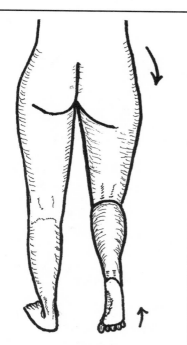

Figure 125. Trendelenberg's Sign.
Have the patient lift the right leg and see if the right hip elevates (normal) or does not, as shown in the illustration (a positive test). Repeat on the other side. A positive Trendelenberg's sign suggests degenerative joint disease, weakness of the gluteus or hip dislocation.

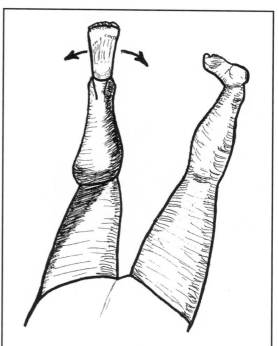

Figure 126. Hip Isolation Test.
With the patient prone, flex the knee to about 90° and move the foot medially and laterally so that the hip is internally and externally rotated. Limited range of motion implies degenerative joint disease of the hip. This test isolates the hip so that extra-articular causes of discomfort are minimized.

the gluteus or hip dislocation. Seeing a compensatory lordosis when the hip is extended suggests hip joint disease (Thomas's sign).

Friedrich Trendelenberg (1844–1924) was the son of philosopher Friedrich Adolf Trendelenberg. Trendelenberg introduced numerous surgical innovations including gastrostomy in patients with esophageal stricture, use of specific position (Trendelenberg) for performance of vascular surgical cases, and surgical embolectomy. He founded the German Surgical Society in 1872, and was greatly interested in surgical history. He wrote an account of ancient Indian surgery as well as an autobiography.

Hip Range of Motion

Next, observe the hip range of motion. With the patient prone, flex the knee to about 90° and move the foot medially and laterally so that the knee swings medially and laterally. Limited range of motion implies degenerative joint disease of the hip. This test isolates the hip so that extra-articular causes of discomfort are minimized.

Palpate Over the Greater Trochanter

Palpate over the greater trochanter. Pain over the greater trochanter on palpation suggests fracture if other signs are present, trochanteric bursitis, or possible referred pain from the knee. Flattening of the thigh when a patient lies supine suggests upper motor neuron disease (Heilbronner's sign).

EVALUATION OF THE KNEE

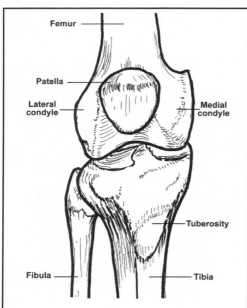

Figure 127. Knee Anatomy.

This illustration shows the relationships among the basic bony structures of the right knee.

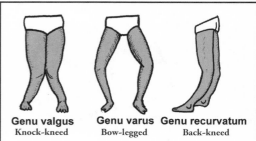

Genu valgus
Knock-kneed

Genu varus
Bow-legged

Genu recurvatum
Back-kneed

Figure 128. Common Knee Deformities.

Normally the knees and the medial malleoli touch when the patient stands. Valgus deformity of the knees produces the knock-kneed deformity where the ankles are further apart than the knees. Bilateral varus knee deformities produce bowlegs where the knees are apart when the ankles touch. Knees that curve backward in the lateral dimension have a genu recurvatum deformity.

Knee Inspection

If the patient is knock-kneed (knees touch but ankles do not) there is a valgus deformity of the knee (see Figure 128). If the patient is bowlegged (ankles touch but knees do not) there is a varus deformity of the knee. It is normal is for both the ankles and the knees to touch. If the knees curve backward in the lateral dimension, that is a genu recurvatum deformity. Look for scars from previous knee surgery. Osteoarthritis will produce bony enlargement sometimes magnified by coincident quadriceps muscle atrophy.

Observe Knee Range of Motion

Observe passive knee range of motion by gently flexing and extending the knee with the patient supine. Decreased range of motion sug-

gests degenerative joint disease. Increased lateral movement suggests damaged ligaments.

Check for Crepitus

Check for crepitus in the knee joint by listening for the crunching, popping sound (or feeling) on joint movement. Finding no crepitus is normal. If crepitus is present it suggests degenerative joint disease. (The location defines the affected compartment.) Anterior crepitus suggests anterior knee degenerative joint disease. Lateral crepitus suggests lateral knee degenerative joint disease. Medial crepitus suggests medial knee degenerative joint disease. Crepitus on extension suggests patellofemoral syndrome.

Evaluate for an Effusion

Now search for a knee effusion. Feel for a spongy movement of the patella or note a bulge between the patella and the condyles. If there is any spongy downward movement of the patella when the leg is fully extended, then an effusion is present. In addition, you can milk the fluid from the medial side with your forefingers and middle fingers, and then push with your thumbs from the lateral side just below the patella. Seeing a medial bulge (bulge sign) suggests effusion. Anesthesia in the popliteal fossa suggests neurosyphilis (Bekhterev's sign).

Vladimir Mikhailovich Bekhterev (1857–1927) was a Russian physician whose lasting work was his research on brain morphology and his original description of several nervous symptoms and illnesses. While studying in Europe he worked with such eminent physicians as Wilhelm Wundt, Paul Flechsig, Karl Westphal and Jean-Martin Charcot. Bekhterev published over 800 original articles and several seminal books on the nervous system. Bekhterev was an academic competitor and faculty colleague of Ivan Pavlov. In December 1927, Joseph Stalin, who at the time suffered from depression, called Bekhterev to the Kremlin for consultation. Persistent rumors in Russia have it that Bekhterev diagnosed Stalin as suffering from "grave paranoia." The same day he had visited the Kremlin Bekhterev suddenly died, presumably murdered in accordance with Stalin's orders.

Note the Relationship of the Tibial and Femoral Condyles

Now check the relative position of the tibial and femoral condyles. Tibial condyles displaced posteriorly to femoral condyles suggest a prior posterior cruciate ligament tear. Tibial condyles displaced anteriorly to the femoral condyles suggest a prior anterior cruciate ligament tear.

EVALUATION OF THE ANKLE AND FOOT

Inspect the Anatomic Landmarks

The examination of the ankle and foot is important because functional problems are common and because the foot can be examined in detail. First, inspect the anatomic landmarks. Atrophy of the anterior muscles (foot dorsiflexors) suggests foot drop. Now inspect

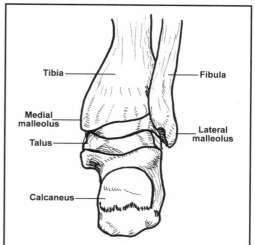

Figure 129. Posterior Ankle Anatomy.

This illustration shows the relationships among the bones involved in the ankle joint as viewed from behind. The ankle joint is basically a hinge between the tibia and superior talus, moving only in one plane.

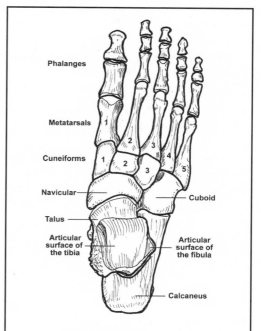

Figure 130. Foot Anatomy.

This figure shows the bones of the foot. The foot shows more complex biomechanics than the ankle. Sources of foot pain can sometimes be inferred from reviewing the anatomy of the painful area.

the toes, foot and arches. Lateral deviation of great toe is hallux valgus. Plantar atrophy is an early sign of thromboangiitis obliterans (Samuel's sign). Medial displacement of the Achilles tendon when viewed from behind suggests pes planus (Helbing's sign).

Check the Skin

Note the skin over the ankles and feet. Wet feet suggest alcoholism (especially in an elderly woman who becomes anxious at night in the hospital). Also note calluses, varicosities and edema. Edema suggests right heart failure or hypoalbuminemia. (You can tell them apart by checking the pit recovery time.) Diffuse edema with redness and warmth suggests deep venous thrombosis, superficial thrombophlebitis, or cellulites. (Check for tinea infection between the toes.) Brawny, hyperpigmented skin suggests chronic venous insufficiency. Seeing a chevron over the lateral malleolus suggests a ruptured Baker's cyst. Lack of capillary refill of the lower leg vasculature in less than three seconds suggests peripheral vascular disease (Moschcowitz's sign).

Check Passive and Active Range of Motion

Check passive ankle range of motion. Decreased inversion or eversion suggests a problem with the subtalar joint. Decreased dorsiflexion or plantarflexion suggests tibiotalar joint dysfunction. Painless bony irregularities around the joint suggest a Charcot joint.

Now check active plantar flexion with knee at 90°. (Have the patient "step on the gas.") Weakness suggests S1 nerve root damage or tibial nerve dysfunction, tibiotalar ankle sprain, gastrocnemius muscle tear, and Achilles tendon damage or tendonitis.

Check active dorsiflexion of the foot against resistance. Weakness suggests foot drop (L5), tibiotalar ankle sprain, and extensor tendonitis. Next, check ankle inversion against

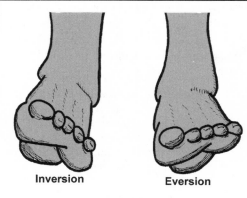

Inversion   **Eversion**

Figure 131. Ankle Inversion and Eversion.

Inversion and eversion of the foot test the subtalar joint which is a functional articulation of the talus and navicular, and the calcaneus and cuboid. Decreased inversion or eversion suggests a problem with these subtalar joint articulations.

resistance. Weakness suggests foot drop (L5), subtalar ankle sprain, and anterior tibialis tendonitis. Check ankle eversion against resistance. Weakness suggests superficial peroneal nerve problem (S1), subtalar ankle sprain, and peroneal retinaculum sprain.

Check dorsiflexion of the great toe. Weakness suggests foot drop or L5 lesion, first metatarsal phalangeal joint problem, and extensor hallucis longus tendonitis.

Evaluate the Pedal Pulses

Check the dorsalis pedis and posterior tibial pulses and capillary refill (see Chapter 18).

Check Foot Sensation

Check foot sensation. Decreased sensation to the dorsal foot suggests foot drop or L5 lesion, while decreased sensation to the plantar foot suggests a tibial nerve or S1 lesion. Chapter 21 contains information on the neurological examination of the foot.

SPECIAL CIRCUMSTANCES

The Elderly Patient with Hip Pain After a Fall

Chapter 23 has an extended section on this evaluation. An abbreviated assessment is given here.

First, inspect the leg. If it is foreshortened and externally rotated, consider fracture of the femoral neck (intertrochanteric fracture). If the leg is externally rotated but not foreshortened, consider fracture of the femoral shaft. If the thigh is externally rotated, flexed and abducted, consider anterior dislocation. If the thigh is internally rotated and adducted with a very prominent greater trochanter, consider posterior dislocation. Feeling a crepitant sensation when palpating over a bone in the absence of infection suggests sarcoma (Dupuytren's sign).

Now check for osteophony (bone sound) which is Hueter's sign. Place the diaphragm of your stethoscope on the pubic symphysis. Gently percuss each kneecap with your forefinger. An intact bone will produce a clear, bright tapping sound. A hip fracture will give a muffled, distant sound. Other approaches use a tuning fork on the patella or listening over each iliac crest as opposed to the pubic symphysis. This test is extremely helpful in evaluating patients on home visits or in the nursing home.

Signs of Sciatica

A way to tell sciatica from a hamstring injury: Flex the hip with the leg straight until it feels painful and then dorsiflex the foot. A hamstring pull will not be painful while the pain will increase in sciatica (Bragard's leg sign). Pain on the contralateral side when the nonpainful side is flexed at the thigh with the leg held in extension suggests sciatica (Fajersztajn's sign). Loss of sensation on the lateral portion of the foot suggests sciatica (Szabo's

Table 17.1. Signs of fracture	
Name	*Clinical Manifestation*
Allis's sign	• Laxity of the fascia lata that connects the greater trochanter to the iliac crest on palpation suggests femoral neck fracture.
Cleemann's sign	• A transverse crease superior to the kneecap suggests a femoral fracture.
Coopernail's sign	• Ecchymosis of the labia in pelvic fracture
Desault's sign	• Limitation in the normal range of motion in the circular arc of the hip suggests proximal femoral fracture.
Hueter's sign	• Bony transmission of sounds is reduced in a fracture.
Keen's sign of Pott's fracture	• Increased diameter of the leg at the level of the malleoli suggests • fibular fracture.
Langoria's sign	• Relaxation of the extensor muscles of the thigh with intrascapular femoral fracture
Laugier's sign	• Swelling along the inguinal ligament in a femoral neck fracture
Ludloff's sign	• Ecchymosis and swelling along the inguinal ligament and inability to raise the thigh when the patient is sitting suggest fracture of the greater trochanter.

sign). Pain on straight leg raise that is relieved with leg flexion suggests sciatica (Lasègue's sign). Pain on adduction of the thigh suggests sciatica (Bonnet's sign). Pain in the buttocks when the great toe is hyperextended suggests sciatica (Turyn's sign). Pain in the lower back or down the leg when the patient is supine suggests sciatica (Linder's sign).

Ernest-Charles Lasègue (1816–1883) initially began his academic career in the study of philosophy. One day he heard a lecture by Armand Trousseau and so changed his course of studies to clinical medicine. For a time as a student, he was too poor to pay his rent, as he and his roommate Claude Bernard would spend their francs procuring rabbits and guinea pigs with which they would perform medical experiments.

He was professor of clinical medicine at the Hôpital Necker, and became a favorite teacher who was considered a "universal specialist," being broadly read and having written across a wide range of medical subject matter. Witty and "free from all outward formalities," Lasègue took part in a classic bit of verbal sparring with celebrated pathologist of the day, Rudolf Virchow.

CHRONIC HIP PAIN OR DECREASED RANGE OF MOTION

Remember the possibility of referred pain from the knee.

Check Patrick's Test

Place patient's ankle on the contralateral knee and then gently press down on the flexed knee (see Figure 78). Pain in the hip suggests DJD of the hip; pain radiating from the back down the leg suggests radiculopathy; and pain in the lower spine suggests compression fracture.

Check Laguerre's Test

With the patient supine, grasp the heel on the symptomatic side and passively flex the knee and hip, and passively rotate the hip. Pain over

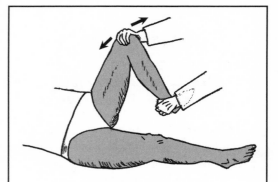

Figure 132. Laguerre's Test.
With the patient supine, grasp the heel on the symptomatic side and passively flex the knee and hip, and passively rotate the hip. Pain over the greater trochanter suggests trochanteric bursitis, while pain in the hip and groin suggests osteoarthritis of the hip.

the greater trochanter suggests bursitis, while pain in the hip and groin suggests osteoarthritis.

Perform Trendelenburg's Test

Have the patient stand and transfer the weight to the non-painful leg (Trendelenburg's test). If the painful buttock drops and becomes flaccid, suspect severe degenerative joint disease, weakness of the gluteus or hip dislocation (see Figure 125).

Feel Along the Anterior Iliac Spine

Check along the anterior iliac spine and inguinal ligament for meralgia paresthetica, which will present as dysesthesia along the anterior thigh that increases with palpation.

ANTERIOR KNEE PAIN

Check for Bony Deformity; Check for Effusion

Check for joint effusion (vide supra) which, if present, will show a patella with spongy bal-

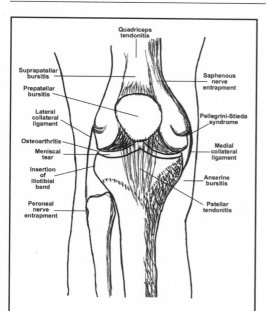

Figure 133. Common Sites for Pain Around the Knee.

This illustration shows the location and possible cause of pain around the knee. Quadriceps tendonitis and suprapatellar bursitis produce pain above or on the kneecap. Saphenous nerve entrapment causes discomfort behind the knee. The Pellegrini-Stieda syndrome is calcification of the medial collateral ligament, producing pain in the medial knee. Anserine bursitis causes pain medially below the knee. Causes of lateral knee pain are damage to the lateral collateral ligament and peroneal nerve entrapment. Tenderness between femur and fibular head suggests lateral collateral ligament sprain. Pain just anterior to the femoral condyles suggests lateral meniscus tear. Tenderness over the lateral tibial condyle radiating over lateral thigh suggests iliotibial band syndrome.

lottement, bulging of the joint, or a fluid wave. Check for tenderness and swelling over the quadriceps muscles. The presence of pain suggests quadriceps rupture or strain.

Search for Patellar Tenderness

Check for tenderness around the patella. Doughy swelling above the patella suggests suprapatellar bursitis (housemaid's knee). Swelling and tenderness on the patella suggests prepa-tellar bursitis (roofer's knee), usually brought on by constant kneeling. Marked tenderness and swelling over the patella suggests patellar fracture. Tenderness below the patella without swelling suggests tendonitis (jumper's knee). Swelling and tenderness below the patella suggests infrapatellar bursitis (pastor's knee).

Patella-Femoral Syndrome

Check for patella-femoral syndrome. Look for quadriceps atrophy, especially the vastus obliquus medialis. Also feel for tenderness behind the patella with palpation.

Perform the Patellar Inhibition Test

Stabilize the patella with your thumb and forefinger and then gently try to push it toward the feet, and have the patient contract the quadriceps to bring patella upward. Pain and relaxation of the quadriceps is a positive test. Now move the patella medially and laterally with knee flexed to 30°. Increased lateral mobility is a positive apprehension test. Voluntary contraction of the quadriceps when moving the patella laterally is also a positive test. Check for lateral patellar displacement with extension that resolves with flexion.

PAIN BEHIND THE KNEE

Search for a Popliteal Mass

A nontender area of bogginess suggests a Baker's cyst. Feeling a pulsatile mass suggests popliteal artery aneurysm. Feeling a tender mass in the popliteal fossa suggests bursitis.

Look for Focal or Diffuse Tenderness in the Popliteal Fossa

Focal tenderness in the medial popliteal fossa without a mass suggests a hamstring muscle strain. Diffuse tenderness and swelling suggests a ruptured Baker's cyst or deep venous thrombosis.

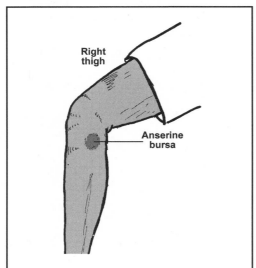

Figure 134. Anserine Bursitis.
The anserine bursa (named because it resembles a goose's foot, pes anserina in Latin) is located just below and medial to the knee. Exquisite tenderness on gentle palpation at this site suggests anserine bursitis.

MEDIAL KNEE PAIN

Palpate for Tenderness

Check for an anatomic deformity and palpate the site of tenderness. Pain behind the knee suggests a hamstring tear. Exquisite tenderness medial and inferior to the tibial plateau suggests anserine bursitis. Tenderness midway between the femur and the tibia suggests medial collateral ligament damage. Tenderness anterior to the condyles suggests a medial meniscus tear.

Check for Joint Laxity

Now test for joint laxity with lateral movement. The degree of laxity defines the extent

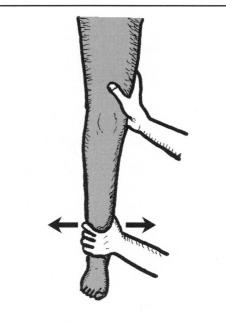

Figure 135. Bohler's Sign.
Test for joint laxity with medial and lateral knee movement. The degree of laxity defines the extent of medial collateral ligament tear. Pain in the lateral knee with this movement suggests lateral meniscus tear (Bohler's sign).

of medial collateral ligament tear. Pain in the lateral knee with this movement suggests lateral meniscus tear (Bohler's sign).

Check for Meniscus Tear

Check for a medial meniscus tear with the McMurray maneuver. With the patient supine, passively flex knee until the heel hits the buttock. Rotate foot laterally and then extend knee. A loud click over the lateral knee suggests a medial meniscus tear. Also check Apley's compression test (see Figure 137). With the patient prone and the knee flexed to 90° (perpendicular to the examining table), push down and gently twist the foot. Pain or crepitus is a positive test. With patient sitting cross-legged, push on the painful knee (Payr's test). Medial knee pain is a positive test.

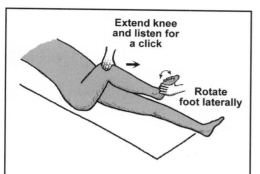

Figure 136. McMurray's Test.

McMurray's test is a maneuver to check for a medial meniscus tear. With the patient supine, passively flex knee until the heel hits the buttock. Rotate foot laterally and then extend knee. A loud click over the lateral knee suggests a medial meniscus tear.

LATERAL KNEE PAIN

Palpate for Tenderness

Check for anatomic deformity. Palpate the site of tenderness with the knee straight and then flexed to 90°. Tenderness over the fibular head suggests fibular fracture. Tenderness between femur and fibular head suggests lateral collateral ligament sprain. Tenderness

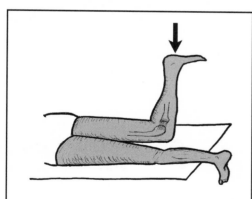

Figure 137. Apley's Compression Test.

With the patient prone and the knee flexed to 90° (perpendicular to the examining table), push down and gently twist the foot. Pain or crepitus is a positive test indicative of a meniscus tear.

just anterior to the femoral condyles suggests lateral meniscus tear. Tenderness over lateral tibial condyle radiating over lateral thigh suggests iliotibial band syndrome.

Check for Joint Laxity

Check for joint laxity by holding the knee and moving the foot medially. The amount of pain and the degree of laxity defines the extent of lateral collateral ligament tear. Pain in the medial knee suggests medial meniscus tear.

Check for Ober's Sign

With patient supine, passively flex and abduct the leg, then gently let go and have the patient maintain the leg position. Pain in anterior thigh (positive Ober's sign) suggests tensor fascia lata syndrome. Pain in lateral knee suggests iliotibial band syndrome.

Look for a Meniscus Tear

Check the McMurray maneuver. With the patient supine, passively flex the knee until the heel hits the buttock. Rotate the foot laterally and then extend knee. A loud click over the medial knee suggests a lateral meniscus tear. Also check Apley's compression test (supra vida).

A KNEE THAT GIVES WAY

Check the Basic Landmarks for Anatomic Deformity

♦ Examine the Anterior Cruciate Ligament

Perform the drawer test (see Figure 138) by pulling out on the tibia to see how far the tibia slides anteriorly over the femur. Noting greater than 2mm movement suggests a tear. Sensing

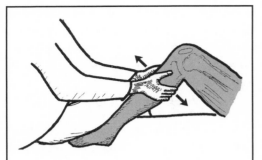

Figure 138. Drawer Test.
Perform the drawer test by sitting on the foot and pulling out on the tibia. The goal is to see how far the tibia slides anteriorly over the femur. Noting greater than 2mm movement suggests a tear. Sensing a sharp stopping point of movement is normal. A boggy stopping point suggests a tear. Rotational movement (where only one condyle moves) suggests tear of the corresponding collateral ligament.

a sharp stopping point of movement is normal. A boggy stopping point suggests a tear. Rotational movement (where only one condyle moves) suggests tear of the corresponding collateral ligament.

Now check the drawer test with the patient prone. Lachman's sign is basically a drawer sign with the posterior knee supported to relax the hamstrings.

Check the Galway-MacIntosh test. With the patient supine, passively flex the hip with the knee extended. Anterior movement of the tibia more than 2mm suggests a tear. Confirm by applying valgus force to the leg while passively flexing the knee. A sharp reduction of the subluxation at 20°–40° flexion is a positive test.

Check the Posterior Cruciate Ligament

Perform the drawer test to see how far the tibia slides posteriorly over the femur. Greater than 2mm movement suggests a tear. A sharp stopping point of movement is normal. A boggy stopping point suggests a tear. Rotational movement, where only one condyle moves, suggests tear of the corresponding collateral ligament.

Check for posterior sag by supporting the distal femur with pillows and seeing if the tibia is posteriorly displaced. With the patient supine and knee flexed at 90°, push posteriorly on tibial plateau. Posterior movement suggests a tear.

Check for Godfrey's sign. With the patient supine, passively flex at the hip with the knee in full extension. Pull up on the distal foot to 90° with varus and external rotation. Posterior movement of the tibia suggests a tear.

Check the Collateral Ligaments

Check for joint laxity with lateral movement. The degree of laxity defines the extent of medial collateral ligament tear. Check for joint laxity by holding the knee and moving the foot medially. The amount of pain and the degree of laxity defines the extent of lateral collateral ligament tear.

Check for Meniscal Tear

Check for a medial meniscus tear by performing the McMurray maneuver. With the patient supine, passively flex the knee until the heel hits the buttock. Rotate the foot laterally and then extend the knee. A loud click over the lateral knee suggests a medial meniscus tear. A loud click over the medial knee suggests a lateral meniscus tear.

Now check Payr's test. With the patient sitting cross-legged, push on the painful knee. Medial or lateral pain is a positive test.

Additional Knee Signs

Decrease in knee pain by forward flexion and lateral rotation of the foot suggests medial meniscus injury (Bragard's sign). Increased anterior-posterior movement of the tibia over the femur with a click or pain suggests damage to the anterior or posterior cruciate ligaments (drawer sign or Rocher's sign). Medial knee pain on downward pressure exerted on the sitting patient's knee suggests either medial meniscus lesion or posterior horn cell lesion (Payr's sign).

ANKLE OR FOOT INJURY

Check Landmarks for Anatomic Abnormality, Ecchymoses or Swelling

Ecchymosis under both malleoli, with a broad appearing heel, suggests a calcaneal fracture. Ecchymosis and focal swelling over the fifth metatarsal suggests fracture of the proximal fifth metatarsal bone (Jones's fracture). Swelling and tenderness over the lateral malleolus suggests a lateral sprain, if anterior and inferior, and a peroneal retinaculum sprain, if on the posterior rim. Swelling and tenderness over the medial malleolus suggests a medial sprain, syndesmotic sprain, or tibialis tendonitis, if posterior to medial malleolus.

Palpate the Lateral Knee

Tenderness suggests proximal fibular fracture.

Check for Anterior Movement of the Calcaneus Over the Distal Tibia

A firm end point and 4mm of movement or less suggest a first-degree lateral sprain. Sensing a boggy end point and more than 4mm movement suggests a second-degree lateral sprain. More than 4mm of movement and no end point suggest a third-degree lateral sprain.

Check the Talar Tilt Test

Passively invert the foot and compare it with the opposite foot. Greater than 10° difference suggest a second-or third-degree lateral ankle sprain.

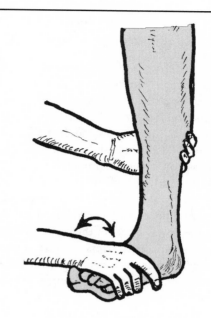

Figure 139. Talar Tilt Test.
This test is helpful to check for an ankle sprain. Passively invert the foot and compare the degree of inversion with the opposite foot. Greater than 10° difference suggests a second- or third-degree lateral ankle sprain.

Squeeze the Malleoli Together

Increased pain produced by squeezing the malleoli together suggests a syndesmotic sprain.

Externally Rotate Foot at the Ankle

Increased pain produced by externally rotating the foot at the ankle also suggests a syndesmotic sprain.

A PAINFUL FOREFOOT

Check for Anatomic Abnormalities

Lateral displacement of the great toe is hallux valgus. Pain on flexing the toes suggests an inflammatory lesion of the arch of the foot (Strunsky's sign).

Palpate the Toes and Metatarsal Heads

Tenderness and swelling next to a hallux valgus suggests bunion, gout, or trauma. Tenderness over the top of the toe after forced dorsiflexion is turf toe. Tenderness of the great toe distally suggests sesamoiditis. Toes with hyperextended MTP and PIP flexion with a corn on top suggest hammertoes. Toes that point upward are cock-up toes.

Tenderness over the plantar aspect of the metatarsal heads is metatarsalgia. Tenderness over the dorsal aspect of the metatarsal heads suggests metatarsal stress fracture. Discrete tenderness over the dorsal aspect of the second metatarsal head is Freiberg's infarction (aseptic necrosis).

Burning pain between the third and fourth toes at MTP joint suggests Morton's neuroma. To test for this, place your thumb between the third and fourth interspace on sole and push in. A click suggests Morton's neuroma (Mulder's sign). Swelling, tenderness and ecchymosis suggest a phalangeal fracture.

Thomas George Morton (1835–1903) was an American surgeon whose father was the dentist who discovered the anesthetic effect of ether. Morton was one of the first surgeons to successfully remove an appendix (with the patient surviving) after a correct diagnosis of appendicitis. He was a prolific medical writer and wrote a classic article on blood transfusion. He is best remembered for his neuroma and his metatarsalgia sometimes producing a sudden cramplike pain in the metatarsal area radiating to the 4th and 5th toe and sometimes to the calf of the leg.

A PAINFUL LATERAL FOOT

Palpate the Lateral Malleolus

Swelling and tenderness of the lateral malleolus suggests sprain, distal fibular fracture or a peroneal retinaculum sprain if the tenderness is at the posterior lateral malleolus.

Check for Tenderness at the Base of the Fifth Metatarsal

Tenderness at the base of the fifth metatarsal bone suggests avulsion fracture, bursitis, Jones's fracture if 2cm from the base, and metatarsalgia if the pain is over the metatarsal head.

Check for Ankle Joint Laxity

Check for anterior movement of calcaneus over tibia. Feeling a firm end point and less than 4mm of movement suggests a first-degree lateral sprain. Feeling a boggy end point and more than 4mm movement suggests a second-degree lateral sprain. Noting more than 4mm of movement and no end point suggests a third-degree lateral sprain.

Perform the Talar Tilt Test

Passively invert the foot and compare it with the opposite side. Noting greater than 10° difference suggests a second-or third-degree lateral sprain. If both the talofibular and calcaneofibular ligaments are ruptured, the talus will tilt but not with rupture of only one ligament (Talar tilt sign).

A PAINFUL MEDIAL FOOT

Check the Foot for Anatomic Abnormalities

Seeing a flat foot with tenderness and swelling at the base of the second metatarsal after a crush injury is Lisfranc's fracture.

Palpate the Medial Malleolus Moving Distally

Swelling and tenderness of medial malleolus suggests medial ankle sprain, and tibialis tendonitis (if posterior to the medial malleolus). Navicular tenderness suggests navicular bursitis. Pain and tingling over the medial and plantar aspects of the foot suggests the tarsal tunnel syndrome. Tap over the posterior-inferior aspect of the medial malleolus to reproduce the sensation (Tinel's sign).

Tenderness just distal and medial to the heel suggests plantar fascitis. Tenderness radiating from the medial arch to the medial great toe suggests flexor hallucis longus tendonitis. Palpate the central sole of foot before and after passive flexion of great toe. If this produces tenderness on flexion, it confirms flexor hallucis longus tendonitis.

Squeeze the Malleoli Together

Increased pain on squeezing the malleoli together suggests a syndesmotic sprain.

Externally Rotate the Foot at the Ankle

Increased pain on rotation of the foot at the ankle suggests a syndesmotic sprain.

A PAINFUL SOLE

Inspect the Sole for Anatomic Abnormalities

Lateral deviation of the great toe is hallux valgus. Thickening of the skin on the sole is a callus. Thickening of the plantar fascia with contractures of the lateral toes suggests a plantar Dupuytren's contracture. Seeing an increased arch suggests pes cavus (associated with congenital abnormalities). Redness, swelling and loss of the longitudinal arch suggest deep foot cellulites. Pain on the sole of the foot in thrombophlebitis is Payr's vascular sign.

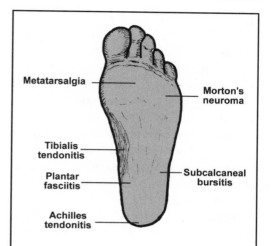

Figure 140. Painful Sites on the Sole.
Discomfort over the metatarsal heads suggests metatarsalgia. Burning pain between the third and fourth toes suggests Morton's neuroma. Tenderness over the medial plantar aspect suggests plantar fascitis. (Pain increases with flexing the toes.) Discomfort along the arch implies tibialis tendonitis. Pain located at the distal aspect of the calcaneus suggests subcalcaneal bursitis or Achilles tendonitis.

Palpate the Great Toe and Then the Metatarsal Heads

Tenderness of the plantar aspect of the metatarsal heads is metatarsalgia. Tenderness over the medial plantar aspect suggests plantar fascitis. (Pain increases with flexing the toes.) You may also palpate a bone spur on the distal aspect of calcaneus. Tenderness at the distal aspect of the calcaneus suggests subcalcaneal bursitis.

A PAINFUL HEEL

Look for Anatomic Abnormalities; Palpate the Achilles Tendon and the Heel

Tenderness and swelling deep to the Achilles tendon between the tendon and the calcaneus suggests retrocalcaneal bursitis. Tenderness of the overlying skin over the distal third of the Achilles tendon suggests tendo–Achilles tendonitis. Diffuse tenderness of the Achilles tendon suggests Achilles tendonitis. A discrete area of tenderness of the Achilles tendon suggests Achilles enthesitis.

Feeling a discrete gap in the Achilles tendon suggests Achilles tendon tear (a risk factor for an old person on fluoroquinolones and steroids). Check to see if the patient can push off toes while walking. Inability to do so confirms the tear. With the patient kneeling, gently squeeze the calf. Lack of passive plantar flexion (Simmond's sign) suggests tear or muscle damage. Tenderness immediately posterior to the medial malleolus suggests tibialis tendonitis. The patient will tend to stand with a slight valgus displacement of the toes.

Leg Signs of Endocrine or Metabolic Disorders

Cramping of the calves can be an early sign of diabetes mellitus (Unschuld's sign). Difficulty walking up stairs or rising from a chair secondary to proximal muscle weakness suggests hyperthyroidism (Plummer's sign).

Henry Stanley Plummer (1874–1937) was an American endocrinologist who worked at the Mayo Clinic. He described the use of iodine to treat hyperthyroidism and the toxic adenoma of the thyroid gland. Plummer's nails are the onycholysis of hyperthyroidism especially involving the ring finger.

Plummer-Vinson syndrome is characterized by an iron-deficiency anemia, atrophic changes in the buccal, glossopharyngeal, and oesophageal mucous membranes, koilonycha (spoon-shaped finger nails), and dysphagia.

Leg weakness, pain on gently squeezing the calves, decreased knee jerk reflexes and anesthesia over the anterior thigh suggests beriberi (Vedder's sign). Thigh flexion that produces knee spasm (Schlesinger) and calf spasm (Pool) suggests hypocalcemia (Pool-Schlesinger's sign). Eversion of the foot when tapping over the peroneal nerve suggests hypocalcemia (peroneal sign), my favorite way to determine hypocalcemia since it seems to be the first to appear and last to disappear.

Tenderness to percussion over the tibia suggests chlorosis (Golonbov's sign). Exquisite pain of the great toe when touching the fifth toe joint suggests gout (Plotz's sign). Loss of hair on the posterior surface of the legs suggests gout (Tommasi's sign).

CHAPTER 18

The Peripheral Vascular Examination

"Since all living things are warm, all dying things cold, there must be a ... seat and fountain, a kind of home and hearth, where the cherisher of nature, the original of the native fire, is stored and preserved; from which heat and life are dispensed to all parts as from a fountain head; from which sustenance may be derived; and upon which concoction and nutrition, and all vegetative energy may depend. Now that the heart is this place, that the heart is the principle of life ... I trust no one will deny."

— William Harvey

"Man is the only animal that blushes — or needs to."

— Mark Twain

The peripheral vascular examination provides valuable information on general health status. It can help us determine the effectiveness of the heart as a mechanical pump and the integrity of the arteries and veins. In addition, some specific systemic diseases have direct affects on the peripheral vascular system. Vascular disease is very common in elderly people and careful assessment of vascular structure, function and integrity is important consideration.

ARTERIAL EVALUATION

Be sure to feel the quality of the vessel as well as the pulse wave. Check the pulse on both sides at the same time (for example, radial, femoral or dorsalis pedis pulses). This is especially important if there is any beat-to-beat variation, such as atrial fibrillation or frequent premature contractions, because otherwise the difference in each side may be missed. Always measure the blood pressure in all extremities if you suspect arterial disease.

Check the capillary refill to ascertain small

vessel integrity. The three-second rule is to press a vascular bed (such as the great toe) and see if the blanching discoloration returns (as it should) in less than three seconds. Disappearance of a bruit with arterial compression suggests stenosis distal to the site of compression. Pulses that disappear with exercise are an indication for angiography (DeWeese's sign).

CAROTID ARTERIES

Inspection

The funduscopic exam provides a mechanism to evaluate distal branches of the internal carotid artery. Noting asymmetric arcus senilis may represent carotid obstruction on the side with the least amount of white pigmentation.

Carotid Artery Palpation

Palpate gently between the sternocleidomastoid and the trachea. Have the patient turn slightly toward you to relax the neck muscles. Do not go above the thyroid cartilage so you do not inadvertently massage the carotid sinus. Check the pulse rate and note the regularity of the pulse. An irregularly irregular rate suggests atrial fibrillation. A regular pulse with alternating strength (pulsus alternans) suggests an important sign of heart failure from any cause.

The Carotid Upstroke

Note whether the carotid upstroke is brisk or delayed, by comparing the pulse timing with the cardiac PMI. A delayed upstroke (pulsus parvus et tardus) suggests aortic stenosis, any left ventricular outflow obstruction or any significant decrease in stroke volume. Vascular stiffness due to aging can reduce the delay, causing a more normal feeling upstroke.

The Nature of the Carotid Pulsation

Note whether the impulse is vigorous or not. Feeling a bounding, vigorous upstroke with a rapid collapse (Corrigan's water hammer pulse) suggests aortic insufficiency due to the increased pulse pressure. Very rarely mitral insufficiency can give a vigorous upstroke.

Note whether the peak of the pulse is single, double or multiple. Feeling a single peak is normal. Feeling two peaks (bisferiens pulse) suggests asymmetric septal hypertrophy or combined aortic stenosis and insufficiency. A confirmatory trick is to listen over the brachial artery while slowly increasing the pressure on the artery. With enough pressure you will hear a systolic bruit that splits into two distinct bruits. Feeling multiple peaks, called a carotid shudder, suggests combined aortic stenosis and insufficiency. A carotid shutter can also be felt in isolated aortic valve lesions, including calcification of the aortic ring.

Note the nature of the collapse of the pulse wave. A rapid collapse suggests aortic insufficiency.

Note the presence of a vascular thrill.

Unequal Carotid Pulses

Unequal carotid pulses suggest carotid stenosis. (Check for asymmetric arcus senilis.) If every other beat feels weak (pulsus alternans), consider severe heart failure.

Auscultation Over the Carotids

The basic practice is to look for surgically correctable disease in symptomatic individuals. Use the bell of the stethoscope and start at the supraclavicular fossa along the sternocleidomastoid to assess the origin. Slowly listen up the neck to the angle of the jaw. The higher up the neck a bruit is heard, the more significant it may be and less likely it is to be a transmitted murmur. Significant bruits are high-pitched and may be loud. Swishing, to-

and-fro, or continuous bruits suggest significant obstruction. Loss of transmitted cardiac sounds with neck turning suggests carotid disease.

SPECIAL TESTS

Carotid Sinus Massage

This is a useful test to know how to perform, but it is even more important to know when not to perform it. When in doubt, don't. Do not perform this if there is evidence of old cerebrovascular disease. Listen for carotid bruits and do not perform this maneuver if a bruit is present. Also be very cautious in patients over age 85.

Have the supine patient turn the head gently away from the side to be massaged. Gently palpate the carotid pulse just below the angle of the jaw. Massage the pulsation for three to five seconds by pushing in and back to compress the artery. Do not exceed five seconds of carotid massage and *do not* massage both sides simultaneously. Massage the left carotid artery to affect the AV node. Massage the right carotid artery to affect the sinus node.

Interpretation

Most elderly patients will drop their systolic blood pressure with carotid sinus massage. In left bundle branch block the massage may transiently restore normal conduction as the rate slows. In suspected digitalis toxicity (digitalis may accentuate the carotid sinus reflex), if the basic rhythm evolves to a digitalis toxic rhythm, such as fixed coupling or high-grade heart block, then digitalis toxicity is likely.

♦ IN THE SETTING OF
A REGULAR TACHYCARDIA

If the tachycardia immediately drops to normal, then the condition was most likely paroxysmal atrial tachycardia. If the rate slows somewhat, then the condition is not ventricular tachycardia. If the rate slows gradually, then the condition is probably sinus tachycardia. If the slowing and recovery is chaotic, then the condition is probably atrial flutter or paroxysmal atrial tachycardia with block.

♦ IN THE SETTING OF
AN IRREGULAR TACHYCARDIA

If the rhythm becomes slow and irregular, then check rhythm with exercise. A rhythm that becomes regular with exercise suggests atrial flutter or paroxysmal atrial tachycardia with block. If the rhythm is slow and regular, then atrial fibrillation has been excluded.

♦ IN THE SETTING OF
A REGULAR BRADYCARDIA

If the slowing is chaotic or irregular, then suspect paroxysmal atrial tachycardia with block or second-degree AV block. If the rate speeds up, then consider 2:1 AV block that has been converted to regular conduction. No change in rate suggests complete heart block.

♦ IN THE SETTING OF
A NORMAL PULSE RATE

If the pulse rate dramatically slows or is one-half the original rate, then consider paroxysmal atrial tachycardia with block or atrial flutter.

Special Uses of Carotid Sinus Massage

♦ CHEST PAIN (LEVINE'S TEST)

Listen over the apex. Make sure the patient still has chest pain and have the patient quantify it on a 10-point scale. Massage the right carotid artery (to slow the sinus node). When you hear the heart slow, ask the patient to rate the pain again. A positive test for angina pectoris is a significant decrease in pain with massage.

♦ CONGESTIVE HEART FAILURE

Carotid massage will not work in the setting of aortic stenosis or atrial fibrillation. It may reverse a surprisingly large number of cases of pulmonary edema.

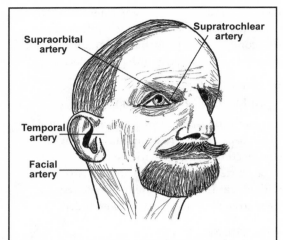

Figure 141. Testing for Internal Carotid Artery Occlusion.

Palpate the supraorbital artery (a branch of the internal carotid) above the mid-portion of the eyebrow (it is not always palpable) and keep your finger on the pulsation. Palpate the temporal artery (a branch of the external carotid) just in front of the tragus on the ipsilateral side. Gently press the temporal artery to obliterate the pulse. If the supraorbital arterial pulse disappears with the temporal artery pressure, then there is internal carotid artery occlusion.

Checking for Internal Carotid Occlusion

Palpate the supraorbital artery (a branch of the internal carotid) above the mid-portion of the eyebrow (it is not always palpable) and keep your finger on the pulsation. Palpate the temporal artery (a branch of the external carotid) just in front of the tragus on the ipsilateral side. Gently press the temporal artery to obliterate the pulse. If the supraorbital arterial pulse disappears with the temporal artery pressure, then there is internal carotid artery occlusion.

An alternative method: Palpate the supratrochlear artery (a branch of the internal carotid) in the inner canthus of the eye and keep your finger on the pulsation. Palpate the facial artery (a branch of the external carotid) along the angle of the mandible on the ipsilateral side. Gently press the facial artery to obliterate the pulse. If the supratrochlear arterial pulse disappears with the facial artery pressure, then there is internal carotid artery occlusion.

Unilateral arcus senilis suggests carotid occlusion on the side without the arcus.

Hearing a bruit over the carotid, eyeball and over the skull suggests contralateral carotid occlusion due to increased flow on the side without the occlusion (Fisher's sign).

> *Charles Miller Fisher (born 1913) was a Canadian neurologist who spent three-and-a-half years in a German prison camp in World War II. He used the time to learn German, which later allowed him to read primary texts on cerebrovascular disease. He described carotid artery stenosis and cardiac arrhythmias as risk factors for stroke, as well as the syndrome of transient ischemic attacks.*
>
> *In 1956 he described a disturbance now thought to be a variant of the Guillain-Barré syndrome. It is characterized by total external ophthalmoplegia, ataxia, and loss of tendon reflexes. Early symptoms include fever, headache, and pneumonia. They are followed by facial paralysis, diplopia, external ophthalmoplegia, and paresthesia of the arms and trunk.*

Determining Internal Carotid from External Carotid Bruits

Compressing the facial and temporal arteries will increase an internal carotid bruit and decrease an external carotid bruit. Hyperventilation increases the bruit of the external carotid artery and decreases the internal carotid bruit. Having the patient hold his or her breath for 20 seconds should increase an internal carotid artery bruit and decrease an external carotid bruit.

TEMPORAL ARTERIES

Palpate the temporal arteries just in front of the tragus of each ear and up along the temple. Always check these pulses in an elderly patient with headache or unilateral visual change, or when polymyalgia rheumatica, giant cell arteritis, or temporal arteritis is being considered. Palpate both sides at the same time. An absent pulse on one side or feeling a nodular or tender temporal artery suggests temporal arteritis.

SUBCLAVIAN ARTERIES

The subclavian arteries are usually palpable along the medial portion of the supraclavicular fossa. A bruit may be heard on the side ipsilateral to a hemodialysis vascular access. Pressing on the branchial artery will extinguish the bruit.

Subclavian Compression Syndromes

Subclavian compression syndromes may produce pain, tingling or cyanosis in the neck, shoulder, arm or hand. They are often associated with a particular movement or activity.

♦ SCALENUS ANTICUS COMPRESSION

Have the patient turn his or her head toward the painful side and raise the chin. If holding the breath after maximal inspiration produces pain or a subclavian bruit, or if the radial pulse disappears, that is a positive test (Adson's maneuver).

Also look for lateral cervical disc compression, since about fifty percent of these cervical discs will produce the scalenus anticus syndrome. Have the patient place his or her ear on the shoulder on the painful side. Gently press on the top of the head. Pain on pressing the head suggests lateral rupture of the intervertebral disc. Confirm by having the patient place a hand on his or her head. If the pain disappears, then nerve root compression is confirmed. Another test of scalenus anticus syn-

drome is to have the patient place both palms on the occiput and rotate the elbows back, as if sleeping on a hammock. Another test is to have the patient squeeze a tennis ball ten times behind his or her head, then feel the radial pulses and listen for a subclavian bruit. For each of these tests, pain, producing a subclavian bruit or losing the radial pulse, is a positive test.

♦ COSTOCLAVICULAR SUBCLAVIAN COMPRESSION

Palpate the radial pulse while the patient moves the shoulders back as far as possible and then down toward the ground. If this maneuver reproduces the patient's symptoms, it is a positive test.

UPPER EXTREMITY ARTERIES

Initial Observations

Inspect the arms from the shoulders to the fingertips, noting skin color, symmetry, venous distension and edema. Abnormal findings include skin pallor, redness, or cyanosis; bilateral or unilateral swelling or atrophy; or edema. In arterial insufficiency the skin becomes very thin, shiny, and atrophic. Fingernails become dusky and develop central depressions (Heller's deformity).

Note the skin temperature on each side. Use the back of your fingers and hands against the patient's fingers, and move up the arm from the hands to the shoulder. Coolness of the arm or localized areas of warmth or coolness are abnormal.

Check the capillary refill of the fingernail beds by lightly pinching the nail beds of the patient's fingers between the pads of the thumb and index finger of your right hand and release. Normally the fingerpad should return to normal in less than three seconds.

Radial Artery

Feel the vessel with two or three fingers. This helps to see if a sclerotic vessel will roll and helps to determine the degree of compressibility. Compare each side and compare with the femoral pulse. Normally the femoral pulse should be palpable just ahead of the radial pulse since the radial artery is further from the heart. If the radial pulse precedes the femoral pulse, then there is aortic obstruction.

Ulnar Artery

Check Allen's test. Have the patient rest the right hand with the palm up. Place your left thumb over the patient's radial artery and your right thumb lightly over the ulnar artery. Have the patient make a tight fist with the right hand. Compress the radial artery and the ulnar artery by pushing down with your thumbs. Now ask the patient to open the fist. The palm should be pale. Now release your right thumb from the ulnar artery. Normally the palm will immediately turn pink; if it does not then there is a lack of patency in the deep palmar arch.

Digital Arteries

Pallor in some digits but not others when the hand is elevated for two minutes suggests digital artery disease. Redness in some digits but not in others when the hand is dependent suggests digital artery disease.

♦ RAYNAUD'S PHENOMENON

Raynaud's phenomenon is a color change in the fingers when cold. There is pallor from ischemic vasospasm, redness from increased blood flow, and cyanosis from deoxygenated blood. It is associated with collagen vascular disease (SLE, scleroderma, mixed connective tissue disease), vascular disease (arterial vasculitis, arterial embolism), blood dyscrasias (cryoglobulinemia, polycythemia rubra vera, multiple myeloma), occupational exposure to vibration, toxic exposures (vinyl chloride, beta-blockers, ergot alkaloids), and many other conditions.

THORACIC AND ABDOMINAL ARTERIES

Aortic Aneurysm

Clues to a thoracic aneurysm include diminished left arm blood pressure, dullness to the right of the sternum (Potain's sign), feeling a tracheal tug, and hearing a new aortic regurgitation murmur. A clue to an abdominal aortic aneurysm is feeling a pulsatile abdominal mass. Feeling a width greater than 3.5cm is abnormal. An aneurysm moves your fingers apart while a mass over the aorta moves the fingers up and down. If you can move the mass up toward the head or down toward the feet, then it is not an aneurysm.

Dissecting Aneurysm

The patient will have tearing pain, often radiating to the back, and will appear restless and clammy. (Patients may say that the pain is so bad that they are afraid they are going to live.) The blood pressure may be elevated. Hypotension suggests a leaking abdominal aneurysm, especially if you find a pulsatile abdominal mass. A double pulse may be felt. Anterior dissection may produce aortic regurgitation and dullness to the right upper sternal border (Potain's sign). A warm, pulseless extremity suggests compromise of the sympathetic chain by the dissection.

Renal Arteries

Check for renal bruits in any elderly person with hypertension. Listen below the costal margin just above the umbilicus and along the paravertebral muscles down the flank (see Figure

117). Use the diaphragm of the stethoscope. The bruit is high-pitched and tends to be asymmetric. A to-and-fro swishing bruit suggests fibromuscular dysplasia.

Aorto-Iliac Disease (Leriche Syndrome)

Aortic-iliac disease, affecting the aortic bifurcation, causes vascular impotence, absent pulses in the groin or leg, fatigue and heaviness of the lower extremities, but does not affect toes and feet.

> *René Leriche (1879–1955) was a French surgeon who studied the control of pain and surgery of the autonomic nervous system during World War I. His classic "The Surgery of Pain" presents a comprehensive study of pain and its treatment in various diseases, and includes an excellent discussion of pain as an abstract concept. Leriche emphasized regarding the patient as a whole rather than concentrating on operative techniques. He was an outstanding technical surgeon, with a great flair for teaching and innovation. He was a superb speaker who never used notes.*
>
> *"Physical pain is not a simple affair of an impulse, traveling at a fixed rate along a nerve. It is the resultant of a conflict between a stimulus and the whole individual."*

LOWER EXTREMITY PULSES

Aneurysms of the abdominal aorta are associated with distal peripheral aneurysm. Atherosclerosis, although a generalized metabolic disorder, tends to build up at bifurcations of major vessels. In the lower extremity, the superficial femoral artery becomes occluded at the adductor hiatus. Diabetics tend to have femoral-tibial occlusions, whereas non–diabetics tend to have ileal-femoral occlusions.

Initial observations

Inspect the legs, from the groin to the feet, noting any asymmetry, skin changes, hair distribution, varicosities or edema. Signs of vascular insufficiency include pallor, coolness, cyanosis, atrophy, loss of hair, pigmentation along the shin or ankles, or ulcers. Check the capillary refill by pinching the great toes and noting the time it takes for the color of the nail beds to return to normal (normally less than three seconds).

Femoral Artery

Palpate the right femoral artery pulse by placing index and middle fingers of your left hand over the patient's right inquinal ligament about midway between the right anterior superior iliac spine and the right symphysis pubis. Feel the opposite side with your right hand at the left inguinal ligament, appreciating both pulses. Inequality of the pulse suggests vascular disease.

Now check the radial and femoral pulses on the right side. The femoral pulse should be felt before the radial pulse. Listen for a vascular bruit. If a bruit is present, then have the patient flex and extend the ankle rapidly to see if this increases the bruit. Also compress the femoral artery high in the femoral triangle near the inguinal ligament in the anterior-medial thigh. If the bruit increases, then consider occlusion of the profunda artery. If the bruit decreases, then consider occlusion of the common femoral artery or the proximal femoral artery. If the patient has a femoral popliteal bypass graft, then compression suggests occlusion of the graft is eminent.

Popliteal Artery

Have the patient supine and place both hands around the knee to feel in the popliteal space. Slowly lift the knee until you get to about 90°. If you cannot feel the pulse, then stop at 90°. Feel the skin temperature over the shin. Normally there is a point of warmth at the upper portion of the anterior thigh. Coolness in this area suggests acute vascular insufficiency. In chronic popliteal disease vascular collaterals may cause the involved knee to feel warmer rather than cooler.

Dorsalis Pedis and Posterior Tibial Arteries

The dorsalis pedis pulse is usually felt along the dorsum of the foot just lateral to the extensor tendon of the great toe. The posterior tibial pulse is usually just behind and slightly below the medial malleolus.

VENOUS EXAMINATION

Jugular Veins
(see also Chapter 15)

Have the patient begin supine, then elevate the examining table until the top of the venous pulse wave is visible. Always examine the patient from the right side, looking at the right neck because there is a more accurate determination since it is a straight shot from jugular veins to the superior vena cava and right atrium. Check to see that the left side is about the same height. Distension only on the left side suggests compression of the left side by aortic aneurysm or extreme ectasia of the aorta.

Have the patient turn the head slightly to the left. Look just lateral to the lateral head of the sternocleidomastoid to see if the internal jugular pulsation is visible. (If so use it.) Look along the right supraclavicular fossa for the external jugular vein. Confirm the vein by gently compressing it at the base of the neck and watching it distend. If you cannot see the jugular veins, have the patient perform Valsalva's maneuver to increase the venous pressure.

Determining the Central Venous Pressure

Note the height of the column of blood by using whichever vein is most distended.

Note the highest level of the pulsation. This may appear as a flicker. Estimate the height of the venous column by going from the height of the pulsation to the fourth intercostal space, about half (or a little less) of the cross-sectional diameter of the body which is the level of the right atrium. The upper limit of normal by this approach is 16cm of water. More than 3cm above the clavicle is abnormal.

Confirm the height by Gartner's maneuver: Raise the right hand very slowly until the veins begin to collapse and note the height of the hand compared to the right atrial reference at the fourth intercostal space.

Also confirm increased venous pressure by von Recklinghausen's maneuver. Have the supine patient place one hand on a thigh and one hand on the bed. If both hands show venous distension, then the venous pressure is elevated. If only the veins on the hand on the bed are distended, then the venous pressure is normal. Confirm increased venous pressure by checking the sublingual veins. Dilation of the sublingual veins suggests elevated venous pressure.

Variations in the Venous Pulse with Respiration

Note the variations in the JVP with respiration. Collapse of the venous column with inspiration is normal. Seeing an increase in JVP with inspiration (Kussmaul's sign) suggests a problem with right atrial filling, such as constrictive pericarditis or right ventricular failure.

Next, study the venous waveforms. This evaluation is covered in detail in Chapter 15.

Arm Veins

Distended arm veins and upper chest veins in an upright patient suggest superior vena cava syndrome. The patient will also have Kussmaul's sign, with an increase in JVP with inspiration. Confirm with additional increase in arm pressure by placing a tourniquet under the arms and across the chest.

Unilateral distension and swelling suggests upper extremity deep venous clot. This is usually caused by malignancy (lung, stomach, pancreas, breast, head and neck, and prostate).

Leg Veins

◆ SIGNS OF DEEP VENOUS OBSTRUCTION

Dilated veins over the tibial plateau in a supine patient that do not collapse with elevating the leg (Pratt's sign) suggest deep venous obstruction. Unilateral warm, stiff feeling skin to a pinch (secondary to edema) suggests deep venous thrombosis (Rose's sign). Measure the difference in circumference of a distended calf. Observing more than 2.5cm difference between the calves suggests deep venous thrombosis (2cm difference in the thigh). Tenderness to percussion of the medial surface of the tibia suggests deep venous thrombosis (Lisker's sign). Cough-induced pain that disappears when the proximal vein is compressed suggests deep venous thrombosis (Louvel's sign). Asymmetric tenderness to blood pressure cuff inflation at less than half the pressure of the opposite side suggests deep venous thrombosis (Löwenberg's sign).

◆ VARICOSE VEINS

Varicose veins with pulsations suggest tricuspid insufficiency. Hearing a murmur over the veins suggests tricuspid insufficiency. Dark purple discoloration of the skin with varicose veins suggests AV fistula.

Inspect the saphenous system for varicosities that will appear as large wormlike, tortuous vessels. Perform the manual compression test by having the patient stand, and then placing your right hand over the distal lower part of the varicose vein and your left hand over the proximal vein. Your hands will be about 15–20cm apart. Compress the proximal

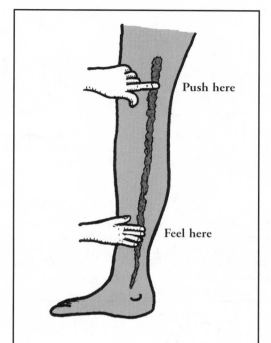

Figure 142. Manual Compression Test.
Have the patient stand, and place your right hand over the distal lower part of the varicose vein and your left hand over the proximal vein. Your hands will be about 15–20cm apart. Compress the proximal portion of the varicose vein with your left hand. If you feel a palpable pulsation in your distal hand, the test is positive, indicating insufficiency of the saphenous venous system.

portion of the varicose vein. If you feel a palpable pulsation in your distal hand, the test is positive.

Now perform Trendelenburg's test. Have the supine patient elevate a leg to 90° until the venous blood has drained from the great saphenous vein. Now place a tourniquet around the upper thigh of the patient's leg, tightly enough to occlude the great saphenous vein but not the arterial pressure. Help the patient stand and look for venous filling. Slow filling (over 30 seconds) from below of the superficial veins, while the tourniquet is applied, is normal. Rapid filling of the superficial veins is abnormal, as is sudden additional filling of the superficial veins after the tourniquet is released.

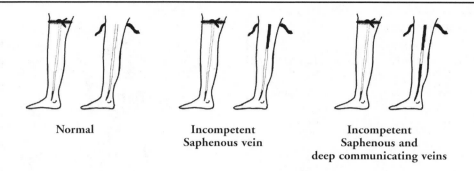

Normal   Incompetent
Saphenous vein   Incompetent
Saphenous and
deep communicating veins

Figure 143. Trendelenberg's Test.

Have the supine patient elevate a leg to 90° until the venous blood has drained from the great saphenous vein. Now place a tourniquet around the upper thigh of the patient's leg, tightly enough to occlude the vein but not the arterial pressure. Help the patient stand and look for venous filling. Slow filling (over 30 seconds) from below of the superficial veins, while the tourniquet is applied, is normal. Rapid filling of the superficial veins is abnormal, as is sudden additional filling of the superficial veins after the tourniquet is released.

SPECIAL TESTS

Buerger's Test of Lower Extremity Arterial Insufficiency

Raise the patient's leg above his or her head. If the sole of the foot becomes pale, then that is a positive test. Now let the legs hang dependent to see if the involved leg becomes cyanotic or hyperemic, to confirm the vascular insufficiency.

Leo Buerger (1879–1943) was an Austria-born American physician and urologist. As professor of urological surgery at Mt. Sinai Hospital, Buerger developed a radium therapy against malignant bladder tumors. In collaboration with F. Tilder Brown he developed a cystoscope.

Bueger's disease is a chronic inflammatory disease of the peripheral vessels forming blood clots that reduce blood flow, and produce ulceration and gangrene. Severe pain of the extremities at rest is the first symptom in four-fifths of cases. The pain resembles intermittent claudication and usually causes insomnia. Other features include cold extremities, sudden sweating, and occasionally Raynaud's phenomenon. Central nervous system involvement may include focal lesions of the cerebral cortex with resulting paralysis, sensory disorders, convulsions, aphasia,

hemianopsia, personality changes, and mental deterioration. It occurs almost exclusively in males. This disease was mentioned already by the late fifth century B.C. Greek historian Thucydides. In modern times it was first described in 1876 by Carl Friedländer (1847–1887) as arteritis obliterans.

Dorsalis Pedis-Brachial Systolic Pressure Ratio

Normally the dorsalis pedis pressure is up to 10mmHg higher than the brachial blood pressure. With exercise-induced symptoms the ratio is 0.5 or more, and the apparent dorsalis pedis resting blood pressure is more than 60mmHg.

Hepatojugular Reflux (Pasteur's Test)

HJR suggests right-sided heart failure, tricuspid regurgitation, pericardial disease, and inferior vena cava obstruction. It is an excellent way to differentiate tricuspid insufficiency from mitral insufficiency.

Position the patient so that you can see the top of the venous pulse. Place your hand over the right upper quadrant and gently push in toward the spine for at least 30 seconds while having the patient relax and breathe normally. A rise in the venous pressure of more than 3cm is a positive test.

Perthes' Test

Apply a tourniquet at the mid-thigh, at a pressure below arterial pressure, and have the patient walk for five minutes. Normally the walk will reduce the caliber of the greater saphenous vein, implying that the deep veins and the communicating veins are competent. If there is deep venous obstruction, the greater saphenous vein will be more distended and often painful. No change in size of the greater saphenous vein suggests that all the leg veins are incompetent.

Georg Clemens Perthes (1869–1927) was a German surgeon who was orphaned early in childhood and raised by an aunt. He chose medicine as a career through family connections with the famous surgeon Friedrich Trendelenburg. His surgical innovations include the method of draining an empyema, the right upper quadrant incision, and a pneumatic cuff for bloodless limb surgery. Perthes performed extensive studies on X-rays and was an early pioneer of radiation therapy for breast cancer. He was the first to radiograph congenital aseptic necrosis of the femoral head.

CHAPTER 19

The Female Genitalia

"Education is an admirable thing, but it is well to remember from time to time that nothing that is worth knowing can be taught."

— Oscar Wilde

"Patience is the companion of wisdom."

— Saint Augustine

Having laid the appropriate groundwork with an attentive history and thoughtful physical examination to this point will make the female genital exam easier and help relax the patient. Review with the patient what you are going to do before you start and allow the patient to empty her bowels or bladder. Make sure the end of the table does not face a door and that the room is warm. Male doctors must always have a female assistant in the room at all times.

Appreciate the patient's sense of vulnerability and act respectfully and carefully. Make sure your gloved hands are warm and the patient is comfortable. Position the patient at the end of the examination table and help her get into the stirrups.

Patients with degenerative joint disease involving the hips can be examined in Sim's position (left lateral decubitus) with her right thigh flexed.

James Marion Sims (1813–1883) was an American gynecologist considered by many to be the father of gynecology. He is chiefly remembered for his vaginal speculum, his operational approach to vesico-vaginal fistula, and the lithotomy position, called Sim's position. Sims continued practicing as a surgeon right up to his death. Within weeks after his death, a suggestion was made in the Medical Record that a statue be erected in his memory. The Sims statue, erected in 1894, was the first ever to be erected in the United States in honor of a physician and stands today in Bryant Park in New York City. "Let man learn to be honest and do the right thing or do nothing."

INSPECTION

Note the Pubic Hair

Absent pubic hair suggests endocrine dysfunction. Look carefully at the hair. Lice eggs attach to the hairs and can be seen.

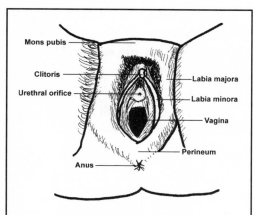

Figure 144. Female External Genitalia.
The female external genitalia is composed of the mons pubis, vulva (which includes the clitoris, urethral orifice and labia), vagina, and perianal areas.

Check for Labial Lesions

♦ LOOK CAREFULLY FOR PIGMENTED AND HYPOPIGMENTED LESIONS

A pigmented macule with irregular borders suggests malignant melanoma or a dysplastic nevus. Symmetric, hypopigmented, shiny, itchy macules suggest lichen sclerosis et chronicus. Look for an underlying vulvar carcinoma. If the introitus is scarred with fissures, then it is kraurosis vulvae. Ecchymoses on the

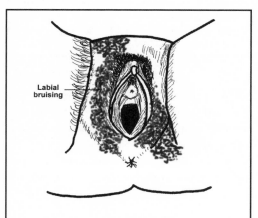

Figure 145. Coopernail's Sign.
Coopernail's sign is ecchymoses observed on the mons pubis, perineum or labia. The sign suggests pelvic fracture.

mons pubis, perineum or labia suggests pelvic fracture (Coopernail's sign).

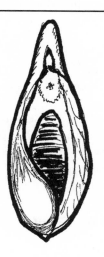

Figure 146. Bartholin's Cyst.
Bartholin's glands are located on the inner labial wall and can develop cysts (when obstructed) or abscess from an infection. Noting a non-tender swelling on the posterior labia majora suggests a cyst. Tenderness implies abscess. Also consider malignancy in the differential diagnosis of a labial mass.

♦ LOOK FOR MASSES

Several non-tender nodules along the outer border of the labia suggests sebaceous cysts. Bartholin's glands are located on the inner labial wall and can develop cysts (when obstructed) or abscess from an infection. Consider possible malignancy in any newly discovered labial mass in an elderly woman. Multiple small cysts that line the inner vaginal wall are Gartner's duct cysts. Raised dome-like papules with a central depression suggest molluscum contagiosum. Multiple, irregular, flesh-colored papules suggest condyloma acuminatum. Plaques with central pearly exudates suggest condyloma latum.

♦ SEARCH FOR GENITAL ULCERS

Painful vesicles suggest herpes infection. A single painless ulcer with a fibrotic rim suggests primary syphilis. A single painful ulcer suggests lymphogranuloma venereum. Seeing an ulcerated plaque with irregular margins suggests vulvar malignancy, Behçet's syndrome, dermatitis herpetiformis, and erythema multiforme.

◆ NOTE ANY GENITAL PLAQUES

Red plaques that itch and have serous oozing suggests contact dermatitis. Red plaques with silver scales and well-demarcated border suggest psoriasis. A plaque resembling psoriasis but darker red and friable suggests Paget's disease of the vulva. A bright red rash that involves the labia suggests candida. A bright red rash that spares the labia suggests tinea cruris.

Look for Fistulous Tracts

Seeing any fistuli suggests Crohn's disease, perirectal abscess, diverticulosis, and malignancy.

Sir James Paget (1814–1899) is considered one of the founders of modern pathology. During his first year as a medical student he noted some white specks in the muscle of a cadaver and found them to be small, encapsulated worms, later named Trichina spiralis by the British anatomist and palaeontologist Richard Owen (1804–1892). This was the first demonstration of trichinosis in humans. Paget made notable scientific contributions as well as writing important books on surgical pathology, tumors and surgery. In 1871, after narrowly escaping death from infection following an accidental cut during a post mortem investigation, Paget restricted himself to consulting practice. His success was phenomenal, resting on his charming personality as much as his anatomical pathological knowledge and surgical skill.

Paget was one of the first to recommend surgical removal of bone marrow tumors (myeloid sarcoma) instead of amputating the limb. If Paget's main field was in surgery, he is now chiefly remembered as an outstanding histologist, one of the first to encourage the study of pathological histology.

His fame rests on his descriptions of several diseases, the most famous of which is osteitis deformans which he described in 1877.

Touch the Patient's Inner Thigh After Informing Her and Then Gently Spread the Labia Majora

◆ NOTE THE LABIA MINORA

This is a common site for malignancy. Look for any ulcers or masses.

◆ EXAMINE THE CLITORIS

Enlargement suggests an endocrine problem.

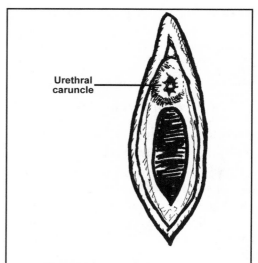

Urethral caruncle

Figure 147. Urethral Caruncle.
Normally the urethra is the same color as the surrounding skin. A cherry-red, slightly enlarged urethral orifice suggests urethral prolapse called a urethral caruncle.

◆ CAREFULLY LOOK AT THE URETHRA

Generally the urethra is the same color as the surrounding skin. A cherry-red urethra suggests urethral prolapse called a urethral caruncle. Polyps, if present, are often on the posterior surface. Seeing a purulent discharge suggests urethral diverticulum, urethritis, or significant urinary tract infection.

◆ EXAMINE THE INTROITUS

Seeing bulging of the anterior superior vaginal roof from above is a cystocele. Seeing bulging of the vaginal floor from below is a

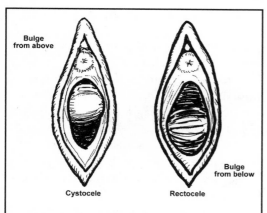

Figure 148. Cystocele and Rectocele.
Seeing bulging of the anterior superior vaginal roof from above and into the introitus is a cystocele. Seeing bulging of the vaginal floor from below is a rectocele. If the cervix is visible at the introitus, there is uterine prolapse.

rectocele. If the cervix is visible at the introitus, then there is uterine prolapse.

PALPATION

Gently Palpate Along the Labia

Bartholin's glands are not normally palpable. Palpable glands suggest inflammation. Skene's glands are on either side of the urethra.

Carefully Palpate the Urethra

Gently insert your gloved finger two inches into the introitus, and feel the posterior urethral margin on the superior vaginal wall. Note any urethral discharge.

Now Check the Pelvic Muscle Tone

Gently insert your forefinger and middle finger together into the introitus and have patient squeeze your fingers. (Do not tell patient to relax, since this is counterproductive, and does not work.) Pay attention to the muscle

tone. Gently separate your fingers laterally and have the patient bear down. Seeing urine flow suggests stress urinary incontinence. Follow this observation by performing the Bonney-Read-Marchetti test. More information on this test is included in Chapter 24.

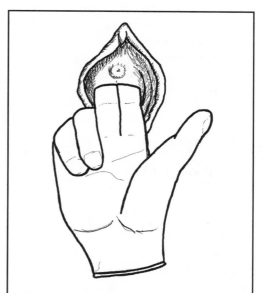

Figure 149. Bonney-Read-Marchetti Test.
This test is performed if urine leakage is observed when pushing on the abdomen during pelvic examination. Perform the test by gently elevating the urethra approximately a centimeter with your forefinger and middle finger, and then pushing on the abdomen again. No urine flow is a positive test and suggests loss of the posterior urethrovesical angle. Chapter 24 discusses the significance of this observation.

Perform the Bonney-Read-Marchetti Test

Perform the Bonney-Read-Marchetti test by gently elevating the urethra approximately a centimeter with your forefinger and middle finger, and having the patient bear down again. No urine flow is a positive test and suggests loss of the posterior urethrovesical angle. Downward bulging of the vagina suggests a cystocele. Upward bulging suggests a rectocele. Protrusion of the cervix suggests uterine prolapse.

Feel the Vaginal Walls for Carcinoma or Fistulae

♦ CHECK FOR SWELLING
AT THE OBTURATOR FORAMEN

Check for swelling at the obturator foramen (on the lateral border between the pubic symphysis and the ischium). Noting a painful swelling suggests a Richter's hernia. Richter's hernia may present as knee pain (Howship-Romberg's sign) and limited range of motion of the hip.

INTERNAL SPECULUM EXAMINATION

Inform the Patient of the Examination

Touch the patient's inner thigh to give the patient the sense that the exam will begin. Gently place your forefinger and middle fingers into the introitus and gently push down. Move the left labia to the side with your left thumb to reduce the likelihood of pinching the labia or getting hair caught in the speculum.

Gently Insert the Closed Speculum

Gently insert the closed speculum horizontally just over your fingers. Have the patient bear down to help relax the perineum. Watch the skin texture and color for stretching or pallor indicating an improper angle. Once inserted, slowly advance the speculum to avoid discomfort. Gently separate the blades of the speculum by moving posteriorly.

Note Any Discharge

A white and bulky discharge suggests monilial infection. A fishy-smelling, foamy discharge suggests trichomonas. A thin, purulent discharge suggests bacterial infection.

Examine the Cervix

Locate and examine the cervix (sometimes easier said than done; experience is key). The size is usually three centimeters. The opening or os is generally a slit. Note any discharge or secretions from the os. Purulent discharge suggests cervicitis.

Check for masses, ulcers or changes in pigmentation. A soft polyp is a cervical polyp. An ulcer on the cervix suggests cervical cancer. Smooth, round, tan-colored lesions are likely to be nabothian cysts.

Examine the Vaginal Mucosa as You Slowly Withdraw the Speculum

Openings in the mucosa suggest rectovaginal fistulae.

BIMANUAL EXAMINATION

Gently Insert Your Forefinger and Middle Finger Posteriorly Into the Vaginal Introitus

Check the vaginal walls, noting any masses or irregularities.

Palpate the Cervix

Deviation from the midline suggests a mass, inflammation or other abnormality. The shape and texture of the cervix should be smooth and not lumpy. Note the cervical mobility by pushing upward. The cervix should easily move a centimeter or so in each direction. Tenderness to movement suggests pelvic inflammation. A rock-hard sensation suggests malignancy. Palpate around the cervix.

Examine the Uterus

Gently push down between the umbilicus and the pubic symphysis with your other hand. Gently push upward with your internal hand to feel the uterus between your hands. Pay attention to the size and texture. Bogginess of the uterus with a purulent discharge from the os suggests endometritis. Feel for any masses along the uterine surface, such as leiomyoma. Note any limitation of movement to palpation. Limited uterine movement suggests adhesions or malignancy.

Palpate the Adnexa

Move lateral to the uterine fundus to the patient's left and lateral with your abdominal hand to the left lower quadrant. Gently push your hands together in a forward pulling movement to feel the left ovary. Ovaries are not generally felt in post-menopausal women. Note any masses, irregularities or other abnormalities. Check the structures on the right side.

Adnexal masses suggest ovarian neoplasm, stool in the sigmoid colon, redundant sigmoid colon, distended cecum, appendiceal abscess and pelvic tuberculosis. A large mass may be an enlarged ovarian cyst. Confirm a large cyst by Blaxland's test: Place a ruler on the abdomen just above the iliac crest. Push down on the ruler. Feeling the aortic pulse with the ruler is a positive test. Ascites or other swelling will not produce the aortic pulsation.

RECTOVAGINAL EXAMINATION

Change gloves. Gently insert your forefinger into the introitus and your lubricated middle finger into the anal opening. Feel between your fingers for atrophy of the perineal muscle. Feel carefully for masses along the rectovaginal septum. Feel the uterus with the bimanual technique. Feel the adnexa with the bimanual technique.

CHAPTER 20

The Male Genitalia

"Youth is easily deceived because it is quick to hope."

— **Aristotle**

"The art of being wise is the art of knowing what to overlook."

— **William James**

Remember the sensitivity of the genitals to pressure, so go slowly and gently. Wear gloves. Some organisms such as spirochetes can be transmitted to you if you have any open skin lesion. The nature of the examination may produce a normal autonomic response of erectile function. Normally the scrotum hangs relaxed unless it is cold.

INSPECTION

Examine the Glans

Examine the glans while holding the penile shaft. If the patient is uncircumcised, look for fissures on the edge of the foreskin. (These suggest infection.) Retraction of foreskin should be smooth and easy. Difficulty in retraction of the foreskin suggests phimosis. Difficulty in reexpansion is paraphimosis. Pur-

ple discoloration with irregular borders on the glans penis suggests urinary extravasation into the corpus cavernosum (Brodie's sign).

Search for Skin Lesions

Ulcers suggest sexually transmitted disease or malignancy. Syphilis (chancre) produces a fibrotic rim to the painless ulcer. A syphilitic chancre may feel like a coin under the skin when examined with the eyes closed. There are often bilateral inguinal lymph nodes. Other (much less common) lesions include chancroid and Herpes simplex (multiple vesicles that are painful). Note any nodules, scars, or signs of inflammation. Ecchymoses on the perineum, or scrotum suggests pelvic fracture (Coopernail's sign).

Sir Benjamin Collins Brodie (1783–1862) was one of the great surgeons in London during the 1800s. Perhaps Brodie's greatest claim to

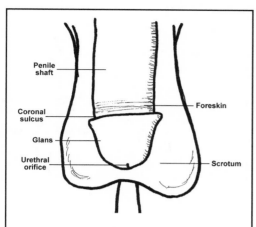

Figure 150. Male External Genitalia.

The male external genitalia include the penis and scrotum. The penis is composed of the penile shaft and the glans penis with the urethral orifice. The corona is the site of the circumcised foreskin.

fame in the field of surgery was the fact that he preferred to do as little of it as possible. His major academic accomplishment was in writing Pathological and Surgical Observations on Diseases of the Joints. *He described case histories of a tuberculous abscess in the head of the tibia (Brodie's abscess), synovitis in the knee, and Reiter's syndrome. Brodie also pioneered the field of varicose vein surgery and developed the Brodie-Trendelenburg Percussion Test for venous valve insufficiency of superficial veins.*

Examine the Urethral Meatus

Normally the urethral meatus is in the middle of the glans. If it is displaced toward 12 o'clock as you look at it (dorsally), this suggests epispadias. If it is displaced toward 6 o'clock as you look at it (ventrally), then it is hypospadias. Note the patency and document any lesion.

Examine Any Penile Discharge

Examine any discharge and be sure to culture it. If the discharge is thick, consider neisseria infection. If the discharge is thin, consider nongonococcal inflammation, such as chlamydia or Reiter's syndrome.

Examine the Penile Shaft

Lichen planus, scabies, psoriasis and secondary syphilis are common causes of penile rashes. Non-tender plaques felt on the lateral margin or along the dorsal midline structures suggest Peyronie's disease.

François de la Peyronie (1678–1747) was the royal surgeon to King Louis XIV. In 1743 he described his famous disease, with the cases of three men with fibrous thickening of the penile shaft, painful erections, and penile curvature. The condition was first described in 1587 by Guilio Cesare Aranzi in his book Tumores Praeter Naturam. *He called the condition "a rare affection of the genitals in people with excessive sexual intercourse: a little penile tumor palpable like a bean in the flaccid penis causing a deformity similar to a ram horn during erection."*

Check the Pubic Hair for Lice

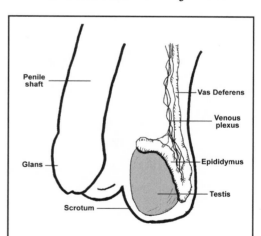

Figure 151. Normal Scrotal Anatomy.

This illustration shows the normal scrotal contents. The epididymus sits on the testis in the most dependent location of the scrotum. The vas deferens, testicular artery and venous plexus all attach to the epididymus.

Examine the Scrotum

Examine the scrotum by lifting the penis up and out of the way. The left side should hang lower than the right. Check the surrounding skin for fungal infection. Candida usually involves the scrotum. (Also check for satellite lesions.) Tinea cruris does not affect the scrotum.

Red, raised, hyperkeratotic lesions suggest Fordyce disease. These are benign and usually do not require treatment or further evaluation. Kaposi's sarcoma produces larger lesions.

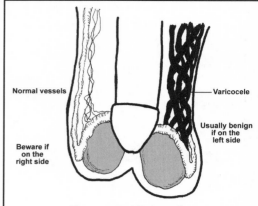

Figure 153. Varicocele.
Painless dilation of the venous plexus is a varicocele. It feels like a bag of worms above the testis. A right-sided varicocele in an elderly man is concerning for malignancy.

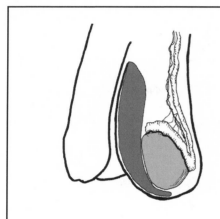

Figure 152. Hydrocele.
A hydrocele is a painless unilateral swelling of clear fluid that transilluminates. The location of the fluid is anterior to the testis.

Note Any Scrotal Swelling, Edema or Inflammation

A swollen left testicle suggests left renal vein obstruction (the vein of the three-paired organs). A large unilateral scrotal mass suggests inguinal hernia or hydrocele; differentiate by transillumination (see Figure 152). A large edematous scrotum suggests right heart failure or any other condition causing significant fluid buildup. A large edematous scrotum with crepitus or eschar suggests necrotizing fasciitis (Fournier's gangrene). This is usually associated with GI or GU pathology. Also consider diabetes or polyarteritis nodosa. A large "bag of worms" appearance on the left side is most likely a varicocele. A right varicocele is unusual and suggests testicular cancer. If the patient has significant proteinuria, strongly consider renal vein thrombosis.

PALPATION

Note Any Plaques or Areas of Fibrosis Along the Penile Shaft

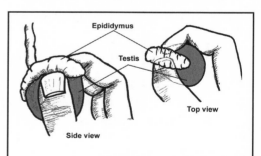

Figure 154. Testicular Palpation.
Gently pinching the sinus of the epididymus can separate the epididymus from the testis. The testis feels smooth, oval and firm. The epididymus normally feels soft and string-like.

Palpate the Scrotal Contents

Be gentle. This obviously avoids discomfort but also minimizes the cremasteric reflex, which can make palpation more challenging. Gently hold each testicle and check the size and consistency. Normally each testicle is about

1.5–2 inches. A large, tender testis suggests or-chitis. A soft consistency suggests atrophy. Each testis should be freely movable. Hypes-thesia of the scrotum suggests neurosyphilis (Pitres' sign).

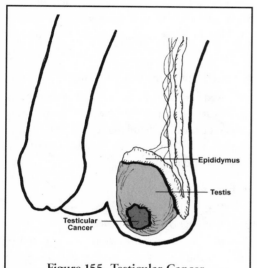

Figure 155. Testicular Cancer.
Testicular cancer usually presents as a hard, painless mass, often on the anterior portion of the testicle.

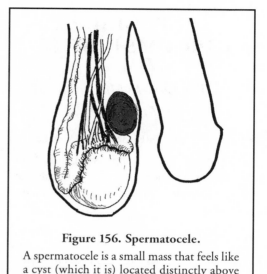

Figure 156. Spermatocele.
A spermatocele is a small mass that feels like a cyst (which it is) located distinctly above the testis. It transilluminates.

Check for Scrotal Masses or Nodules

If a mass is present, note whether it is at-tached to the testis and is distinct from the testes. Note its position on the testis if it is at-tached. A location opposite the epididymis suggests testicular cancer (see Figure 155).

Feel the Epididymis

Feel the epididymis along the top and side of each testicle. It feels like a firm piece of string. Hold the testicle with one hand and palpate the epididymis with the forefinger of your other hand. Feeling a small cystic nodule behind the epididymis suggests a spermato-cele (see Figure 156). Feeling a small, tender nodule at the top of the epididymis suggests epididymitis.

Examine the Spermatic Cord and the Vas Deferens

Note the spermatic cord and the vas def-erens exiting from the epididymis. Trace the spermatic cord to the inguinal canal.

Transilluminate Any Swelling or Mass

Darken the room. Gently pull the scro-tum and shine a bright light from behind the scrotum. Hematoceles will not show any transillumination. Hydroceles will transillu-minate.

Define the Top of the Testicle in Any Swelling

Testicular enlargement should still allow the examiner to feel the upper border of the testicle by palpating along the epididymal sinus. If you cannot feel the upper border of the testicle, consider the possibility of an in-guinal hernia.

SPECIAL CIRCUMSTANCES

The Elderly Man with a Penile Lesion

♦ CHECK FOR FORESKIN INVOLVEMENT

Redness of the foreskin is balanitis. Foreskin that cannot be retracted is phimosis. Retracted foreskin that traps the glans is paraphimosis.

♦ CHECK FOR SKIN LESIONS

Painful vesicles suggest herpes infection. Dome-shaped papules with central depression suggests molluscum contagiosum. Warty lesions suggest condylomata acuminata. Ulcers beside condyloma acuminata suggest penile carcinoma. A painful ulcer or plaque suggests lymphogranuloma venereum. A painless ulcer with fibrotic rim suggests primary syphilis.

The Elderly Man with a Painful Scrotum

♦ CHECK THE CREMASTERIC REFLEX

Check the cremasteric reflex by stroking the inner aspect of the thigh. Seeing a normal reflex (elevation of testis) suggests epididymitis. No cremasteric reflex suggests testicular torsion.

♦ CAREFULLY INSPECT THE SKIN

Redness that spares the scrotum suggests tinea cruris. Redness that involves the scrotum suggests candida. Plaque-like redness suggests erythrasma. (Look for coral red fluorescence under Wood's light.)

♦ ELEVATE THE SCROTUM

Pain relief by elevating the scrotum suggests orchitis or epididymitis, as opposed to testicular torsion (Prehn's sign). Failure to distinguish the epididymis from the body of the testes suggests testicular torsion (Rocher's sign). Failure to extend the testes by gently pulling on it suggests fibrosis and testicular atrophy (Kantor's sign).

CHAPTER 21

The Neurological Examination

"If ... the commencement of the affection be below the head, such as the membrane of the spinal marrow, the parts which are homonymous and connected with it are paralyzed: the right on the right side, and the left on the left side. But if the head be primarily affected on the right side, the left side of the body will be paralyzed; and the right, if on the left side."

— **Aretaeus the Cappadocian**

"The peculiar charm of neurology lies in fact in the satisfaction implicit in its logical structure, and perhaps even more in the essentially clinical nature of the discipline.... The physical signs of a neurological disorder are for the most part unequivocal: the pathognomonic significance of the extensor plantar response is inevitably more clear-cut than that of the basal rale or the suspicion of ankle edema."

— **Henry George Miller**

The neurological examination evaluates the central and peripheral nervous system by observing the patient's responses to specific stimuli. Sometimes these stimuli are natural phenomena such as light or light touch. At other times the stimuli are somewhat unusual, such as placing a tuning fork on the foot. Sometimes the responses searched for are normal responses, while at other times pathological responses are the focus of inquiry.

The neurological examination described in this chapter is a reasonable screening examination. Virtually every phase of it can be expanded, and should be expanded if specific neurological findings suggest the need.

MENTAL STATUS EVALUATION

This evaluation is covered in more detail in Chapter 22 which is devoted to evaluating the patient with possible dementia. In overview, the goal of the mental status examination is to determine whether the patient is able to perceive and act on risks in the environment. This is the clinically relevant question. In order to answer this question, the entire clinical encounter becomes the physical examination of the intellect.

The key to appreciating a memory impairment or subtle dementing illness is to perceive incongruities among the patient's appearance, dress, language and behaviors (see Chapter 3). Other important areas for the clinician to focus on are the patient's level of consciousness, degree of orientation, affect, mood and cognition. Important elements of cognition are attention span, memory (immediate, short-term, and long-term), calculation and judgment.

A critical early feature is that elderly people with early dementing illness often have very limited ability to use their imagination. Patients with distortions in time or space, or dream-like illusions (Alice in Wonderland sign), may have a parietal lobe process.

MOTOR EXAMINATION

Basic Strategy

The basic approach to muscle testing of motor function is to oppose the muscle group being tested. Compare each side by testing the sides simultaneously where it is practical (having the patient rise up on the toes) and each side sequentially when it is not so practical (testing biceps strength).

The fundamental observations are muscle strength, muscle tone, and the presence of adventitious movements. Weak muscles release very smoothly compared to pain-limited breakaway weakness or clasp knife rigidity (vide infra).

Patterns of Muscle Weakness

Patterns of weakness are also important to recognize. If one side of the body is weak that is hemiparesis. One side of the body being paralyzed is hemiplegia. If both lower extremities are weak, that is paraparesis; both lower extremities being paralyzed is paraplegia. If all four extremities are weak, that is quadriparesis; all four extremities being paralyzed is quadriplegia.

Proximal muscle weakness, such as shoulder girdle and quadriceps weakness, is a sign of myopathy, often due to an endocrine or metabolic abnormality, while distal muscle weakness suggests lower motor neuron disease or peripheral neuropathy. (Check distal reflexes and proprioception.)

UPPER EXTREMITY STRENGTH

The basic approach is to start centrally and move distally, testing the flexors and extensors of each joint. This provides information on muscle strength as well as the integrity of the corresponding nerve root.

Table 21.1. Scoring system for muscle strength	
Grade	*Criteria*
5 (normal)	Motion against gravity and full resistance
4	Motion against gravity and some resistance but diminished from normal
3	Movement against gravity but not against resistance
2	Horizontal motion but not against gravity
1	Minimal contraction but no joint movement
0	No muscle contraction is felt

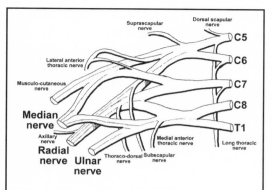

Figure 157. Brachial Plexus.

This illustration shows the brachial plexus with the ultimate destinations of the various nerve components. Lesions affecting the plexus are rare.

Check for Pronator Drift

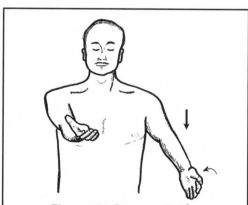

Figure 158. Pronator Drift.

This is a useful test of shoulder or arm weakness. Have the patient stand with both arms extended, palms upward (as if balancing a glass of water on each palm). Have the patient close the eyes. Shoulder or arm weakness will cause the paretic arm to drift downward and pronate, as shown in the figure.

Have the patient stand with the arms extended, palms upward. Have the patient close the eyes. Shoulder or arm weakness will cause the paretic arm to drift and pronate.

Check Shoulder and Deltoids (C4-C5)

With the patient's arms resting at the sides, have the patient raise them without bending

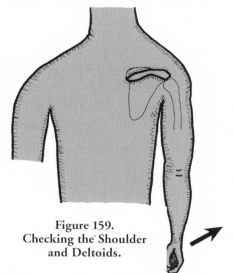

**Figure 159.
Checking the Shoulder
and Deltoids.**

With the patient's arms resting at the sides, have the patient raise them without bending the elbow. Supraspinatus weakness (C4-C5) causes the involved shoulder to rise as the trapezius tries to compensate. The patient may use the hip to begin arm abduction by bouncing it upward.

the elbow. Supraspinatus weakness (C4) causes the involved shoulder to rise as the trapezius tries to compensate, or the patient may use the hip to begin arm abduction.

Check Upper Arm Flexion (C5-6)

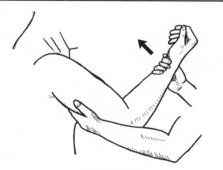

**Figure 160.
Checking Upper Extremity Flexion.**

Upper extremity flexion tests the C5-C6 nerve roots. With the patient's elbow at 90°, have the patient try to touch the shoulder as you try to straighten the arm.

With the patient's elbow at 90°, have the patient try to maintain the angle as you try to straighten the arm.

Check Upper Arm Extension (C6-T1)

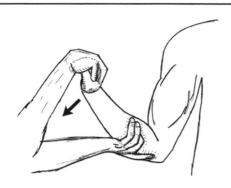

**Figure 161.
Checking Upper Arm Extension.**
With the patient's elbow at 90°, have the patient try to straighten the arm against resistance. This tests the C6-T1 nerve roots.

With the patient's elbow at 90° and, ideally, the upper arm parallel to the floor, have the patient try to straighten the arm against resistance.

Check Wrist Flexion and Extension (C6-C8)

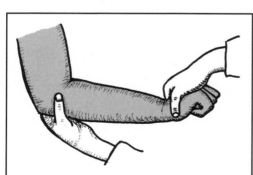

Figure 162. Checking Wrist Flexion and Extension.
With the patient's wrist at 180°, have patient move wrist down (flexion) against resistance and then up (extension) against resistance to test the C6-C8 nerve roots.

With the patient's wrist at 180°, have patient move wrist down (flexion) against resistance and then up (extension) against resistance.

Have the patient simultaneously squeeze your forefingers and middle fingers bilaterally and note any difference in strength.

Check Finger Flexion (C7-T1)

Have the patient move all four fingers from the straight position down toward the palm.

Check Finger Extension (C6-C8)

With the patient's fingers flexed to 90°, have patient straighten them against resistance.

Check Finger Abduction (C8-T1)

Have the patient keep fingers spread apart as you squeeze pairs of fingers together.

Check Finger Adduction C8-T1)

Have the patient squeeze fingers together as you keep them apart.

Check Finger Opposition (C7-T1)

Have the patient oppose the thumb and little finger to make a ring. Try to break the ring with your forefinger.

UPPER EXTREMITY PERIPHERAL NERVES

Testing the Radial Nerve (Wrist Drop)

Check wrist extension and also thumb extension since there are two branches of the radial nerve. Possible causes of weakness include lead poisoning, alcoholism, polyneuritis, trauma, polyarteritis, and neurosyphilis.

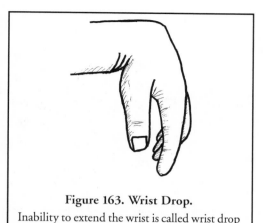

Figure 163. Wrist Drop.
Inability to extend the wrist is called wrist drop and signifies radial nerve palsy.

Testing the Ulnar Nerve (Claw Hand)

Check finger abduction, and look for hypothenar atrophy, interosseous atrophy, and a hollow-appearing palm.

Check Froment's sign. Have the patient pinch a piece of paper on each side (like reading a newspaper) and pull the paper tight. In ulnar neuropathy the paper will slip from the involved side.

Perform the paper-cutting test. Have the patient hold a piece of paper between the forefinger and middle finger as if trying to cut it like a pair of scissors. Try to pull out the paper. Weakness in holding the paper suggests ulnar neuropathy.

If ulnar neuropathy is present, then check for atrophy of flexor carpi ulnaris. If there is none, then there is probably entrapment in the wrist (ulnar tunnel syndrome). Atrophy of the flexor carpi ulnaris suggests C8 radiculopathy or entrapment at the elbow (cubital tunnel). Possible causes of ulnar neuropathy include polyneuritis, trauma, and entrapment syndromes, as mentioned above.

Testing the Median Nerve (Benediction Palsy)

Check the "OK" sign. Have the patient make an "OK" sign by opposing the thumb and forefinger. Check the strength of the "O" with your fingers. Weakness indicates a median nerve abnormality. Also have the patient make a fist to check finger flexors, and look for thenar atrophy. Finger flexor weakness or thenar atrophy suggests median neuropathy.

If median neuropathy is present, then check for atrophy of the flexor carpi radialis. No atrophy suggests median nerve entrapment at the wrist (carpal tunnel syndrome). Atrophy of the flexor carpi radialis suggests entrapment at the elbow (pronator syndrome with the ligament of the pronator teres). Check sensation by testing the tip of the index finger. The benediction hand of median and ulnar paralysis is Charcot's hand sign.

Carpal tunnel syndrome can be caused by rheumatoid arthritis, tenosynovitis at the wrist, amyloidosis, gout, myxedema, plasmacytoma and acromegaly.

UPPER EXTREMITY TONE

Shake hands with the patient, supporting the elbow to unload the biceps. Supinate and pronate the forearm. Normally the range of motion is smooth and fluid. (Test on a colleague to appreciate how minimal the resistance to movement normally is.) Any resistance to movement is abnormal.

Jean-Martin Charcot (1825–1893) was the French neurologist considered to be the founder of modern neurology. Charcot was a great clinician and teacher, and although he taught George Albert Edouard Brutus Gilles de la Tourette and Sigmund Freud, his favorite student was Joseph Jules Babinski. As an educator, Charcot was theatrical in the classroom and was not above the dramatic presentation of patients spotlighted on the stage of the amphitheater, often pausing for minutes in total silence while his students would observe the displayed patient. "If the clinician as observer," Charcot commented, "wishes to see things as they really are, he must make a tabula rasa of his mind and proceed without any preconceived notions whatever." A neurologist whose list of more than 15 eponyms reflects the academic stature he attained. He also described Charcot's Joints, a complication of tabes dorsalis causing a degenerative destruction of the bones and joints in the foot; gave a classic clinical and anatomic description of multiple sclerosis, and completed important work in the study of amyotrophic lateral sclerosis. His academic career was interrupted by the Franco-Prussian war in 1870 and, during the years after it, Charcot focused on the control of typhoid and smallpox epidemics.

Abnormalities of Tone

Rigidity, spasticity, and dystonia are all abnormal resistances to passive movement. Lead-pipe rigidity feels as if the joint is moving through cold molasses. (It implies a basal ganglion problem.) Cogwheel rigidity feels jerky, with a tremor superimposed on the movement. Spasticity feels like opening or closing a clasp knife, with increased resistance followed by sudden release of resistance. (It implies an upper motor neuron problem.) The resistance in dystonia feels rubbery. Decreased tone seems floppy.

Strümpell's sign is involuntary pronation of the forearm with passive flexion and extension of the elbow. It indicates upper motor neuron disease.

LOWER EXTREMITY STRENGTH

Have the Sitting Patient Stand Up from Chair Without Using Hands for Support

The timed stands test measures the time to stand and then sit down ten times. Timing is done with a stopwatch. The greater the impairment, the longer the elderly person takes to perform the test.

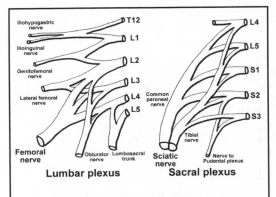

Figure 164. Lumbosacral Plexus.
The lumbar plexus is situated in the psoas muscle. The most important branches are the femoral and obturator nerves. The sacral plexus is positioned in the posterior pelvis. The common and peroneal nerves leave together as the sciatic nerve and then split in the popliteal fossa.

Hip Flexion (T12-L4)

Have the sitting patient raise a knee against resistance.

Hip Extension (L4-S3)

Have the prone patient raise a leg off the examining table and then against resistance.

Hip Adduction (L2-L4)

Try to push the sitting patient's knees apart while the patient resists.

Hip Abduction (L4-S1)

Try to push the sitting patient's knees together while the patient resists.

Knee Flexion (L4-S3)

Have the sitting patient flex a bent knee against resistance.

Knee Extension (L2-L4)

Have the sitting patient straighten a bent leg against resistance.

Have the Patient Rise Up on Tiptoes (L5-S2)

Have the Patient Rock Back on Heels (Soleus and S1)

For the bedfast patient, have them dorsiflex and plantarflex their feet against resistance, with the leg flexed to 90° to remove the contribution of the gastrocnemius.

Lower Extremity Hemiparesis Can Be Brought Out by Barré's Sign

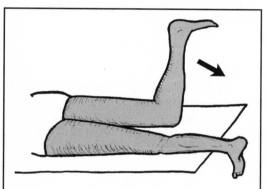

Figure 165. Barré's Sign.
Barré's sign is an indication of lower extremity weakness. With the patient in prone position, passively flex the knees to 90°; the weak leg will flex further or extend, unable to maintain position.

With the patient in prone position, passively flex the knees to 90°; the weak leg will flex further or extend, unable to maintain position.

Jean-Alexandre Barré (1880–1967) was a French neurologist who studied under Babinski and continued the work of Charcot. During World War I he served with the neurological unit of the 6th Army, headed by Guillain. They developed a collaboration including the description of the Guillain-Barré syndrome. Barré wrote more than 800 original articles and enjoyed listening to Verdi.

ADVENTITIOUS MOVEMENTS

Tremors

Bilateral tremor suggests toxic exposure, infection, metabolic disorder, and demyelinating illness. Muscle weakness can also produce a tremor.

Resting Tremor

Seeing a slow tremor (roughly 3 tremors per second) when the hand is otherwise resting suggests Parkinsonism (basal ganglion disorder). For example, if a patient with a resting tremor is asked to drink a sip of water from a glass, the resting tremor will disappear with the movement to the lips and back, and then will resume when the hand returns to rest.

James Parkinson (1755–1824) was initially more active as a political radical than as a physician. He was a strong advocate for the underprivileged and was a member of several secret societies that advocated universal suffrage and broader representation in the House of Commons. In 1799, he published Medical Admonitions which was aimed at improvement of the general health of the population. In 1811 he became an advocate for the mentally ill by crusading for safer management of madhouses, as well as legal protection for mental patients, their families, and their physicians. Parkinson is best remembered for his 1817 work, "An Essay on the Shaking Palsy." Four decades after its publication, Charcot attached Parkinson's name permanently to this syndrome after adding rigidity to the spectrum of manifestations of Parkinson's disease.

Parkinson also fostered an interest in nature and enjoyed traveling with his six children to collect and observe fossils. He published Organic Remains of the Former World in three volumes from 1804–1811, while still practicing medicine in his father's old business. While this work was not the defining work of British paleontology, it stands as one of the first.

Intention Tremor

A coarse tremor with intention suggests cerebellar disease. An intention tremor is a tremor that becomes more pronounced when the hand (or foot) approaches the target. For example, if a patient with an intention tremor is asked to slowly take a sip of water, the hand will start to shake more erratically as it reaches toward the glass. A unilateral intention tremor suggests a cerebellar or brain stem problem.

Rubral Tremor

A tremor with an extended elbow with a rocking wrist movement, like unscrewing a jar, is a rubral tremor and suggests disease of the superior cerebellar peduncle.

Physiological Tremor

A continuous fine tremor not affected by movement or rest suggests physiological tremor.

Essential Tremor

A continuous coarse tremor suggests an essential tremor. This tremor frequently involves the head and trunk.

Fasciculations

Fasciculations are intermittent muscle twitching as the corresponding nerves fail to innervate them. They are rhythmic in nature and are seen at rest or during sleep. Fasciculations are not significant alone but are more ominous if atrophy or muscle weakness is present in the same muscle group. Note the muscle group and the intensity of the fasciculations.

Signs of trouble are muscle atrophy or weakness, and fasciculations that always affect the same muscle group. Conditions to consider include amyotrophic lateral sclerosis (Lou Gehrig's disease) and spinal cord atrophy.

Chorea

Ask the patient to extend his or her tongue and keep it extended. Patients with chorea cannot keep the tongue extended. Significant grimacing and body movement suggests rheumatic fever (Sydenham's chorea). Apparent movement on only one side is chorea mollis, a variant of Sydenham's chorea. Chorea of a body part that worsens over time suggests Huntington's chorea. In Huntington's chorea a strong family history will be present. Paternal inheritance tends to have an earlier age of onset.

Table 21.2. Tremors

Tremor	Characteristic	Pathology	Comments
Resting	Slow, pill rolling, disappears with movement	Basal ganglion	Parkinsonism is most likely
Intention	Coarse, irregular, gets worse approaching target	Cerebellum or brain stem	
Rubral	Rocking motion	Superior cerebellar peduncle	Movement like unscrewing a jar
Physiological	Fine tremor	Increased sympathic tone	Consider anxiety, thyroid disease, alcoholism
Essential	Coarse, continuous	Basal ganglion	Involves head and trunk

Thomas Sydenham (1624–1689) is the English physician considered to be the father of modern medicine. He revived the Hippocratic methods of observation and experience. He was one of the principal founders of epidemiology, and his clinical reputation rests upon his firsthand accounts of gout, malaria, scarlatina, measles, dysentery, and numerous other diseases.

Sydenham himself suffered with renal stones and gout, and apart from his accurate descriptions of these disorders he described a number of other disorders accurately for the first time. He noted the link between fleas and typhus fever. Sydenham introduced opium into medical practice and was the first to use iron in treating iron deficiency anemia, and helped popularize quinine in treating malaria. His treatment of fevers with fresh air and cooling drinks was an improvement on the sweating methods previously employed.

His renown came chiefly from the fact that he alleviated the suffering of the sick and made ill people well. Ironically, the only eponymous use of his name that still remains common, "Sydenham's chorea," refers to two paragraphs interjected into one of his treatises, more or less as an aside.

George Huntington (1850–1916) was an American physician who worked for some time with his father who was also a physician. During this period he was able to observe cases of hereditary chorea which he had first seen on rounds with his grandfather and father. In a review article in 1908, Sir William Osler wrote: "In the history of medicine there are few instances in which a disease has been more accurately, more graphically or more briefly described."

Huntington had a happy family life, five children, and a great fondness for music, often playing the flute to his wife's accompaniment. Moreover, he was an ardent student of nature and guns. Drawing was one of his lifetime interests and he often made sketches of game birds during his trips through the woods.

Hemiballismus

Hemiballismus is a distorted throwing movement of the shoulder implying damage to the subthalamic nucleus of Luys.

Evidence of Muscle Atrophy

Note the hands, arms, shoulders, thighs, legs, and palpate for characteristic flaccid consistency. (Atrophy plus decreased muscle tone equals flaccidity.)

SENSORY EXAMINATION

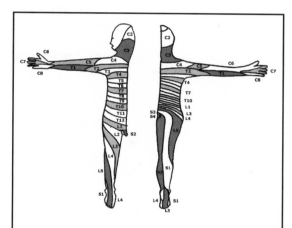

Figure 166. Sensory Dermatomes.
This figure illustrates the sensory dermatomes. Note the boundary in the upper chest between C4 and T2 (since C5-T1 supply the arm). The nipple line in men is about T4 while the umbilicus is at T10. The genitalia are within the S2-S3 dermatome.

General Points

The sensory examination requires significant patient cooperation. If the patient has a specific sensory complaint, then have them draw it or outline it, and begin testing in the center of the area defined.

The Three Types of Sensation

Light touch is transmitted through the anterior spinothalamic tracts and is tested with an artist's paintbrush. Vibration and position sensation travel up the posterior columns and are tested by using a tuning fork and by proprioception. Pain and temperature travel up the lateral spinothalamic tracts and are tested by pinprick and temperature sensations (hot or cold).

Location of the Sensory Abnormality

The location of the sensation depends on the sensory dermatome or the area supplied by a spinal accessory nerve. The sensory examination of the neck tests the C3 nerve root. The sensory examination of the nipple line tests the T4 nerve root. The sensory examination of the umbilicus tests the T10 nerve root.

Sensory loss implies interruption of the sensory fibers below the sensory level. Loss in a saddle distribution (where a saddle would touch the body in the perineal area) suggests lumbosacral disc herniation or cauda equina syndrome. Stocking and glove sensory loss suggests peripheral neuropathy. The sensory examination of the sacrum is important if the patient has diabetes. Test vibration sense with a tuning fork to check for myelopathy.

There is no neurological illness that produces an area of sensory loss that stops exactly at the midline because midline structures have bilateral innervation. If there is a combined motor and sensory loss, then the pattern can help to localize the site of the lesion. Generally, distal sensation is tested first unless the patient has a specific sensory complaint. When testing vibration, use a 128 Hz tuning fork (a 256 Hz tuning fork may be more sensitive for pernicious anemia). According to Sapira, Meissner's fibers first lose the 64 Hz sensations.

THE SENSORY EXAMINATION

The Sensory Examination of the Hand of an Elderly Person

The innervation of the thumb is C6, the forefinger and middle finger are C7, and the

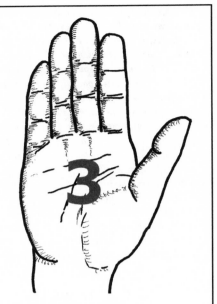

Figure 167. Graphesthesia.
Graphesthesia tests the function of the contralateral parietal lobe as well as several sensory pathways. Using a cotton swab, write a digit on the palm and ask the patient to identify it. Do not let the patient see what you are writing. The numeral "3" for one palm is shown as an example.

pinky is C8. Check pinprick and light touch and place the tuning fork over the second MCP.

Check for graphesthesia that tests the contralateral parietal lobe. Using a cotton swab, write a digit on the palm and ask the patient to identify it. Use "7" and "3" for one palm and "4" and "8" for the other. Do not let the patient see what you are writing. If graphesthesia is abnormal, try stereognosis (identifying objects by touch). Try using a coin, key and pen since they are usually available and have different tactile characteristics.

The Sensory Examination of the Foot of an Elderly Person

Lack of sensation to pinching the Achilles tendon (Abadie's sign) suggests neurosyphilis. The innervation of the medial foot and great toe is L4; the dorsum of the foot is L5; and the lateral foot is S1.

Check pinprick and light touch over the dorsal, medial and lateral foot. Check vibration sense by placing the tuning fork on the great toe. (Sometimes it is useful to first touch the tuning fork on a bony prominence at the patient's elbow or wrist to give them a sense of the vibration.) Let the patient's toes warm if the weather is cold. Decreased vibration sense at the great toe suggests peripheral neuropathy. If the sensation is abnormal, move up the leg to the ankles and then the patella. Vibration can only reliably be tested over bony prominence.

Check great toe proprioception. Have the patient close his or her eyes. Hold the toe by the sides, move the toe toward the head in a large movement (up), and then move the toe away from the patient's head (down). Have the patient say the direction of movement (up or down). Now perform the test by moving the toe about 2mm and noting the response. The small movements and holding the toe by the sides are worth stressing.

CEREBELLAR EXAMINATION

General Points

If the patient can perform a task with eyes open but cannot do so with eyes closed, then this suggests dorsal column disease (impaired proprioception). If the patient cannot perform the task with eyes open, that suggests cerebellar or vestibular tract dysfunction.

Observe the Patient's Gait

More information on balance and gait is contained in Chapter 23. The key components of gait evaluation are balance, initiation of movement, arm swing, speed, and smooth foot rise and follow through. Often this assessment boils down to "Does the gait look safe or not?" Limited arm swing suggests Parkinsonism or basal ganglion disorders. Absent arm swing (Wartenberg's sign) suggests cerebellar disease. Hip stability and ankle stability play crucial roles.

Specific Gait Tests

The tandem walk (walking heel to toe) can bring out most gait problems. Patients with cerebellar disease or hemiparesis will fall to the side. Patients with alcohol-induced vermal cerebellar degeneration will show truncal sway.

Walking with eyes closed is the compass test. Have the patient walk eight steps forward and then eight steps back. With cerebellar or vestibular disease the patient will veer away from the path (toward the side of the lesion). Worsening of the gait with eyes closed suggests the need for sensory input implying sensory ataxia. If the gait is abnormal but not worse with eyes closed, that suggests motor ataxia or cerebellar disease.

Have the patient walk tiptoe. Inability to do so implies Parkinson's disease, lower leg weakness, peripheral neuropathy, spastic hemiplegia, and cerebellar disease.

Have patient walk on heels. Inability to do so suggests foot drop, motor ataxia, and paraparesis.

Gait Patterns in Neurological Illnesses

A bizarre, modern dance-like gait suggests Huntington's chorea. A broad-based gait suggests cerebellar, frontal lobe or dorsal spinal column disease. Patients with cerebellar disease tend to jerk or lurch in an erratic manner and they tend to keep their feet apart as they walk.

Patients with frontal lobe disease tend to walk as if their feet were stuck to the floor (magnetic gait). Patients with dorsal column disease or peripheral neuropathy tend to strike the floor with their feet and have difficulty walking with their eyes closed. A marching gait with high steps suggests foot drop. Short festinating steps suggest Parkinsonism. A waddling gait suggests proximal hip weakness.

Romberg's Test

The patient stands with feet together and eyes open. Note any unsteadiness with eyes open. This suggests cerebellar disease (ataxia). Now have the patient close the eyes. Shifting of the feet is a positive test, suggesting a sensory problem. Movement to one side suggests an ipsilateral cerebellar lesion.

Moritz Heinrich Romberg (1797–1873) was a German neurologist who worked unselfishly as physician to poor people during the Berlin cholera epidemics of 1831 and 1837. Said he:

"Every social group has its own type of health and disease, determined by the mode of living. They are different for the courtiers and noblemen, for the soldiers and scholars. The artisans have various diseases peculiar to them, some of which have been specially investigated by physicians. The diseases caused by poverty of the people and by the lack of the goods of life, however, are so exceedingly numerous that in a brief address they can only be discussed in outline."

Eventually, Romberg relinquished his post as physician to the poor, in favor of teaching and scientific work. Known for his sign of static ataxia in tabes dorsalis, Romberg wrote the three-volume classic, "Lehrbuch der Nervenkrankheiten der Mensch" (A Manual of the Nervous Diseases of Man) from 1840 to 1846. It was the first structured compilation of previously scattered information on neurological physiology, disease groups, and directed therapies.

The Finger-to-Nose Test

The patient touches your forefinger tip (held initially at eye level), then his or her own nose, and back and forth. Move your target finger to the various quadrants (upper outer, lower outer, etc.). Watch for tremor and past pointing (dysmetria) as signs of cerebellar dysfunction.

Thomas's Sign

When patient's hand is raised over the patient's head and let go, it drops unto the head and bounces.

The Heel-to-Shin Test

Have the supine patient move a heel up and down along the opposite shin in a straight line. Patients with cerebellar disease will have difficulty with this test. Have the patient perform the test with eyes closed to check the dorsal columns.

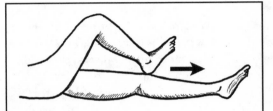

Figure 168. Heel to Shin Test.
This test of cerebellar and dorsal column function complements the finger-to-nose test. Have the supine patient move a heel up and down along the opposite shin in a straight line. Patients with cerebellar disease will have difficulty with this test. Have the patient perform the test with eyes closed to check the dorsal columns.

Rapid Alternating Movements (Dysdiadochokinesia)

Have the patient pat his or her hand as rapidly as possible. Have the patient repeat the test, hand-patting and then rotating palms and patting with the backs of the hands. Also have the patient oppose the thumb to each of the fingers in rapid sequence.

Next, test lower extremity movements with foot tapping. Follow this test with alternate foot tapping (alternating feet).

Rapid Tongue Movements (Especially "K" and "T")

Have the patient say "Topeka, Topeka, Topeka" rapidly.

EXAMINING THE CRANIAL NERVES

Testing CN I (Smell)

Have the patient smell cloves, coffee, cinnamon, nutmeg, allspice or vanilla. The key is appreciating the smell not necessarily being able to identify it. Avoid powerful odors like ammonia, pepper or rubbing alcohol, since mucosal stimulation is innervated by CN V. Make sure that the nasal passages are open.

Check each side separately by having patient smell the open container while occluding one nostril. Repeat with another smell on the other side. A hyperacute sense of smell suggests Addison's disease.

Unilateral loss of smell is significant if the airway is not occluded and suggests a frontal lobe tumor. Bilateral loss of smell is seen in normal aging, Alzheimer's disease, Parkinson's disease, zinc deficiency, renal failure, cirrhosis, pernicious anemia, hypothyroidism, drugs, and toxic exposure.

Testing CN II (Vision)

See Chapter 8.

Testing CN V (Trigeminal Nerve)

The trigeminal nerve is the largest cranial nerve, arising from the mid-pons and traversing the subarachnoid space. The nerve divides into three divisions over the tip of the petrus bone. It does not affect any of the facial muscles of expression.

♦ EVALUATING THE MOTOR PORTION

The motor portion of the trigeminal nerve is supplied by the mandibular nerve, the largest branch (the third division) of CN V.

Masseter strength: Have the patient bite down while you feel the masseter muscle. Masseter weakness can be part of myasthenia

---

Table 21.3. Eye signs of neurological dysfunction

Sign	*Manifestation*
Behr's	A lesion in the optic tract that produces hemianopsia and contralateral pupillary dilation
Bordier-Frankel	The eye rolling upward and outward in peripheral facial nerve paralysis
Cantelli's	Doll's-eye movements
Eyelash	Stimulating the eyelashes of an unconscious patient will not produce movement in brain injury but can produce movement in psychiatric patients
Legehdre's	Inability to keep the buried eyelids closed to resistance, suggesting central facial nerve paralysis
Magendie's	Acute disconjugate gaze, where one eye looks down and in while the other eye looks up and out, suggesting acute cerebellar hemorrhage
Prevost's	Conjugate deviation of the eyes toward the diseased side and away from a paretic side
Revilloid's	Inability to close the eye on the affected side of the face except by closing both eyes simultaneously, suggesting hemiplegia
Weber's	Ipsilateral CN III palsy and contralateral facial paralysis, suggesting a lesion in the internal ventral cerebral peduncle

gravis. The masseter is spared in Guillain-Barré's syndrome. Masseter claudication suggests temporal arteritis.

Temporalis strength: Check the temporalis muscle while patient bites down or clenches the teeth. This may be minimal in an edentulous patient.

Pterygoid strength: Have patient protrude jaw and then push against resistance on each side. Do not test this if the masseter is weak, because the jaw can dislocate. Have the patient bite down gently on a vertically oriented tongue blade and wiggle it back and forth with his tongue to test the internal pterygoids.

♦ Evaluating the Sensory Portion

There are three sensory branches of the trigeminal nerve. The ophthalmic branch runs from the tip of the nose diagonally up to the eye, including the forehead. The maxillary branch goes from the corner of the mouth to the top of the ear. The mandibular branch runs from the jaw line up to the maxillary branch.

Double simultaneous stimulation. Have the patient stare at your nose and tell you which side of the face is touched. With both forefingers gently touch both sides of the upper cheek (maxillary branch), then touch just the right cheek. Then move to the forehead (ophthalmic branch) and repeat the double, then single, touching. Then move to the lower jaw line (mandibular branch) and again repeat the double and single touching.

The corneal reflex tests the ophthalmic branch of CN V afferent and CN VII efferent. This is the most sensitive test of trigeminal nerve dysfunction. Have the patient look up. Touch the cornea between the limbus and the pupil with a *moist*, sterile wisp of cotton, noting blink reflex in *both* eyes. Another approach is to use a 10cc syringe and push a jet of air at the side of the eye. The corneal reflex can be lost in a comatose patient if the corneas become dry. Lateral movement of the lower jaw is the corneomandibular reflex and reflects an intact brain stem in a comatose patient.

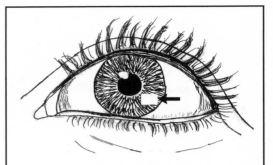

Figure 169. Where to Touch for the Corneal Reflex.

The corneal reflex is the most sensitive test of trigeminal nerve dysfunction. Have the patient look up. Touch the cornea between the limbus and the pupil with a *moist*, sterile wisp of cotton, noting blink reflex in *both* eyes. The corneal reflex tests the ophthalmic branch of CN V afferent and CN VII efferent.

Testing CN VII (Facial Nerve)

Cranial nerve VII is the primary innervation of the muscles of facial expression (passing through the parotid gland) and to the stapedius in the inner ear. The sensory components communicate taste from the anterior two-thirds of the tongue and sensation to the skin of the external ear.

♦ Evaluating Motor Function

Note the facial symmetry. Check the lateral palpebral area and the nasolabial folds.

Have the patient raise the eyebrows. Look for symmetrical forehead wrinkling.

Have the patient tightly close the eyes. Check for muscle strength by gently trying to raise the supraorbital rim.

Have the patient purse lips while you gently press on the cheeks.

Have the patient show the teeth.

♦ Interpreting the Tests

A patient with a supranuclear (cortical) lesion will be able to wrinkle the forehead (since the enervation is bilateral in 95% of the population) but cannot puff out cheeks or show the teeth. Patients with peripheral or brain

21. The Neurological Examination

stem nuclear lesions will have weak forehead and eyelid responses.

Bell's palsy is a facial palsy due to lesions distal to the geniculate ganglion. Ask the patient to close one eye at a time. In very early Bell's palsy the patient will not be able to close the paretic eye without closing both eyes.

Ramsey-Hunt syndrome is caused by herpes virus involvement of the geniculate ganglion. The patient has severe pain, facial palsy with herpetic vesicles on the pinna.

Potentially Confusing Patterns of Facial Abnormality

The patient cannot voluntarily move the facial muscles but shows normal movement on laughing or crying. This pattern suggests intact frontal lobes and a lesion just above the nucleus in the pons. This is called volitional palsy.

The patient has a normal cranial nerve examination but shows clear facial asymmetry during laughing or crying. This suggests a frontal lobe lesion or its projections into the pons.

The patient can smile but cannot puff out cheeks. This suggests fascioscapulohumeral muscular dystrophy (Landouzy-Dejerine disease). CN VII is okay but the orbicularis oris muscle is affected.

♦ EVALUATING VISCERAL MOTOR FUNCTION (TEARING AND SALIVATION)

Unilateral loss of lacrimation may suggest a CN VII lesion, although bilateral loss suggests end-organ failure. Generally lacrimation is not stimulated.

♦ EVALUATING SENSORY FUNCTION (TASTE ON THE ANTERIOR TWO-THIRDS OF THE TONGUE)

The sensory portion of the facial nerve detects sweet, sour, and salty sensations on the anterior tongue. (Bitter is on the posterior tongue and is part of CN IX.)

Make solutions of one-fourth teaspoon table salt in one cup of water (salty), one-fourth teaspoon sugar in one cup of water (sweet), one-fourth teaspoon quinine in one cup of water (bitter), and one teaspoon of white vinegar in one cup of water (sour). Use a sterile cotton swab to place a drop of solution on one side of the tongue, then on the other side. Have the patient point to words written on a piece of paper (sweet, sour, salty, bitter, plain water).

Horenstein's electrical technique. Wire two 9-volt batteries in series to make an 18-volt power source. Touch the leads on the tongue about 3mm apart. Start on each side of the tongue and then move to the back. If the patient senses a metallic taste, then taste sensation is intact.

♦ INTERPRETATION OF SENSORY LOSS

Unilateral loss of taste suggests a lesion in the chorda tympani or geniculate ganglion.

Bilateral loss of taste suggests chronic liver or renal disease, hypothyroidism, diabetes mellitus, medication effect, niacin deficiency, Sjögren's syndrome, radiation effect, influenza, and Dengue fever.

Unilateral Increased Hearing (Not Just CN VIII)

Unilateral increased hearing may result from impairment of the muscle that controls the stapedius muscle that is innervated by CN VII.

Testing CN VIII

♦ EVALUATING THE COCHLEAR COMPONENT

(see also Chapter 9)

♦ EVALUATING THE VESTIBULAR COMPONENT

(usually not tested on an awake person)

♦ ICE WATER CALORICS

Have the patient supine with the head at 30° elevation. Instill ice water into one ear.

Within 30 seconds nystagmus should appear, with the fast component going away from side of stimulus (remember COWS: Cold Opposite, Warm Same). Do not attempt this within one hour after a meal (or tube feeding). Seeing no nystagmus (Bárány's sign) implies vestibular damage.

Robert Bárány (1876–1936) was a Viennese physician who was a student of Sigmund Freud. He later received his surgical training at Vienna General Hospital and entered service at the University of Vienna ear clinic under Adam Politzer. Bárány is mainly known for his contributions to the study of vestibular apparatus. He was able to investigate the relationship between the latter and the nervous system, thus laying the foundation for an entirely new field — otoneurology. His most important discovery was the caloric nystagmus.

In 1914 Bárány volunteered for military service to test his ideas on the treatment of brain wounds. He was captured the same year and, while a Russian prisoner of war, he was awarded the Nobel Prize for Physiology or Medicine. Prince Carl of Sweden persuaded the czar to release him and he received his prize in Sweden in 1915.

Testing CN IX and CN X (These Usually Are Tested Together)

Look for palate symmetry. Note the uvula in the midline (CN X). If it is not, then it points to the normal side or slides over to the normal side. This indicates CN X palsy on the affected (opposite) side.

♦ GAG REFLEX

The afferent limb is CN IX and the efferent limb is CN X. Touch the posterior portion of the tongue or one of the tonsillar pillars to cause the reflex. The uvula will deviate to the "good" side, indicating an incomplete or partial CN X palsy.

No movement at all suggests bilateral paralysis. So stroke the uvula with a cotton swab. If there is no movement of the uvula, then that suggests bilateral lower motor neu-

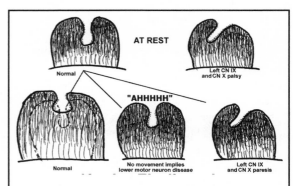

Figure 170. Uvular Findings in Cranial Nerve IX and X Lesions.

The position and movement of the uvula can help differentiate lesions involving CN IX and CN X. The upper panel shows the normal midline uvula and the asymmetrical drop of a left CN IX and CN X palsy. On saying "Ahhhh," the normal response, illustrated in the lower left panel, is symmetrical elevation of the uvula. No movement implies lower motor neuron disease, while a resting midline uvula that raises asymmetrically suggests CN IX and CN X paresis. Note that old tonsillectomy scars may sometimes produce asymmetry.

ron lesion. Symmetrical upward movement suggests upper motor neuron lesion (CN IX, CN X, or both).

♦ SENSATION OF THE TRAGUS

This area is usually innervated by the somatosensory branches of CN X. Loss of sensation suggests CN X lesion.

♦ OCULO-CARDIAC REFLEX

Slowing of the heart rate normally occurs when you gently push on the closed eyes. Absence of this reflex suggests CN X lesion.

Testing CN XI

Note the trapezius muscles for symmetry. Have the patient shrug the shoulders. Check the sternocleidomastoid by having the patient push the jaw against resistance. The direction of head movement is opposite to the sternocleidomastoid being tested.

Trapezius and SCM weakness suggests

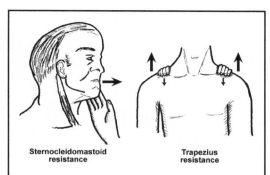

Figure 171. Testing Cranial Nerve XI.

Note the trapezius muscles for symmetry. Have the patient shrug the shoulders against resistance. Check the sternocleidomastoid (SCM) by having the patient push the jaw against your hand for resistance. The direction of head movement is opposite to the sternocleidomastoid being tested. Trapezius and SCM weakness suggests brain stem disease. Trapezius weakness with normal SCM function suggests a lesion above the brain stem or a nerve root abnormality. SCM weakness with normal trapezius function suggests myopathy. Lack of SCM weakness rules out myopathy.

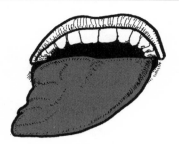

Figure 172.
Right Cranial Nerve XII Palsy.

Test CN XII by having the patient stick out the tongue and wiggle it from side to side. Have the patient push tongue into cheek. Inability to push the tongue to one side suggests a chronic CN XII palsy on the opposite side. In an acute CN XII nerve palsy, the tongue will deviate to the paralyzed side, as shown in the figure. The paralyzed side will be round and full compared to the normal side (Dinkler's sign).

brain stem disease. Trapezius weakness with normal SCM function suggests a lesion above the brain stem or a nerve root abnormality. SCM weakness with normal trapezius function suggests myopathy. Lack of SCM weakness rules out myopathy.

Testing CN XII

Check the patient's tongue for atrophy or fasciculations. Have the patient stick out the tongue and wiggle it to each side.

In an acute CN XII nerve palsy, the tongue will deviate to the paralyzed side. The paralyzed side will be round and full compared to the normal side (Dinkler's sign).

Occipital pain and tongue paralysis suggests malignancy. (Lung, prostate and breast cancer are most likely.)

Have the patient push tongue into cheek. Inability to push the tongue to one side suggests a chronic CN XII palsy on the opposite side.

REFLEXES

Basic Physiology

The reflex arc only involves a couple of spinal segments, so reflex abnormalities can help to localize neurological lesions. The corticospinal tract modulates the intensity of the arc (since most of the tonic descending input from the cortex is inhibitory), so disruption of this pathway (upper motor neuron disease) produces hyperreflexia. Lower motor neuron disease, either involving the spinal cord or the peripheral nerves, will diminish the reflex.

Jendrassik's maneuver (to bring out a diminished reflex). Have the patient interlock fingers and then try to pull them apart; or have the patient clench teeth tightly; or have the patient push knees tightly together.

Grading the Reflex

See Table 21.4 for grading deep tendon reflexes.

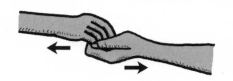

Figure 173. Jendrassik's Maneuver.

Jendrassik's maneuver is a way to amplify a diminished reflex. Have the patient interlock the fingers, as shown in the figure, and then pull them apart while you recheck the reflex. A reflex cannot be graded as zero unless it is absent while Jendrassik's maneuver is being performed.

**Table 21.4.
Grading deep tendon reflexes**

Reflex Grade	Criteria
0	• No reflex, even with Jendrassik's maneuver
1	• Diminished from normal, no joint movement
2	• Normal reflex with joint movement
3	• Brisk reflex with increased joint movement
4	• Brisk reflex with some clonus

Note the Contraction Phase and the Relaxation Phase of the Reflex

The contraction phase is delayed in hypothermia while the relaxation phase is delayed in hypothyroidism. Both phases are delayed in myxedema coma with hypothermia.

Absent reflexes suggest diabetes mellitus, pernicious anemia, peripheral neuropathy, and Eaton Lambert syndrome. (The reflexes in Eaton Lambert syndrome can temporarily appear after a ten-second maximal contraction (Doi's sign). Loss of all reflexes with upper spinal cord damage is Bastian-Brun's sign. The production of goose flesh above the level of a spinal cord lesion on pinching the trapezius is Thomas' sign.

Evaluating the Jaw Jerk

This reflex is critical to evaluate in the patient with hyperreflexic upper and lower extremities because in this setting a normal jaw jerk reflects upper spinal cord compression.

Method 1: Have the patient relax the jaw and place your forefinger on the chin. Tap your finger gently with your reflex hammer and note any jaw contraction (mouth closure). An absent or minimal jaw jerk is normal.

Method 2: Place a tongue blade over the molars on one side and have the patient lightly bite down. Lightly tap the tongue blade with your reflex hammer and note the reflex. Recheck the reflex on the opposite side.

Evaluating the Finger Flexion Reflex (C8)

Slightly extend the patient's fingers with your fingers. Tap your fingers and note the flexion reflex.

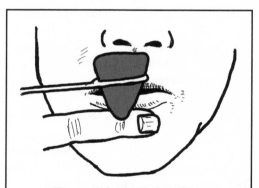

Figure 174. Jaw Jerk Reflex.

Have the patient relax the jaw and place your forefinger on the chin. Tap your finger gently with your reflex hammer and note any jaw contraction (mouth closure). An absent or minimal jaw jerk is normal. This reflex is critical to evaluate in the patient with hyperreflexic extremities because in this setting a normal jaw jerk reflects upper spinal cord compression. A hyperactive jaw jerk with peripheral hyperreflexia suggests a generalized hyperactive state, such as anxiety or hyperthyroidism.

Evaluating the Biceps Reflex (Tests C5-C6 Segment)

Have the patient sit quietly with hands in lap. With a bedfast patient, have the hands draped over the abdomen. Palpate the biceps tendon with your forefinger or thumb. Hit your forefinger with the reflex hammer and evaluate the intensity of the reflex.

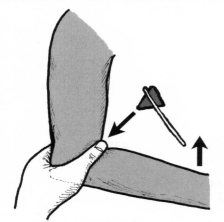

Figure 175.
Checking the Biceps Reflex C5-C6.

Have the patient sit quietly with hands in lap. With a bedfast patient, have the hands draped over the abdomen. Palpate the biceps tendon with your forefinger or thumb. This should be easy, since it is the major tendon spanning the antecubital fossa. Hit your thumb or forefinger with the reflex hammer and evaluate the intensity of the reflex.

Evaluating the Triceps Reflex (Tests C7-C8 Segment)

Support the arm so that the forearm swings down or have the patient place hands on hips. With a bedfast patient, support the arm over the chest. Palpate the triceps tendon just above the elbow.

Tap the tendon with your reflex hammer and note the movement of the forearm. The tendon is short, so tapping too far from the olecranon will miss the tendon and hit the muscle. Evaluate the intensity of the reflex.

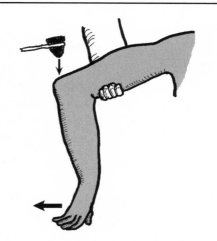

Figure 176.
Checking the Triceps Reflex C7-C8.

Support the arm as shown in the figure so that the forearm swings down. With a bedfast patient, support the arm over the chest. Palpate the triceps tendon just above the elbow. Tap the tendon with your reflex hammer and note the movement of the forearm. The tendon is short, so tapping too far from the olecranon will miss the tendon and hit the muscle. Having the patient turn head toward the side being tested can intensify the reflex.

Having the patient turn head toward the side being tested can intensify the reflex.

Upper Extremity Signs

See Table 21.5 for upper extremity signs.

Abdominal Reflexes (T8-T12)

The patient should be supine and relaxed. Perform the test at the end of expiration. Stroke the upper abdomen (T8-T10) from the outer edge toward the umbilicus. (The umbilicus should move toward stimulus.) Stroke the lower abdomen (T10-T12) from the outer portion toward the umbilicus. (Again the umbilicus should move toward stimulus.) An abnormal test is a difference from one side to the other, or lack of some but not all abdominal reflexes.

Table 21.5. Upper extremity signs

Sign	Manifestation
Chaddock's	• Stimulating the distal ulnar border of a hemiplegic forearm produces wrist flexion and finger extension.
Gordon's	• Extension and spreading of the fingers when pressure is placed on the radial portion of the pisiform bone while supporting the elbow suggests hemiplegia.
Hoffmann's reflex	• Flicking of the fingernails producing a pincer-like movement of the thumb and forefinger suggests diffuse frontal lobe disease.
Leri's	• Inability to flex the elbow when the fingers and wrist are passively flexed suggests organic hemiplegia.
Neri's arm sign	• Supination of a forearm when both pronated forearms are flexed suggests hemiplegia. Pronation that produces flexion of the forearm suggests hemiparesis.
Radialis	• Extreme wrist extension required to make a fist suggests hemiparesis.
Raimiste's	• Releasing the arm being held upright and causing wrist flexion and pronation suggests hemiparesis.
Raimiste's finger sign	• Hand posture with elevation of the forefinger suggests CNS paralysis; loss of this sign indicates a favorable prognosis.
Rossolimo's	• Flexion of the fingers on tapping the palm, or toe flexion with tapping the sole, suggests upper motor neuron disease.
Weil's	• Thumb flexion and adduction when the fingers are passively extended suggests disease of the pyramidal tracts.

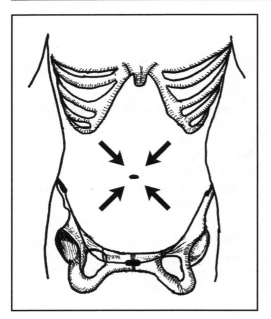

Cephalad moving of the umbilicus when testing abdominal reflexes suggests lower rectus abdominis muscle paralysis (Beevor's sign). Contraction of the lower abdominal muscles normally occurs on stroking the inner thigh

Left: **Figure 177.**
Checking Abdominal Reflexes (T8-T12).

Perform the test at the end of expiration. Stroke the upper abdomen (T8-T10) from the outer edge toward the umbilicus. (The umbilicus should move toward stimulus.) Stroke the lower abdomen (T10-T12) from the outer portion toward the umbilicus. (Again the umbilicus should move toward stimulus). An abnormal test is a difference from one side to the other, or lack of some but not all abdominal reflexes. These reflexes may be difficult to appreciate in obese patients.

(Bekhterev's sign). The bulbocavernosus reflex is Onanoff's sign. Abdominal reflexes can be lost in severe scleroderma (Muller's sign). Abdominal reflexes may be absent on the affected side in hemiplegia (Rosenbach's sign).

Knee Jerk (L3-L4)

Have the patient sit with legs swinging freely. With a bedfast patient, place your hand under the knee being tested and extend it to the opposite knee so you are supporting the tested knee. Tap the patellar tendon just below the knee and evaluate the intensity of the reflex.

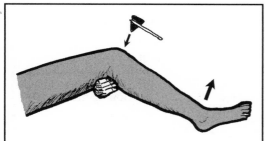

Figure 178.
Checking the Knee Jerk Reflex (L3-L4).
Have the patient sit with legs swinging freely. With a bedfast patient, place your hand under the knee being tested and extend it to the opposite knee so you are supporting the tested knee as shown in the figure. Tap the patellar tendon just below the knee and evaluate the intensity of the reflex. An alternative method is to push the quadriceps tendon downward with your forefinger and tap the forefinger to feel the contraction.

Ankle Jerk (S1-S2)

Have the patient kneel on a chair or the examining table. For a bedfast patient, cross one knee over the opposite knee, slightly dorsiflex the foot and tap the Achilles tendon. Watch for downward movement of the foot.

Ankle Clonus

Actively dorsiflex the patient's foot after two or three rapid flexions and extensions.

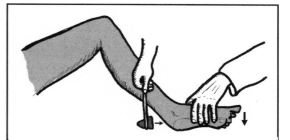

Figure 179.
Checking the Ankle Jerk Reflex (S1-S2).
Have the patient kneel on a chair or the examining table (for a bedfast patient, cross one leg over the opposite knee). Slightly dorsiflex the foot and tap the Achilles tendon. Watch for downward movement of the foot, indicative of the reflex.

Clonus will be a rhythmic beating of the foot for three or four beats (and sometimes several more). Clonus is never normal and implies either sympathetic excess (such as alcohol withdrawal) or pyramidal tract disease. The response may be obtained from other locations such as the jaw, wrist, knee (any tendon to be stretched such as a deep tendon reflex). Sharp dorsiflexion of the foot producing clonus is Charcot-Vulpian sign.

Lower Extremity Signs

Wilhelm Erb (1840–1921) was a German physician who pioneered the use of electricity in the diagnosis and treatment of nervous disorders. He was the first clinician to use the reflex hammer routinely in examinations. Of the many German neurologists who flourished during the late 1800s, he was likely the most significant. Erb was to Germany what Jean-Martin Charcot was to France. Erb had the appearance of a cultured gentleman; he was always immaculately dressed and kept his professorial beard trimmed to the last hair. He was punctual to the minute, and always on alert. Erb was an excellent teacher although somewhat short-tempered. One of his favorite sayings to his students was, "Pray every morning before you get out of bed, 'O Lord let me not idle my life away today.'"

Table 21.6. Lower Extremity Signs

Sign	Manifestation
Bekhterev's reflex	Passive plantar flexion of the toes producing dorsiflexion of the foot and knee flexion
Claude's	Painful stimulation of a paralyzed limb producing reflex contraction
Erb's leg sign	Loss of knee jerk reflex in ataxic disease
Hirschberg's	Adduction and inversion of the foot to medial foot stroking, suggesting pyramidal tract disease
Huntington's	Cough producing knee extension and contralateral hip flexion, suggesting upper motor neuron disease
Mendel's	Hitting the dorsum of the foot causing plantar flexion in upper motor neuron disease
Neri's leg sign	Involuntary bending of the knee when the leg of a supine patient is raised, suggesting hemiplegia
Oppenheimer's	Pushing down on the medial tibia and producing an extensor great toe response
Piotrowski's anticus sign	Excessive dorsiflexion and foot supination on tapping the anterior tibialis muscle, suggesting upper motor neuron disease

Babinski's Reflex

Support the patient's ankle and stroke the sole of the foot from the lateral aspect across the base of the toes. A normal response is plantar movement of the great toe. An abnormal response is dorsiflexion of great toe and fanning of other toes. Bilateral cortical, spinal or pyramidal tract lesions may produce a crossed response where both toes react.

Joseph Jules François Félix Babinski (1857–1932) was the favorite student of Jean-Martin Charcot. Charcot quickly recognized the observational ability of his pupil and aided in launching his career.

As a clinician, Babinski was extremely laconic. While performing his detailed neurological exams, he often would not utter a word, sometimes remaining quiet even afterward. When he did speak, it was to describe the findings of his exceptional observational powers, and their clinical correlation to his thorough understanding of neurological systems. Modern neurology is now based on Babinski's idea of precise localization of the level of a lesion.

In 1896, he reported in a 26-line presentation his "phénomène des orteils" and its pathological correlation. This finding is the now famous "Babinski's sign." Félix Alfred Vupian first reported extension of the great toe in certain types of brain damage half a century before Babinski's presentation. However, it was not until Babinski that the pathological correlate to lesions of the pyramidal tract was known.

Other Reflexes

◆ PHILLIPSON'S REFLEX

Stroking the lower extremity causes withdrawal and contralateral extension in severe spinal cord disease.

◆ FRONTAL RELEASE SIGNS

Grasp reflex. Run your hand along the patient's palm. A grasp, as a handshake, is an abnormal response (positive grasp reflex). This response is frequently misinterpreted as a positive response to "squeeze my fingers." It is never a normal reflex and may be caused by

Table 21.7. Babinski equivalents with same great toe response, except Brissaud's

Sign	Technique
Brissaud's	• Stimulating the foot and seeing contraction of the tensor fascia lata (good for amputation)
Chaddock's	• Stroking the lateral part of the foot
Gordon's	• Pinching the calf
Oppenheimer's	• Running your knuckles down the shin
Schaeffer's	• Pinching the Achilles tendon
Stransky's	• Pulling of little toe laterally away from the great toe
Strumpell's	• Flexing the thigh
Throckmorton's	• Tapping the dorsum of the foot
Williams's	• Gently squeezing the metacarpal bones

parietal lobe dysfunction, as well as frontal lobe processes. Grasp reflex is also called Kleist's sign.

Suck reflex. Touching the lips with a tongue blade causes the lips to pucker like a kiss. The suck reflex/lip pouting when the lips are tapped is Theimich's lip sign.

Root reflex. Stroking the side of the mouth causes the head to turn toward the side of the stroking.

Palmomental reflex. The palmomental frontal release sign is Radovici's sign. Stroking the palm with the handle of the reflex hammer causes the ipsilateral side of the mouth to twitch.

Parietal lobe sign. Stroke the ulnar side of the hand from the wrist to the fingers. A positive sign is having the hand move away or the arm rise.

Bulbocavernosus reflex (S3, S4) is useful for evaluating the elderly man with impotence. Squeeze the glans penis and note the contraction of the bulbocavernosus muscle (just behind the scrotum).

Anal wink (S2–S5). Touching the anal opening produces an anal contraction. This is a key test in some forms of low back pain since it tests the integrity of the distal spinal cord (cauda equina).

AUTONOMIC NERVOUS SYSTEM

Examination of the autonomic nervous system is a major component of the geriatric neurological examination. The relevance of this evaluation derives from numerous conditions, such as diabetes mellitus, that predispose to autonomic dysfunction, as well as the vast number of medications that can influence autonomic activity.

The clinical evaluation of the autonomic nervous system can be remembered by four responses: sweating, pupillary, cardiovascular, and sexual. As a useful rule of thumb, bizarre sounding symptoms, such as a limb that itches on standing, may be due to autonomic dysfunction.

Sweating

Sweating can be segmental or generalized. Segmental sweating on the face suggests Horner's syndrome. Sweating along a dermatome suggests underlying malignancy.

Generalized sweating signifies sympathetic overactivity. One important place to check for moisture is the feet. The feet of an elderly person, or any patient who has had diabetes mellitus for five or more years, should be dry. An elderly person with wet feet has sympathetic overactivity and probable alcoholism.

Skin moisture can be quantified by measuring skin electrical resistance. This can be performed with a simple voltmeter and probes taped at a constant distance. A quick test uses a plastic soup spoon. Hold the spoon and run the bowl of the spoon along the arm, from the medial portion of the biceps, across the antecubital fossa, and along the medial forearm. The plastic spoon will stick to moist (sweaty) skin and will slide without resistance on dry skin. Dusting the patient with powders that change color with sweating is generally not done.

Pupillary Cycling

Hippus is the rhythmic cycling of the pupillary contraction. This tonic dilation and constriction is normally 60 cycles per minute (120 individual beats per minute if you count dilation and then contraction). Slowing of this rhythm suggests involvement of the CNS and the cervical autonomic segments. You can bring out the hippus by shining a bright light on one-third of the pupil. The challenge is to determine the rate of the hippus while you are intently watching the eye. Horenstein's pearl is to hum to yourself a John Phillip Sousa march since they are all set at 120 beats per minute. If the march seems faster than the hippus, then the hippus is too slow.

Cardiovascular Responses

There are four cardiovascular autonomic responses. Two involve the heart rate and two affect the blood pressure. The heart rate responses test the vagus nerve and the upper thoracic sympathetic segments. Since they each test different aspects of the sympathetic arc, the comprehensive evaluation includes all

of the following tests. For example, some patients may have considerable autonomic dysfunction on one test, such as Valsalva ratio, but normal orthostatic blood pressure responses.

The Valsalva ratio. The Valsalva ratio tests the normal variation in heart rate with respiratory (Valsalva) activity. With the patient attached to an EKG machine, start a rhythm strip and have the patient perform Valsalva's maneuver. Immediately mark the start of the maneuver on the EKG. After about 15 heart beats (the maximum increase in heart rate), have the patient release the Valsalva and count another 15 beats. Compare the shortest R-R interval (usually at the 15th beat) with the longest R-R interval (usually at the 30th beat). You can compare either the R-R interval in millimeters or the calculated heart rate. Perform the test three times and average the results. A ratio of the 30th beat interval divided by the 15th beat interval of 1.21 or more is normal. A ratio close to 1.0 (indicating no reactivity) suggests autonomic insufficiency.

Deep breathing test. Again with the patient attached to an EKG machine, have the patient take one deep breath every ten seconds (so that the respiratory rate is six breaths per minute). Compare the slowest heart rate with the most rapid heart rate. A ratio of 1.0 suggests autonomic insufficiency.

The orthostatic pulse. The orthostatic pulse test evaluates the lower thoracic, lumbar and adrenal medullary function. Check the patient's EKG supine and then standing. Compare the ratio of the heart rate at the 15th beat with the 30th beat after standing. A ratio of 1.0 or less is abnormal.

Orthostatic blood pressure. The orthostatic blood pressure test measures the difference in blood pressure supine and standing. Normally the diastolic blood pressure will rise a little and the systolic blood pressure will drop a little. A drop in systolic blood pressure of 20mm of mercury or more, *or* a drop in diastolic blood pressure of 10mm of mercury or more, suggest orthostatic hypotension. If the pulse rate increases with standing, then consider volume depletion. If the orthostatic pulse does not increase (vide supra), then there is autonomic dysfunction.

Blood pressure increase with hand grip. Normally the systolic blood pressure should increase by 10mm of mercury or more with isometric handgrip. An abnormal response is less than a 10mm of mercury response.

Sexual Responses

Sexual responses test the lower lumbar and sacral sympathetic segments. They are not easy to demonstrate clinically and are usually determined from the history. In men, penile erection implies intact autonomic tone, while in women the response is clitoral enlargement. Nipple erection is not very helpful to test, since the mid-thoracic segments that are fully tested in the cardiovascular responses control it.

SPECIAL TESTS

Red Glass Test for Diplopia

Place a red piece of cellophane or a red glass filter over the patient's right eye. Holding a light source at least an arm's length away, move the eye through the basic positions of cardinal gaze. The image of the weak muscle is the most lateral image. The direction of maximum separation indicates the paretic muscle.

Test for Agnosia (Object Recognition)

Place a common object (coin, key, pencil) in the patient's hand without letting it be seen. Ask the patient to name the object. Inability to do so is an agnosia.

Meningeal Signs

With the patient supine, flex the hip and knee to 90° (if this is not already the preferred position of the patient). With knee extension, the neck flexes and patient feels discomfort (Kernig's sign).

Vladimir Mikhailovich Kernig (1840–1917) was a Latvian-born physician and neurologist who is best known in contemporary medical circles for a physical exam sign known as "Kernig's Sign" or "Kernig's Phenomenon." Because it is often explained incorrectly, here is Kernig's original (translated) description:

"I have observed for a number of years in cases of meningitis a symptom which is apparently rarely recognized although, in my opinion, it is of significant practical value. I am referring to the flexion contracture in the leg or occasionally in the arms, which becomes evident only after the patient sits up ... the stiffness of neck and back will ordinarily become much more severe as only now will a flexion contracture occur in the knee and occasionally also in the elbow joints. If one attempts to extend the patient's knees one will succeed only to an angle of approximately 135°. In cases where the phenomenon is very pronounced the angle may even remain 90°."

Medical historian and physician Robert T. Manning adds:

"Medical physicians have forgotten the major causes of meningitis in Kernig's days were pneumococcus and tuberculosis which both produce an intense pachymeningitis around the brain stem — thus the pathophysiology of the sign. These days, viral meningitis is the most common form seen — no pachymeningitis — and a negative Kernig's sign."

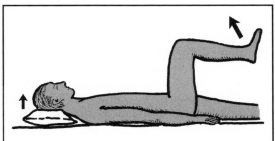

Figure 180. Kernig's Sign.
Kernig's sign is a clue to meningeal irritation or inflammation. With the patient supine, flex the hip and knee to 90° (if this is not already the preferred position of the patient). With knee extension, the neck flexes and patient feels hamstring discomfort in a positive test.

	Table 21.8. Meningeal signs	
Sign	**Manifestation**
Brudzinski's	Passive neck flexion producing bilateral hip, knee and ankle flexion
Brudzinski's second sign	Lowering a flexed leg, followed by contralateral flexion
Guilland's	Contraction of the contralateral leg with pinching of the quadriceps
Kernig's	Neck pain and stiffness when the knee is extended
Leichtenstern's	Pain on light tapping on several long bones
Signorelli's	Facial tenderness just in front of the mastoid process
Squire's	Alternating dilation and contraction of the pupils with the pulse

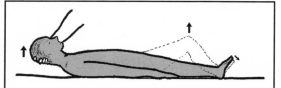

Figure 181. Brudzinski's Sign.
Brudzinski's sign is another manifestation of meningeal irritation. Passively elevate and flex the neck of the supine patient. A positive sign is flexion of the hips with a little flick of the foot.

Josef Brudzinski (1874–1917) was a Polish pediatrician who was a colleague of Antoine Bernard-Jean Marfan. During his career, he helped establish several children's hospitals, and in 1910, with the help of a Polish philanthropist, he designed and built a children's hospital in Warsaw according to his own plan. He also established the first Polish pediatric journal in 1908.

Although Brudzinski also carried out important work regarding intestinal flora and the prophylaxis of infectious diseases, as well as the establishment of a hospital system for children, he is best remembered for the sign that carries his name. Classically, the sign is positive in cases of meningitis, but may also be seen in association with subarachnoid hemorrhages and encephalitis. Meningeal signs described by Brudzinski include:

Brudzinski's reflex: Passive flexion of a supine patient's knee into the abdomen results in reflexive flexion of the contralateral hip and knee and, conversely, a forced extension of the previously flexed leg results in reflexive extension of the contralateral leg.

Brudzinski's symphyseal sign: Pressure on the symphysis pubis elicits reflexive knee and hip flexion and abduction of the leg.

Brudzinski's cheek phenomenon: Pressure on the cheek below the patient's cheekbone elicits a reflexive raising and simultaneous flexion of the forearm, in approximate analogy to the symphyseal sign for the leg.

Signs of Neurosyphilis

Syphilis produces a contracted pupil on the affected side (Seeligmüller's sign). Loss of the knee jerk in tabes dorsalis is Westphal's sign. Difficulty going down the stairs due to proprioceptive loss suggests tertiary syphilis (stair sign). Analgesia along the distribution of the peroneal nerve suggests tabes dorsalis (Sarbo's sign). The marching gait due to loss of proprioception is Charcot's gait. This gait can produce Charcot joints, particularly the ankle, with hypermobility and instability, usually without pain. It results from repeated trauma, 2° loss of proprioception, and lack of the pain pathways that would provide protection. Forced flexion of the toes producing leg withdrawal suggests long tract disease (Marie-Foix's sign). Dissociation of loss of pain and touch suggests polyneuritis or tabes dorsalis (Remak's sign).

Signs of Polio

Floppy neck in a paralyzed patient suggests poliomyelitis (Hoyne's sign). A patient with polio will resist all attempts to raise to a sitting position from a supine position unless the knees are flexed (Morquio's sign). A patient with pain on spinal flexion, such as poliomyelitis, will sit up by extending the arms far behind them for support (Amoss's sign). In polio only the great toe moves since the other toe muscles are paralyzed.

Neurological Signs of Metabolic Disorders

See Table 21.9 below.

Determining Cerebral Dominance

Check the thumb; often it is larger and squarer on the dominant hand. Note the diameter of the wrist (larger on the dominant side). Check the diameter of the biceps. Look for occupational calluses on the hands.

SPECIAL CIRCUMSTANCES

The Elderly Person with an Abnormal Gait
(see also Chapter 23)

A waddling gait suggests proximal muscle weakness. A festinating gait, with small steps and a shuffling quality, suggests Parkinsonism. A stiff straight back (poker gait) suggests a primary back problem. A scissors gait, where the thighs scissor across each other, suggests basal ganglion disease. A marching gait suggests foot drop or damage to the peroneal nerves. A wide-based gait with feet stuck to the floor suggests frontal lobe disease, such as normal pressure hydrocephalus. A wide-based gait with lots of sway suggests cerebellar or vestibular disease.

Table 21.9. Neurological signs of metabolic conditions

Sign	Manifestation	Condition
Chvostek's	Facial twitching on tapping on the facial nerve just anterior to the ear	Hypocalcemia in 25% of normal people
Hoffman's sensory sign	Increased sensitivity of the ulnar and trigeminal nerves	Hypocalcemia
Kashida's	Muscle spasms on heat or cold stimulation of a muscle	Hypocalcemia
Lust's	Eversion of the ankle and dorsiflexion of the foot on tapping along the peroneal nerve	Hypocalcemia
Marie's	Fine tremor	Hyperthyroidism
Quinquaud's	Asterixis	Alcoholism
Trousseau's	Carpopedal spasm on taking the blood pressure	Hypocalcemia
Vedder's	Leg weakness, pain, on gently squeezing the calves, with decreased knee jerk reflexes and anesthesia over the anterior thigh	Beriberi

The Elderly Patient with Muscle Weakness

Perform the basic neurological exam with these considerations.

♦ NOTE THE DISTRIBUTION OF WEAKNESS

Check the distribution of weakness by comparing one side to the other.

♦ LOOK CAREFULLY FOR HEMIPARESIS

Anterior tibial sign of spastic hemiplegia: Hip flexion of the thigh on the abdomen causes reflex contraction the anterior tibial muscle.

Check Barré's sign: With the patient prone, flex the leg onto the thigh. If the leg flops back to extension, that is a positive test.

♦ COMPARE THE STRENGTH OF THE UPPER EXTREMITIES TO THE LOWER EXTREMITIES

Bilateral lower extremity weakness suggests lower spinal cord disease.

♦ CHECK PERIANAL SENSATION AND THE ANAL WINK

Check for perianal sensory loss by gently touching a pin to the perianal tissue. (Sensory loss is a neurological emergency.) Check the anal wink by stimulating anal area with your gloved finger and noting contraction. Lack of anal contraction in this setting is a neurological emergency. Either of these signs in this setting suggests lower spinal cord compression.

♦ DETERMINE IF THE WEAKNESS IS PROXIMAL VERSUS DISTAL

Can the patient stand from a chair without using the arms? Difficulty suggests proximal muscle weakness caused by steroid excess, thyroid disorder or a spinal cord lesion. Going from supine to standing requiring the use of the arms is Gower's sign.

♦ NOTE MUSCLE STRENGTH, TONE AND ADVENTITIOUS MOVEMENTS

Note any atrophy or fasciculations that suggest a lower motor neuron problem.

♦ CONSIDER A PRIMARY MUSCLE DISORDER

Check for muscle tenderness by squeezing the muscle. Tenderness suggests polymyositis or dermatomyositis. (Look for an underlying malignancy.)

♦ CHECK FOR WRIST AND ANKLE CLONUS

Wrist and ankle suggest clonus upper motor neuron damage.

♦ CONFIRM THE BABINSKI REFLEX

♦ CHECK FOR HOFFMAN'S SIGN

Check for Hoffman's sign by clicking patient's middle fingernail. Noting a pincer movement of the thumb and forefinger is a positive test, indicating increased tone.

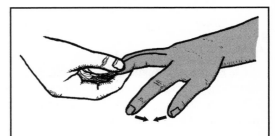

Figure 182. Hoffman's Sign.
Hoffman's sign indicates increased tone. Perform the test by clicking patient's middle fingernail with your fingertip. Noting a pincer movement of the thumb and forefinger is a positive test.

The Elderly Patient with Resting Tremor, Slow Movements and Rigidity (Parkinsonian Features)

♦ CONSIDER TOXIC EXPOSURE

Note any history of toxic exposure, such as neuroleptic drugs, illegal drugs, manganese exposure, and carbon monoxide.

♦ SEARCH FOR A HISTORY OF CNS INFECTION

Note any history of CNS infection, such as neurosyphilis, Jakob-Creutzfeldt disease (associated with eating beef from Britain, Canada and possibly the US), or post-encephalitis.

◆ LOOK FOR ANY LIVER DISEASE

Note any liver disease, such as Wilson's disease, and hepatolenticular degeneration (which affects basal ganglia).

◆ SEARCH FOR ANY OTHER NEUROLOGICAL SYMPTOMS

Note any other neurological symptoms. Myoclonic jerks suggest Jakob-Creutzfeldt disease. Impaired downward gaze suggests progressive supranuclear palsy. Focal neurological signs suggest subdural hematoma, basal ganglion strokes, and neoplasm. Orthostatic hypotension suggests Shy-Drager syndrome. Cerebellar signs (ataxia, dysmetria, dysarthria) suggest Olivo pontine cerebellar degeneration.

◆ CONSIDER A TRIAL OF A DOPAMINE-ENHANCING DRUG

Note the patient's response to a dopamine-enhancing drug. Symptom resolution or significant improvement suggests idiopathic Parkinson's disease.

The Elderly Patient with Writhing, Twisting Movements (Dystonia)

Unilateral movement suggests a basal ganglion (usually putamen), vascular event or malignancy. Generalized movements suggest medication effect, Huntington's chorea (check family history), and Wilson's disease (check liver function and slit lamp examination).

The Elderly Patient with Possible Aphasia

◆ EVALUATE THE PATTERN OF SPEECH

Lack of speech (mutism) is not aphasia. The key to the evaluation of a patient with aphasia is to check fluency, comprehension and repetition.

◆ DETERMINE THE FLUENCY OF THE SPEECH

Fluent speech sounds normal but the words are not correct. Paraphasias are words generally in the same category. Paranymy is use of words that rhyme or sound similar but are way off the mark.

Yes, the patient's speech is fluent. (This implies a parietal or temporal lobe lesion.) Next, see if the patient can follow a simple command ("Close your eyes"), to test comprehension.

If the patient can follow a command, then see if the patient can repeat a simple phrase ("UVA is number One"). If so, the patient probably has anomic aphasia. (Suspect an inferior frontal, parietal, or temporal lesion.) You can confirm this by giving the patient a list of objects to name, which should cause them difficulty.

If the patient cannot repeat a simple phrase, the patient probably has conduction aphasia caused by a lesion in the posterior Sylvian fissure.

Table 21.10. Types of aphasia

Type	Fluency	Comprehension	Repetition
Wernicke's	Fluent	No	No
Anomic	Fluent	Yes	Yes
Conduction	Fluent	Yes	No
Transcortical sensory	Fluent	No	Yes
Transcortical motor	Nonfluent	Yes	Yes
Broca's	Nonfluent	Yes	No
Mixed transcortical	Nonfluent	No	Yes
Global	Nonfluent	No	No

If the patient cannot follow a command, then see if the patient can repeat a simple phrase. If so, the patient has transcortical sensory aphasia due to a watershed infarct. These patients can repeat like parrots but cannot comprehend.

If the patient cannot repeat a sentence on command, then they have Wernicke's aphasia due to a lesion in the superior temporal lobe. (They may also have right superior quadrantanopsia.)

No, the patient's speech is not fluent. (It is coarse and harsh.) Next, see if the patient can follow a simple command ("Close your eyes"), to test comprehension.

If the patient can follow a command, then can the patient repeat a simple phrase? If so, the patient probably has transcortical motor aphasia. Suspect a watershed lesion.

If not, the patient probably has Broca's aphasia caused by a lesion in the frontal lobe (often with right hemiplegia and facial paresis).

If the patient cannot follow a command, then, can the patient repeat a simple phrase? If so, the patient has mixed transcortical aphasia due to a watershed infarct. If not, the patient has global aphasia.

The Elderly Person with a Gaze Palsy

◆ HORIZONTAL GAZE PALSY

Inability of the patient to conjugately shift gaze in a particular direction suggests CNS disease. Cortical lesions may cause the eyes to deviate toward the side of the lesion. A transient gaze preference suggests frontal lobe disease. Persistent gaze preference suggests a parietal lesion. Lesions below the cortex tend to cause the eyes to deviate away from the side of the lesion. Bilateral frontal lobe lesions may compromise the person's ability to follow a command but still allow tracking of a moving object.

◆ VERTICAL GAZE PALSY
(PARINAUD'S SYNDROME)

Parinaud's syndrome suggests midbrain dysfunction near the posterior commissure, such as from pinealoma. Also consider Wernicke's encephalopathy. Check the pupillary reflexes. Accommodation is greater than light stimulation (the opposite of the Argyll Robertson pupil).

Carl Wernicke (1848–1905) was a German neurologist who studied under Theodor Hermann Meynert who influenced him greatly. Meynert was virtually the only name Wernicke mentioned in his lectures and only his portrait hung on the wall in Wernicke's clinic.

Wernicke's work was mainly concerned with brain anatomy and pathology and with clinical neuropsychiatry. Wernicke was a taciturn and reserved man, not easy to deal with. He did not have much contact with his younger pupils, but his way of examining patients and his demonstrations were so lucid and stimulating that those who had the good fortune to attend his clinics were deeply influenced in their further consideration of neurological and psychiatric problems.

The Elderly Patient with Diplopia

◆ HAVE THE PATIENT CLOSE ONE EYE

If the diplopia disappears when the patient closes one eye, then consider a refraction problem, cataract, or dislocated lens.

◆ CHECK FOR PROPTOSIS

If proptosis is present, then consider an orbital lesion (lymphoma, thyroid disorder, cavernous sinus problem).

◆ PERFORM THE TENSILON TEST
(EDROPHONIUM CHLORIDE)

If positive, this finding suggests myasthenia gravis.

◆ CHECK THYROID FUNCTION TESTS

◆ CHECK FOR ISOLATED EYE MUSCLE WEAKNESS

Finding a partial CN III palsy that spares the pupil suggests diabetes mellitus, thyroid disorder, or vascular disease.

Finding a superior oblique palsy (CN IV) suggests thyroid disorder, trauma or vascular disease.

Finding lateral rectus palsy (CN VI) suggests diabetes mellitus, thyroid disorder, trauma, increased intracranial pressure, and demyelinating disease.

♦ CHECK FOR MULTIPLE WEAK MUSCLES

Weakness in the proximal limb girdle suggests myopathy or mitochondrial problem. Weakness in the bulbar muscles with diplopia suggests oculopharyngeal muscle dystrophy.

♦ CHECK FOR A COMPLETE CN III PALSY

A complete CN III palsy suggests diabetes mellitus, thyroid disorder, and aneurysm.

♦ CHECK FOR BRAIN STEM SIGNS

If brain stem signs are present in a patient with diplopia, this suggests vascular disease.

♦ CHECK FOR SIGNS OF PARKINSONISM

If parkinsonian features are present, consider progressive supranuclear palsy and paraneoplastic syndromes.

The Elderly Patient with CN IX, CN X, and CN XI Palsy Suggests Disease at the Foramen Magnum (Vernet's Syndrome)

ADDITIONAL NEUROLOGICAL PEARLS

Charles-Édouard Brown-Séquard (1817–1894) was creative and curious. He took an early interest in digestion and would swallow sponges attached to strings and then pull them up in order to analyze the gastric juices they contained. Later, he injected himself with an extract taken from the testicles of freshly killed guinea pigs and dogs, and thereby claimed to have been "rejuvenated." Considered outlandish at the time, his work stimulated great interest in the study of hormones and endocrinology. He understood that the interdependence of cells within the body was also based on mechanisms of "internal secretions" that influenced remote organs. It was Brown-Séquard who discovered that the adrenal glands are essential for life, perhaps his greatest achievement.

Brown-Séquard's syndrome, or Brown-Séquard's hemiplegia, is based on his experiments involving the surgical division of the dorsal columns of the spinal cords of "cold-blooded vertebrates, birds and mammals." He observed that hemisection of the spinal cord resulted in ipsalateral paralysis and ataxia, as well as contralateral loss of pain and temperature sensitivity.

Table 21.11. Additional Neurological Pearls	
Sign	*Manifestation*
Bonhoeffer's	• Decreased muscle tone in thalamic or basal ganglion disease
Brissaud-Marie's	• Spastic paralysis of the lips and tongue in the setting of hemiplegia, suggesting a pontine lesion
Brown-Sequard's	• Paralysis and loss of proprioception with contralateral complete loss of sensation, suggesting a unilateral spinal cord lesion
Brun's	• Vertigo, headache, nausea and vomiting on sudden head movement, suggesting cerebellar tumor or tumor in the third or fourth ventricles
Charcot's	• The characteristic gait of a patient with hemiplegia, with extension and circumduction of the paralyzed leg

Table 21.11. Additional Neurological Pearls *(continued)*

Sign	*Manifestation*
Courtois'	• When the neck of a comatose patient is flexed, unilateral flexion of the hip and knee, ipsilateral to the lesion
Crichton-Browne's	• Bilateral lip tremors seen in multi-infarct dementia
Dejerine's	• Radicular pain increasing with laughing, coughing, straining or sneezing
Dissociation	• Loss of temperature and pain sensation with intact touch and position sense, suggesting a problem in the spinothalamic tract, such as syringomyelia or deep brain lesion
Froment's	• Flexion of the distal phalanx of the thumb to hold a piece of paper between the thumb and forefinger, suggesting ulnar nerve paralysis
Grasset's	• Preservation of the sternocleidomastoid contraction in hemiplegia
Grasset-Gaussel	• A supine patient with hemiparesis who can raise either leg separately, but cannot raise them together; if the paralyzed leg is raised, it will fall when the unaffected leg is passively raised
Grasset-Hoover	• Feeling increased pressure on the hand placed under the foot while the patient raises the weak foot, suggesting hemiparesis
Holme's	• Inability of a patient to quickly adjust to a jarring movement, suggesting cerebellar disease
Horsley's	• Higher axillary temperature on the hemiparetic side, suggesting middle meningeal artery hemorrhage
Joffroy's	• Decreased ability to calculate simple arithmetic in early dementia
Kerr's	• With spinal cord disease, the skin feeling softer below the sensory level
Lhermitte's	• Electric shock feeling down the back with neck flexion, suggesting cervical spinal cord irritation
Lichtheim's	• Patient with aphasia who can demonstrate the number of syllables of a word with fingers, suggesting subcortical disease
Marinesco's	• Coldness, redness and edema of the hand, suggesting syringomyelia
Myerson's	• Blinking that is not extinguished with tapping on the forehead or over the temple, suggesting basal ganglion disease, especially Parkinsonism
Negro's	• Cogwheel rigidity in Parkinsonism
Neri's leg sign	• Knee flexion with trunk flexion and contralateral extension on standing, suggesting sciatica

Table 21.11. Additional Neurological Pearls *(continued)*

Sign	*Manifestation*
Parkinson's	• Masked face
Raimiste's movement	• Abnormal involuntary movement of one side when the opposite limb is moved, suggesting spasticity
Souque's	• Loss of reflex leg extension when a seated patient is quickly leaned backward, suggesting a problem in the corpus striatum
Vermel's	• Visible unilateral temporal artery pulsation in the setting of migraine headache
Villaret's	• Plantar flexion of the great toe when the calcaneus is squeezed, suggesting sciatic nerve involvement
Tinel's	• Paresthesia of a peripheral nerve distally when tapping on the nerve in the setting of injury, suggesting partial recovery
Wartenberg's arm sign	• Absence of arm swinging with walking, suggesting extrapyramidal tract disease
Wartenberg's leg sign	• Decreased leg swinging on the examining table, suggesting extrapyramidal disease

CHAPTER 22

Evaluation of Mental Status

"You can tell whether a man is clever by his answers. You can tell whether a man is wise by his questions."

— **Naguib Mahfouz**

"Be what you would seem to be — or, if you'd like it put more simply — never imagine yourself not to be otherwise than what it might appear to others that what you were or might have been was not otherwise than what you had been would have appeared to them to be otherwise."

— **Lewis Carroll**

Evaluating the elderly person with possible memory impairment is an important medical responsibility. Because independent living depends so much on adequate mental functioning, accurate assessment of mental performance is an essential component of geriatric care; errors or oversights can produce unfortunate and far-reaching consequences. This chapter will offer some observations, with the basic premise that the clinical interview and examination is the "physical examination" of the intellect. This approach is still a work in progress and is presented to stimulate additional thinking.

DEMENTIA DEFINED

Dementia is a loss of intellectual ability that occurs over a long period of time and affects many areas of cognitive functioning. Memory loss is one feature, but at least one other impairment must be present: linguistic ability, orientation, visual-spacial skills, and calculating with numbers. The key elements of the definition are severity, duration, and the presence of multiple deficits.

Dementia is really a symptom rather than a diagnosis. Aging does not cause dementia, although aging and dementia are related in subtle and complex ways. Many conditions can produce dementia. Its course is unpredictable. No one, in my experience, has the skill to consistently and confidently predict the precise course of the illness and the specific sequence of behavioral and functional change.

Additional clues for the course of mental impairment are available from determining the onset. In addition to delirium, a rapidly progressing change in mental function over days to weeks suggests encephalitis. A course of impair occurring over weeks to months suggests normal pressure hydrocephalus and subdural hematoma. There is a lot of variability in the presentation and these observations are mainly meant as rules of thumb.

How to Tell Dementia from Delirium

Dementia and delirium can coexist, and having impaired mental function is a risk factor for delirium. Dementia is differentiated from delirium by its onset. Delirium occurs suddenly with rapid fluctuations in mental status. The delirious patient often has reduced attention span, agitation, disorganized thinking, and perceptual disturbances. Asterixis is pathognomonic for delirium. Delirium is a medical emergency requiring prompt evaluation of its cause. Some possible differentiating features are shown in Table 22.1.

The Goal in Evaluating Mental Function

The fundamental clinically relevant question regarding mental status is "Can this older person appreciate and act on risks?" Note that this statement does not imply risk reduction, since a person may choose to take a risk. The key is whether the person acts with knowledge

of the implications of his or her decisions. However we approach mental status evaluation, this is the question we need to answer. Secondary questions: "What is the degree of mental resiliency and flexibility? How well are unpredictable circumstances handled? How large is the sphere of activity?"

Patients worried about their memory have several implicit concerns. What is happening to me? What can be done about it? How will things progress? No matter how we approach mental status testing, we need to address these questions.

Mental Status Questionnaires

The most widely accepted method of mental status assessment is the use of mental status questionnaires. An older person is asked a series of questions, or is given a task to perform such as copying a geometrical figure, and the total number of correct or appropriate responses is compared to a standardized scale. This approach has several advantages; most importantly, it ensures that mental function is addressed during the evaluation. Questionnaires are quick, convenient, reliable and inexpensive to administer, and the numerical results seem familiar and meaningful, like laboratory test values.

Despite these advantages, mental status questionnaires are often inadequate in clinical practice. Patients and families, having noticed changes in mental ability, ask questions about

Table 22.1. Differentiating features between dementia and delirium

	Dementia	*Delirium*
Onset	Months to years	Hours to days
Movements	Generally normal	Asterixis, tremor
Speech	Usually normal	May be slurred
Attention span	Usually normal	Fluctuates
Perception	Hallucinations uncommon	Hallucinations common
Mood	Disinterested	Fear, suspicion, hypervigilance
EEG	Mildly slow	Always abnormal

the cause, significance, and likely course of these changes. Underlying these concerns is the hope that the process can be reversed or slowed. In addition, the physician must consider the patient's safety and the safety of others. Fundamental issues are raised about activities, like driving and cooking, that demand constant attention to avoid the risks of injury or death. Not surprisingly, traditional mental status scales offer little help in answering these challenging questions.

A Different Approach

Fortunately, the clinician has a wealth of relevant information, gathered from subtle observations, careful questioning, and the physical examination, that greatly help in making specific diagnostic and management decisions. Discounting the value of these direct observations purely in favor of information gathered with a questionnaire can lead to serious errors.

The sensitive clinician, paying careful attention to the patient, generally reaches an impression of the person's mental function and the reliability of their information early in the interview. This impression is not a final judgment, but a preliminary integration of numerous subtle observations. This observational strategy complements more conventional methods and is surprisingly underreported in geriatric assessments.

When determining mental function, the clinician must accurately size up the elderly patient as a person, to be able to place the subsequent information in context. The premise is that everything about an individual, including appearance, dress, language, and behaviors, represents a unified presentation of self (see also Chapter 3). Each of us presents a unified sense of self that is revealed to others through the choices we make. None of the expressions is random. We can use the static features of physical characteristics, grooming, and dress as a backdrop for comparison with the active responses of language and behavior.

In essence, as long as the patient's present-ation of self seems unified and congruent along these multiple dimensions, the physician tends to assume normal mental functioning. Any apparent incongruity, that may reflect anything from a simple eccentricity to a sign of illness, tends to trigger further inquiry. The physician must begin the assessment without preconceived notions of the person's mental function. An open, unbiased state of mind allows the clinician to gather necessary information and avoids premature closure regarding mental functioning.

There are some limitations and points of caution. Naturally, the environment may modify the specific clues of this presentation of self. For example, the patient's home, the clinic, the hospital, and the long-term care facility have very different influences on personal expression. Also, the processes of making and interpreting observations happen almost simultaneously. The physician routinely forms judgments about patients, but must always be cognizant of the difference between what the patient means by what he or she says or does, versus what the doctor would mean if he or she said or did the same. Finally, making accurate and detailed observations requires motivation, careful attention, and an understandable language of perceptive description.

OBSERVATIONS OF MENTAL FUNCTION

Appearance and Grooming

Observations of the patient's appearance and grooming form the basis of the evaluations. The person's apparent age should be compared to his or her chronological age. Facial symmetry and expressiveness may reflect illness or drug effect, or the degree of interest in interacting. An example is a woman who moves slowly and has a slight hand tremor, and whose facial expression does not seem to change.

◆ Patient's General Attitude

Another observation is the patient's general attitude. Sometimes people with early mental impairment seem overly polite and a little too folksy and cooperative. This lack of inhibition may seem incongruous with other observations. Likewise, a flat, depressed or suspicious attitude communicates useful information.

◆ Hygiene and Facial Grooming

Hygiene and facial grooming may show areas of neglect, application of makeup, shaving, or other facial features. These clues reflect personal tastes, manual dexterity, joint range of motion, eyesight, degree of interest in appearance, and cognitive level, including the level of awareness, concentration, memory, and apraxia. An example of this type of observation is an elderly woman with mascara and eye shadow applied more heavily around the left eye and with uneven lipstick on the right side of her mouth. Observations of the hair, including the style, coloring, cleanliness, or the use of a hairpiece, are also useful in appreciating mental status. The mouth may show signs of dental decay, gum abnormalities, and adventitious movements. These can suggest illness or drug effect, manual dexterity, susceptibility to injury, degree of interest in self-care and cognitive function. For example: an elderly man with a few loose, yellowed teeth in the front of his mouth, and wrinkled or cracked skin at the corners of his mouth.

◆ Clues from Exposed Skin

Clues from exposed skin are also informative in evaluating mental function. Skin texture, cleanliness, lesions (such as fresh scars or burns), calluses and tattoos can reflect vocational and avocational activities, financial circumstances, illness, manual dexterity, joint range of motion, eyesight, susceptibility to injury, interest in appearance, and overall awareness. An example of this type of observation would be an elderly man, who lives alone, with rough, dry and calloused hands which also have numerous small healing cuts and scars.

Dress

Observation of dress comprises the second dimension of mental status observations. These observations can reveal personal tastes, ethnic or cultural influences, weight change, eyesight, seasonal variations, degree of interest in appearance, susceptibility to injury (for example: accidental hypothermia), and the ability to make choices compatible with social norms.

The patient's sense of style is shown in the color, material, designs, and ornamentation. The fit of the clothing can reflect weight change and the state of the fastenings can suggest a change in cognitive function. For example, seeing an elderly man whose pants are unzipped and whose shirt is misbuttoned raises questions of mental acuity. The degree of cleanliness also reflects the function of instrumental activities of daily living. An extensive list of observations related to dress is included in Chapter 3.

Language

Language provides the third dimension of the observational mental status evaluation. In analyzing language there are some initial considerations while interviewing. The first observation is whether you can capture and maintain the patient's attention. If you cannot capture and maintain the patient's attention, then strongly consider delirium or psychiatric illness.

◆ Look for Potential Barriers to Communication

Potential barriers to communication include vision, hearing, receptive and expressive aphasia, language, and too much ambient noise, such as in a busy emergency room. These communication difficulties can be misinterpreted as mental dysfunction and must be fully compensated for before mental function can be evaluated. An example is an elderly man who continually looks puzzled when the physician talks, and frequently looks at family members.

◆ BE ALERT TO LINGUISTIC MODIFICATIONS

Analyze the delivery as well as the content of language. As outlined in Chapter 3, key observations are the speech rate, pauses, tonal quality, volume, pitch and articulation. These observations can reflect general physical status (voice strength as a marker of overall vitality), personality, self-confidence, self-esteem, emotional or affective status, and cognitive function (level of awareness, concentration, memory, dysphasia). An example of a paralinguistic observation is a woman who talks very rapidly and loudly, at a feverish pitch, rarely pausing for more than a few seconds.

◆ ANALYZE THE LANGUAGE COMPLEXITY

Pay attention to word choices, clearness, sensibility, appropriateness, sentence complexity, descriptive richness and pronoun use. Linguistic simplicity or complexity reveals personality, self-confidence, level of intellectual sophistication, and cognitive function. An example of this area is a man who uses very technical and impersonal terms when talking about his life's work, using many words repetitively.

◆ ANALYZE THE LOGIC OF THE CONTENT OF THE PATIENT'S STATEMENTS

Consider the clearness and completeness of the thoughts communicated and the precision of the answers. Pay attention to sensibility, consistency and level of sophistication. In performing this analysis consider digressions from the main theme and whether the conversation returns to the point. Notice the flow of ideas, the patient's level of anticipation and insight, and evidence of judgment and abstract thinking.

People with early dementia may have difficulty in using their imagination. Try having the person take you on a "mental walk" through the house by asking them to meet you at the front door and showing you through the house. Another area to pay close attention to is the precision of the answers. The boundaries of the answer to a question are contained in the question (a concept of context specificity). A person with dementia may quickly answer a question, but not within the implied boundary. For example, a gardener with early dementia was asked specifically what plants she planted last weekend. The answer, "Annuals and perennials," was too abstract. Likewise an elderly realtor was asked where specifically to buy a house. The answer, "Buy a single-family dwelling in a good neighborhood," did not exactly answer the question.

Behaviors

Behaviors are the fourth category of mental status observations. Level of consciousness can reflect sleep patterns, illness or medication affect. An example is a man who does not have his eyes completely open and who slurs his words.

◆ POSTURE

The posture shows general physical status, illness or drug effect, self-confidence, self-esteem, personality, degree of interest in interacting, and cognitive function. For example, the elderly woman who sits hunched over, with her arms tucked close to her body, may be signaling vulnerability.

◆ THE DEGREE OF INTERACTION

The degree of interaction is another important area of behavioral observation. This interaction toward the physician and others is revealed through eye contact, body language, and sense of intensity (see Chapter 3). Interaction suggests general physical status, illness or drug effect, self-confidence, self-esteem, personality, degree of interest in interacting and cognitive function. An example is an elderly man who looks directly at you and listens attentively, but raises his eyebrows and avoids eye contact with his wife when she talks about how he is doing.

♦ WATCH THE PERFORMANCE OF
  SIMPLE TASKS OR ACTIONS

These actions include how the person walks into the room, takes a seat, and so on. Pay attention to the amount of time and the degree of effort required. The performance of simple tasks is intimately related to the person's future needs for care. (The slower you are in task performance, the greater your risk of needing help within the next year or two.) Movement reflects general physical status, illness or drug effect, eyesight, manual dexterity, range of joint motion, degree of interest or motivation, and cognitive level. An example is an elderly man who slowly shuffles into the examining room and almost drops backwards into a seat, but who rises more decisively and confidently when the visit is over and walks out of the room more quickly.

SUMMARY

This observational approach to exploring mental function involves an active mental process employed by the clinician to appreciate any incongruities in the person's presentation of self. From this perspective the clinical encounter becomes the physical examination of the intellect. This strategy does not seem to take longer than the usual careful medical history and may represent a subset of the clinician's general information gathering skills. Nevertheless, it is useful to refine your approach.

The physician's capacity to know and understand his or her patients is firmly grounded in the ability to make, describe, and interpret observations. This is especially true of an integral and complex domain such as mental functioning that consists of multiple, interacting dimensions. Effective mental functioning cannot be fully defined by existing approaches that focus on specific standardized sets of questions. Mental functioning is too dynamic, and its manifestations are too variable, to fully assist patients and their families by using a fixed, static, content-oriented "pencil and paper" approach.

The framework shared in this chapter is crude and rudimentary, and must be considerably refined and tested. To paraphrase Sir William Osler's basic tenet, "If you carefully observe the patient, he will tell you the diagnosis," and you can learn a lot more in the process.

CHAPTER 23

Assessment of Balance and Gait

"Wisdom stands at the turn in the road and calls upon us publicly, but we consider it false and despise its adherents."

— **Kahlil Gibran**

"The power of moving in every part of the body by means of the muscles which obey the will, or by means of others the actions of which are involuntary; the various perceptions by the five external senses; and lastly those mental powers named memory, imagination, attention, and judgment, together with the passions of the mind; all these seem to be exercised by the ministry of the nerves; and are impaired, disturbed, or destroyed, in proportion to any injury done to the brain, the spinal marrow, and nerves, not only by their peculiar diseases, of which we know little, but by contusions, wounds, ulcers, and distortions, and by many poisons of the intoxicating kind."

— **William Heberden**

Balance and gait assessment is difficult to teach, especially in a book. Sequential logic works but seems cumbersome. Pattern identification is difficult to communicate because of the nuances and subtleties of the observations. In addition, multiple neurological and musculoskeletal conditions can occur in the elderly patient, producing a complex picture.

THE GAIT CYCLE AND COMMON PATTERNS

The gait cycle is divided into stance and swing phases. In the stance phase the body weight is accepted and the single limb supports the body weight as the opposite leg swings through. In the swing phase the limb is moved forward.

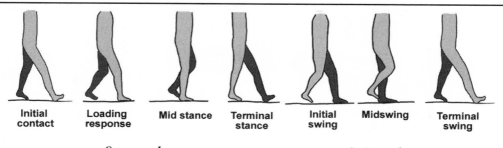

Stance phase   Swing phase

Figure 183. Gait Cycle.

This illustration shows the components of the gait cycle. The gait cycle is divided into the stance and swing phases. These phases are shown for the right leg. Each component of the gait cycle will be illustrated.

The stance phase begins with initial contact of the foot. The biomechanical goals are to position the foot, slow down the leg, absorb the shock of contact and continue the progression of movement. The muscles most active during the initial contact are the hip extensors, knee flexors and the ankle dorsiflexors.

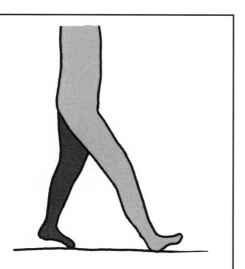

Figure 184. Initial Contact.

The stance phase begins with initial contact of the foot. The biomechanical goals are to position the foot, slow down the leg, absorb the shock of contact and continue the progression of movement. The muscles most active during the initial contact are the hip extensors, knee flexors and the ankle dorsiflexors.

The line of body weight is normally medial to the subtalar center, creating an eversion force that is normally countered by the pretibial muscles.

Abnormal contact patterns are the shuffle, flatfoot contact and forefoot contact. Shuffling occurs when there is a low heel strike usually caused by weak ankle dorsiflexors or a plantar flexion contraction. Flatfoot contact can be caused by spastic hamstring muscles, or weak or spastic quadriceps muscles. Knee problems can also produce a flatfoot contact. When the forefoot strikes first, that is foot drop. There are three patterns of foot drop. Neutral foot drop is when the 2nd and 5th metatarsals hit equally, implying ankle and knee dysfunction, such as in cerebral palsy. Equinovarus foot drop is when the 5th metatarsal hits first, implying peroneal nerve weakness or stroke. Equinovalgus foot drop, when the 2nd metatarsal hits first, suggests a bedfast patient with inactivity of the inverting muscles.

The loading response is the initial period of double stance support (when both legs are on the ground). The biomechanical goals are to absorb the body weight, stabilize the pelvis and slow the leg. The active muscles during the loading response are the hip abductors, knee extensors and ankle plantar flexors.

Abnormal loading response patterns are

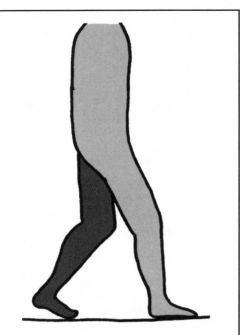

Figure 185. Loading Response.
The loading response follows the initial contact and is the first period of double stance support (when both legs are on the ground). The biomechanical goals are to absorb the body weight, stabilize the pelvis and slow the leg. The active muscles during the loading response are the hip abductors, knee extensors and ankle plantar flexors.

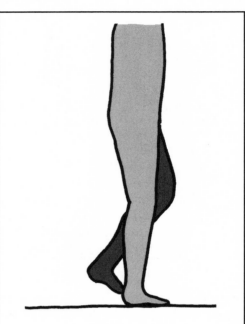

Figure 186. Mid-Stance.
The mid-stance follows the loading response. The biomechanical goals are to stabilize the trunk by the hip muscles to limit pelvic tilting and to stabilize the knee. In addition, the ankle rocker action preserves momentum and allows progression over the stationary foot. The ankle plantar flexors are the primary active muscles. Problems with the knee or ankle produce abnormal mid-stance patterns.

either stiff or excessive knee motion. Stiff or minimal knee motion can be caused by weak quadriceps muscles or problems with plantar flexion, such as spasticity, contractures or weakness.

Once the loading response is complete, the mid-stance portion of the gait cycle occurs. The biomechanical goals are to stabilize the trunk by the hip muscles to limit pelvic tilting and to stabilize the knee. In addition, the ankle rocker action preserves momentum and allows progression over the stationary foot. The ankle plantar flexors are the primary active muscles. Problems with the knee or ankle produce abnormal mid-stance patterns. Knee problems such as quadriceps muscle weakness or polio with flexion contractures require ankle compensation, usually with a fore-

foot stance. Ankle problems require knee compensation. Spasticity of the plantar flexors causes premature heel lifting, while restricted ankle motion produces knee hyperextension (genu recurvatum).

The last part of the stance phase is when the heel normally rises. (Watch for this.) Weak ankle plantar flexors prevent efficient heel rise. The biomechanical goals are to accelerate the body mass beyond the stationary foot. The passive hip extenders (psoas muscles) and knee extenders allow the trunk and pelvis to move forward, generating ankle dorsiflexion.

The limb now prepares for the swing through, with the goals preparing to clear the foot and transfer body weight to the other limb. The critical action is knee flexion which is compromised by joint disease, quadriceps

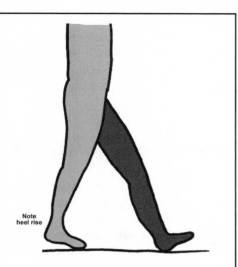

Figure 187. Terminal Stance.

The terminal stance phase is when the heel normally rises. (Watch for this.) Weak ankle plantar flexors prevent efficient heel rise. The biomechanical goals are to accelerate the body mass beyond the stationary foot. The passive hip extenders (psoas muscles) and knee extenders allow the trunk and pelvis to move forward, generating ankle dorsiflexion.

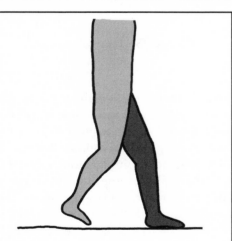

Figure 188. Initial Swing.

The initial swing clears the foot and completes the transfer of body weight. The key motions are hip flexion, knee flexion and ankle dorsiflexion. Abnormal patterns in initial swing result in relative limb lengthening. To compensate, the patient may drag the toes, or show excess trunk movement, excess knee flexion or increased ankle dorsiflexion.

spasticity and slow speed. The active muscles are the hip flexors, knee flexors and ankle dorsiflexors.

The action continues with the initial swing which clears the foot and completes the transfer of body weight. The key motions are hip flexion, knee flexion and ankle dorsiflexion. Abnormal patterns in initial swing occur with weak contralateral hip abductors, spastic quadriceps muscles or weak ankle dorsiflexors. These problems result in relative limb lengthening. To compensate, the patient may drag the toes, or show excess trunk movement, excess knee flexion or increased ankle dorsiflexion.

As the swing moves to the mid-swing, the biomechanical goals are to continue the leg forward movement and clear the foot. During

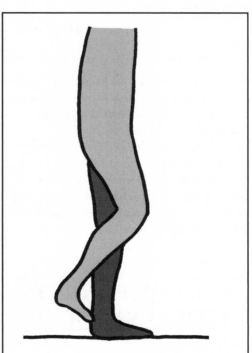

Figure 189. Mid-Swing.

The biomechanical goals of the mid-swing are to continue the leg forward movement and clear the foot. The critical actions are knee extension and ankle dorsiflexion, with the active muscles being the hip flexors, knee extensors, and the ankle dorsiflexors.

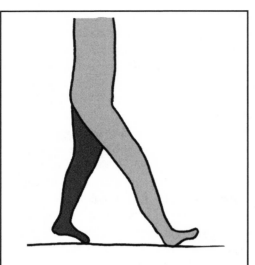

Figure 190. Terminal Swing.
The goals of the terminal swing phase are to slow the leg, stabilize the knee, position the foot, and prepare to contact the ground. The active muscle groups are the hip extensors, knee extensors, knee flexors, and the ankle dorsiflexors.

mid-swing, the critical actions are knee extension and ankle dorsiflexion, with the active muscles being the hip flexors, knee extensors, and ankle dorsiflexors.

At the end of the cycle, the goals of the terminal swing phase are to slow the leg, stabilize the knee, position the foot, and prepare to contact the ground. The active muscle groups are the hip extensors, knee extensors, knee flexors, and ankle dorsiflexors.

KEY COMPONENTS OF THE EVALUATION

In overview, there are three parts to the assessment. The lower extremity examination looks for mechanical issues. The complete neurological examination (from toe to head) focuses on muscle weakness, impaired proprioception, cerebellar signs, basal ganglion dysfunction, and frontal lobe disease. The func-

tional evaluation assesses the person's fall risk. Elements of the functional examination include the Tinetti variation of the "up and go" test, with sitting, standing, walking, and turning; the functional reach test; and toe tapping.

Examine the Lower Extremities

The first part of the evaluation of balance and gait is to carefully examine the lower extremities. Additional information is contained in Chapter 17. The initial search is for mechanical problems in the legs. Look carefully for orthopedic problems, vascular disorders, rheumatic conditions, podiatric concerns (especially shoes), and prostheses. Systematically examine the range of motion of the hips, knees, ankles and feet. Palpate the femoral, popliteal, dorsalis pedis, and posterior tibial pulses, and look for skin lesions. Do not forget to check the shoes for potentially useful signs of wear (see Figure 3).

Check for Leg Weakness

Once your overall survey is complete, check the muscle strength for any signs of leg weakness. If leg weakness is present, carefully note the distribution. Proximal weakness suggests myopathy, and the patient will have difficulty rising from a sitting position. Distal leg weakness implies neuropathy, and the patient will have difficulty walking on the toes and heels.

If there is a monoparesis, the patient will drag and circumduct the leg. In this case (monoparesis), note the deep tendon reflexes. If the reflexes are hyperreflexic, this suggests a CNS lesion, such as an anterior cerebral artery stroke or a parasagittal lesion. Normal or decreased reflexes imply sacral plexus radiculopathy or peripheral nerve problems. Paraparesis (scissors gait) implies a spinal cord, foramen magnum or parasagittal lesion.

Review the Neurological Considerations

Reviewing the presence of neurological symptoms and signs can help to focus the differential diagnosis.

Ask About Dizziness

If the patient complains of dizziness or vertigo, then consider evaluation for vascular, brain stem, vestibular, or medication problems.

Check Romberg's Sign

The presence of Romberg's sign implies proprioceptive abnormality. If the spinal cord is involved, the Babinski sign should also be present. If Romberg's sign is due to neuropathy, then the patient's ankle jerks should be absent.

Look for Cerebellar Signs

If the patient has unsteadiness with eyes open, ataxia, or incoordination, then evaluate the rapidity of the onset of symptoms. Sudden onset of gait abnormality implies a posterior fossa stroke. Progressive or subacute onset suggests a mass, demyelinating disease, degenerative disease, drug effect or metabolic disorder.

Note Any Adventitious Movements

If the patient has a resting tremor and difficulty in initiating gait, consider basal ganglion dysfunction and Parkinsonism.

Check the Lower Extremity Muscle Tone

If the patient has increased lower extremity muscle tone (resistance to extension or tonic foot response) and a gait as if feet are stuck to the floor, consider normal pressure hydrocephalus or frontal lobe dysfunction.

If the patient has an unsteady gait with none of the neurological features listed above, then consider a senile gait or psychiatric illness.

Perform the Tinetti Functional Assessment

The sequence of the Tinetti evaluation includes sitting balance, neck turning, arising from a chair, standing balance, balancing on one leg (then the other), standing balance with eyes closed (Romberg's test), sternal nudge, tandem walk, walking on heels, walking on toes, observing the gait, and sitting down. The utility of this assessment is that specific observations of abnormality suggest various treatment options.

♦ SITTING BALANCE AND ARISING FROM CHAIR

If the patient has difficulty balancing in the chair or cannot rise without using hands on the arms of the chair, consider proximal muscle weakness, arthritis, or neurological disease. Treatment options for this area of impairment include raising the height of the seat, muscle strengthening exercises, and treatment of specific conditions such as arthritis.

♦ NECK TURNING AND EXTENSION

If the patient has limited neck range of motion or symptoms with neck movement, then consider cervical arthritis, cervical spondylosis, or vertebral-basilar insufficiency. Treatment options include avoidance of quick head-turning, turning the body with the head (en bloc) and storing objects low to avoid looking up into high cabinets.

♦ STANDING BALANCE

The patient who is unsteady standing may have orthostatic hypotension, cerebellar disease, sensory deficits, muscle weakness, or pain. Treatments or adaptations include changing position slowly (with leg pumps before standing, by raising up on the toes to pump the gastrocnemius), muscle strengthening, using an assistive device, improved foot care, medication adjustment, and treatment of specific diseases.

♦ STANDING WITH EYES CLOSED (ROMBERG'S TEST)

As mentioned earlier, if the patient has a positive Romberg's test, then there is a sensory deficit (either decreased vision or vestibular function) or decreased position sense (dorsal column spinal cord disease). The lesion implies spinal cord disease if Babinski's sign is present or neuropathy if the ankle jerks are absent. Treatment options include improving the lighting, using night lights, prescribing assistive devices, and changing footwear.

♦ STERNAL NUDGE

Gently nudge the patient's sternum to see how he or she responds. Make sure the patient is well protected before giving the nudge. If the patient staggers and becomes unstable, consider neurological disease and back disease. Treatment options include removing obstacles, using assistive devices, avoiding slippers, and treating specific conditions. These are patients to observe closely during acute illness.

♦ UNSTABLE TURNING AROUND

If the patient is unstable turning around, consider cerebellar disease, hemiparesis, visual field cut, or reduced proprioception. Treatment possibilities include assistive devices, proper shoes, gait training, and reducing obstacles.

♦ UNSAFE SITTING DOWN

The elderly person who crashes down in the chair may have proximal muscle weakness, poor vision, or apraxia. Treatment options include muscle strengthening, raising the height of the seat, and visual assessment.

Gait Observations and Clinical Pearls

Table 23.1 lists some basic observations to make while watching the patient walk down a hall, turn around and walk back.

There are a number of gait observations, but the fundamental question to answer is, "Does the gait look safe?"

A walk with toes turned out implies fallen arches.

Waddling like a duck suggests proximal muscle weakness or hip dislocation.

A marching gait implies foot drop (anything that affects the tibialis anterior muscle).

Walking as if on hot coals implies dysesthesia of the feet.

Short steps that do not leave the floor and both legs stiff, slow and scraping is called scissoring and implies spastic paraplegia. This gait suggests a lesion in the spinal cord, foramen magnum or a parasagittal lesion.

Broad-based gait implies dorsal column or cerebellar dysfunction.

In dorsal column conditions the feet slap the floor and the patient does very poorly blindfolded.

Cerebellar disease causes irregularly irregular steps with truncal instability, swaying and lurching.

Weakness causes a broad-based, tremulous gait.

People with difficulty starting and stopping tend to have basal ganglion or frontal lobe impairment. Note the improvement in gait once it is established.

Short shuffling steps with en bloc turning suggest Parkinsonism.

The patient with decreased step height and dragging feet suggests neurological disease, poor vision, fear of falling, and habit.

Marching implies foot drop. Note the foot placement pattern and exaggerated knee rise. The foot placement will either be neutral, due to knee and ankle dysfunction, equinovarus (caused by peroneal weakness), or equinovalgus, from inactive foot invertors (vide supra).

Table 23.1. Gait observations and possible clinical implications

Movement Feature	Clinical Implication	Comments
Delayed initiation of movement	Integrity of sensory and locomotor coordination	
Delayed initiation with freezing or short steps	Parkinson's disease Frontal lobe disease Low pressure hydrocephalus Subcortical white matter disease	Step length tends to normalize after several steps in frontal lobe disease and low pressure hydrocephalus
Delayed initiation with no freezing or short steps	Hearing impairment Depression Hypothyroidism	
Broad-based gait	Frontal lobe, sensory (dorsal spinal column disease or peripheral neuropathy) or cerebellar dysfunction	
Abnormal cadence	Cadence implies overall motor coordination	Normal is between 100 and 120 steps per minute and symmetrical
Too fast	Hyperthyroidism Anxiety Competitive personality	Greater than 120 steps per minute (the higher the number the more abnormal the cadence)
Too slow	Hypothyroidism Parkinsonism Postural instability Low pressure hydrocephalus	Less than 100 steps per minute (slow cadence denotes frailty and increased risk of falling)
Highly variable	Cerebellar ataxia Subcortical white matter disease Progressive supranuclear palsy	Also implies perceptual problem, attention problem or poor judgment
Asymmetrical	Spastic hemiparesis Peripheral nerve injury Spinal nerve root (radiculopathy) Focal orthopedic concern (joint, bone, muscle or connective tissue) Amputation Vascular disease	Orthopedic problems include hip, knee, ankle, foot or leg muscle, tendon or bursa problems
Abnormal turn-around	Cerebellar diseas Parkinsonism	Subtleties may appear here since it is more demanding than walking straight
Abnormal arm swing		
Reduced	Parkinsonism Hemiparesis (usually from a stroke)	
Adventitious movements	Parkinsonism, chorea, dystonia	

One stiff leg dragged around in a semi-circle suggests upper motor neuron disease (spastic hemiplegia). Look for equinovarus foot placement. Increased deep tendon reflexes suggest anterior cerebral artery stroke or a parasagittal lesion. Normal or decreased reflexes imply sacral plexus radiculopathy or peripheral nerve problems.

With a painful hip, the patient will often place a hand on the hip and attempt to minimize weight on the hip by knee flexion, pelvic tilt and trunk compensation.

A painful knee is suggested when the knee is flexed and the ankle is flexed to minimize knee movement. The gait may have a hopping quality.

BALANCE AND GAIT ASSESSMENT AFTER A FALL

Risk Factors for Falling

Risk factors for falling are increasing age, having previous falls, muscle wasting, poor overall health, being on multiple medications, and having lower extremity arthritis. Factors *not* associated with falls include alcohol ingestion, past vigorous physical activity, blood pressure (or postural changes), the number of environmental hazards, living alone, or education level.

Causes of Falls

Predisposing factors account for about 40% of falls. These factors include accidents (slips and trips) and environmental hazards such as walking surface, lighting, and obstacles.

Precipitating factors for falls are sentinels of illness. Conditions that precipitate falls include acute illness; weakness, balance and gait disorders; syncope and drop attacks; dizziness and vertigo; and orthostatic hypotension.

Sequelae of Falls

Often the impact is minimal, as most falls do not result in injury. However, a major concern is the subsequent loss of confidence or fear of falling. A vicious cycle can be established, beginning with loss of confidence, increased anxiety, limited excursions, social isolation, deconditioning, depression, further loss of confidence, increased unsteadiness, and so on.

A major concern is sustaining a fall-related injury such as a soft tissue injury or fracture. Approximately 3%–6% of falls result in a fracture. Hip fractures are common. The hip fracture rate is 0.5% for 65–69 year olds and 10% for those over 85. Arm fractures are roughly one-third of fractures, rib fractures are 20% of fractures, and vertebral, pelvic, and facial fractures are about 5% each.

Decreased bone density is a significant factor in fall-related injury. Bone mass is reduced by 25%–30% in women over the life span and by 15%–20% in men. The fracture likelihood is *traumatic intensity x frequency / bone strength*.

Table 23.2.
Risk factors for injurious falls in independent-living people

Risk Factor

- Advanced age (over 90 triples the risk)

- History of a previous fall

- Impaired mental function

- Short step length

- Use of assistive device such as a cane or walker

- Medications, especially psychoactive drugs, sedatives, nonsteroidal anti-inflammatory drugs, vasodilators, anticonvulsants, benzodiadepines, antidepressants, cardiovascular drugs

Table 23.3. Risk factors for injurious falls in institutionalized people

Risk Factor

- Increasing age
- History of falling
- Cognitive impairment
- Being ambulatory
- Visual impairment
- Antihypertensive medication

Fracture Implications

For the physician: The fall was probably severe, so look for other injuries.

For the patient: More than 50% of injured fallers are discharged to long-term care and more than 50% of these will stay.

Evaluation of the Elderly Person at the Site of a Fall

◆ KEY ISSUES

If you are called to see an elderly person who has just fallen, you have two fundamental questions: 1) Has the patient had a catastrophic event? and 2) Has the patient sustained an injury? Look carefully for any evidence of myocardial infarction, pulmonary embolus, stroke, arrhythmia, hemorrhage, or any other acute catastrophe. Next, evaluate the extent of any injuries, such as fracture, internal injury, or soft tissue injury.

◆ BASIC OBSERVATIONS

Pay careful attention to the patient's level of consciousness, vital signs (especially respiratory rate, pulse and postural BP, and temperature), pallor or ecchymoses. The cardiac evaluation may show arrhythmia, a new murmur, signs of aortic stenosis, or cardiac ischemia.

The extremities may show bony deformity, swelling or ecchymosis, pain on use or weight-bearing, and decreased range of motion.

Carefully inspect the leg. If it is foreshortened and externally rotated, consider fracture of the femoral neck (intertrochanteric fracture). If the leg is externally rotated but not foreshortened, consider fracture of the femoral shaft. If the thigh is externally rotated, flexed and abducted, consider anterior dislocation. If the thigh is internally rotated and adducted with a very prominent greater trochanter, consider posterior dislocation.

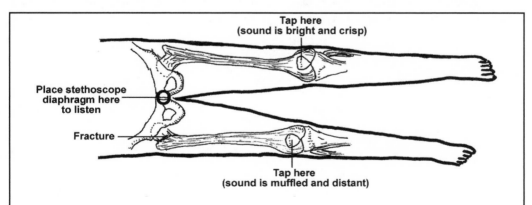

Figure 191. Checking Osteophony (Heuter's Sign).

This test is extremely helpful in evaluating patients on home visits or in the nursing home, and in experienced hands may be more sensitive than a simple hip radiograph. Place the diaphragm of your stethoscope on the pubic symphysis. Gently percuss each kneecap with your forefinger. An intact bone will produce a clear, bright tapping sound. A hip fracture will give a muffled, distant sound.

Now check for osteophony (bone sound) and Hueter's sign. Place the diaphragm of your stethoscope on the pubic symphysis. Gently percuss each kneecap with your forefinger. An intact bone will produce a clear, bright tapping sound. A hip fracture will give a muffled, distant sound. Other approaches are using a tuning fork on the patella or listening over each iliac crest as opposed to the pubic symphysis. These tests are extremely helpful in evaluating patients on home visits or in the nursing home, and in experienced hands may be more sensitive than a simple hip radiograph.

For any possible fracture stabilize the extremity and check the neurovascular bundle distal to the probable fracture site.

Now perform a careful neurological evaluation. Again note the level of consciousness, mental function, focal neurological signs, muscle strength, tone, adventitious movements, and cerebellar findings.

Evaluation of the Patient in the Office Who Has Experienced a Recent Fall

♦ KEY FEATURES IN THE HISTORY

Evaluating the elderly person who has experienced a fall is a key aspect of geriatric assessment. Historical points include medications taken, history of previous falls, and the circumstances of the fall. Important considerations include the location, time of day, presence of witnesses and their account of the fall, and the relation of the fall to cough, position, urination, or head turning. Another useful inquiry is the patient's thoughts on the cause.

♦ SPECIFIC QUESTIONS TO CONSIDER

Did the patient have any awareness of falling or was it totally unexpected? Did the patient slip or trip? Was there any loss of consciousness? Did the patient have immediate recall after the fall? Could the patient get up and walk? Was there any incontinence of urine or stool? Can a witness verify any loss of consciousness? Were there any associated symptoms, such as dizziness or vertigo, palpitations, chest pain, dyspnea, aura or a sudden focal neurological event?

♦ KEY PHYSICAL FINDINGS

Key things to examine include level of consciousness, mental function, vital signs, skin, cardiovascular abnormalities, the extremities, and neurological function. Functional testing should include toe tapping, functional reach, and Tinetti's functional assessment test.

CHAPTER 24

Evaluation of Urinary Incontinence

"Everyone has been made for some particular work, and the desire for that work has been put in every heart."

— **Rumi**

"Be careful about reading health books. You may die of a misprint."

— **Mark Twain**

"There is nothing so stupid as the educated man if you get him off the thing he was educated in."

— **Will Rogers**

Urinary incontinence is the involuntary loss of urine that can cause a social or hygienic problem. Approximately one-third of community-living elderly people experience some degree of urinary incontinence; its prevalence is twice as high in women as in men. Because the majority of people with urinary incontinence can be cured, there is room and need for considerable education about treatment options. This chapter will review relevant neurology and physiology, develop a simple clinical taxonomy, outline an approach to the patient with urinary incontinence, and review general and specific treatment options.

RELEVANT CNS CONNECTIONS

Four neurological loops play a key role in communicating bladder status to the brain and in providing control over urinary storage and elimination.

Stretch receptors in the bladder wall communicate (through Loop 2) to the brain stem detrusor nucleus located at the juncture of the pons and the midbrain. When a critical degree of bladder distension is reached, bladder contractions of increasing force occur. These contractions must be inhibited (by Loop 1 in the brain) to avoid the abrupt and un-

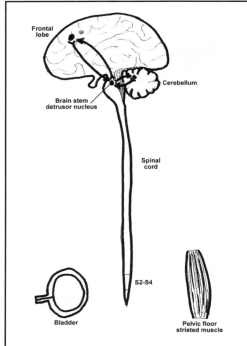

Figure 192. Loop 1.

Loop 1 is an intracranial loop with fibers originating in the frontal lobes, thalamus, and cerebellum, and modulating the response of the brain stem detrusor nucleus. Damage to this loop causes the urinary control system to revert to a more primitive state.

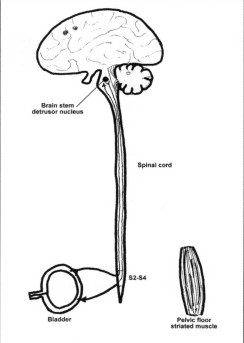

Figure 193. Loop 2.

Loop 2 is the primary reflex arc of detrusor (bladder) innervation. Stretch receptors in the bladder wall communicate directly to the brain stem detrusor nucleus located at the juncture of the pons and the midbrain. When a critical degree of bladder distension is reached, the brain stem detrusor nucleus sends signals down the spinal cord to produce bladder contractions of increasing force. These contractions must be inhibited (by Loop 1 in the brain) to avoid the abrupt and unwanted emptying of the bladder.

wanted emptying of the bladder. Loop 2 is the primary reflex arc of detrusor innervation. Loop 1 modulates Loop 2 activity through cortical, thalamic, and cerebellar inputs.

Loop 3 allows passive relaxation of the pelvic floor muscle during bladder filling to make room for the expanding bladder.

Loop 4 provides volitional control over the pelvic floor muscles and the external urethral sphincter.

Localization of Autonomic Receptors in the Bladder

The second important piece of neurological information to understand is the localization of the autonomic receptors in the bladder. Cholinergic receptors are distributed through-

out the bladder and their stimulation produces bladder contractions.

Alpha-adrenergic receptors are located primarily along the bladder outlet and urethra; stimulation of these receptors causes smooth muscle contraction and increases bladder outlet resistance. Beta-adrenergic receptors are located along the body and dome of the bladder; stimulation of these receptors allows bladder relaxation.

The basic implication of this localization is that storing urine is predominantly an adrenergic event, with bladder relaxation (beta

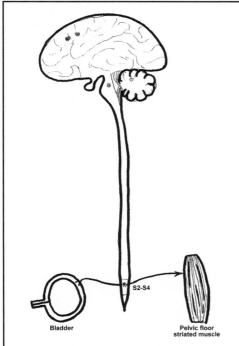

Figure 194. Loop 3.

Loop 3 originates with the stretch receptors within the bladder and, through a purely sacral arc, communicates with the pelvic floor striated muscles. Loop 3 allows passive relaxation of the pelvic floor muscle during bladder filling to make room for the expanding bladder.

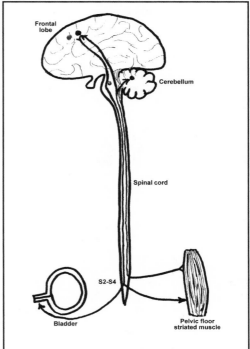

Figure 195. Loop 4.

Loop 4 supplies volitional control over the pelvic floor muscles and the external urethral sphincter, and provides the awareness of the need to void. The loop originates with the stretch receptors in the pelvic floor striated muscle and communicates this information to cells adjacent to loop 1 neurons in the frontal lobes, thalamus and cerebellum. Motor fibers pass down the spinal cord to the external urethral sphincter allowing the conscious stopping of urine flow.

receptor stimulation) and increased outlet resistance (alpha receptor stimulation). Voiding is predominantly a cholinergically mediated event by inhibiting the adrenergic system and stimulating bladder contractions.

THE PHYSIOLOGY OF NORMAL MICTURITION

To maintain urinary continence, the pressure inside the bladder must remain below the intraurethral pressure (or else urine would flow). So let us review the factors influencing bladder pressure and urethral resistance.

Factors Influencing Bladder Pressure

Two factors influence bladder pressure: the muscle tone and intra-abdominal pressure. Detrusor tone is augmented by cholinergic stimulation, beta-adrenergic inhibition, and bladder filling (at high volumes). Decreased detrusor tone results from beta-adrenergic stimulation, cholinergic inhibition and muscle relaxants. Intra-abdominal pressure directly affects bladder pressure, since the bladder is an intra-abdominal organ. Anything that increases abdominal pressure, such as coughing,

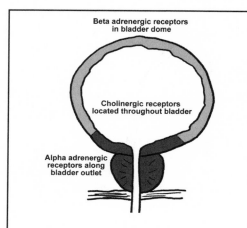

Figure 196. Localization of Autonomic Receptors in the Bladder.

Cholinergic receptors are distributed throughout the bladder and their stimulation produces bladder contractions. Alpha-adrenergic receptors are located primarily along the bladder outlet and urethra; stimulation of these receptors causes smooth muscle contraction and increases bladder outlet resistance. Beta-adrenergic receptors are located along the body and dome of the bladder; stimulation of these receptors allows bladder relaxation.

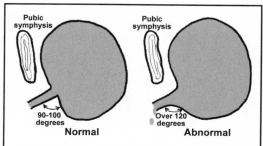

Figure 197. Posterior Urethrovesical Angle.

The posterior urethrovesical angle is a critically important factor that reflects how increases in abdominal pressure are transmitted to the bladder neck. Normally this angle is 90° which causes increases in abdominal pressure to close the bladder outlet. An increase in this angle (such as to 180°) does not allow the transmission of intra-abdominal pressure to pinch the bladder neck shut when abdominal pressure acutely increases. The integrity of this angle is evaluated by the Bonney-Read-Marchetti test.

jogging, laughing, sneezing or bending over will increase bladder pressure.

Four Factors Affect Urethral Resistance

Intra-abdominal pressure directly influences urethral pressure since the proximal portion of the urethra is within the abdominal cavity. So when we cough, jog, laugh, sneeze, or bend over the urethral resistance increases (so the increase in bladder pressure and urethral resistance tend to cancel each other).

Geometric factors are important to allow increases in abdominal pressure to be transmitted to the bladder neck. Especially critical is the posterior urethro-vesical angle. Normally this angle is 90°. An increase in this angle (to 180°) does not allow the transmission of intra-abdominal pressure to pinch the bladder neck shut when abdominal pressure acutely increases. *Urethral smooth muscle tone*

is increased with alpha-sympathetic stimulation and prostatic hypertrophy. Muscle relaxants and alpha-adrenergic blockade reduce bladder outlet resistance. Finally the *thickness of the urethral mucosa* is especially important in postmenopausal women and depends on the quantity of circulating estrogens.

THE PATHOPHYSIOLOGY OF INCONTINENCE

Regardless of the underlying disease, bladder pressure sufficient to overcome sphincter resistance is a prerequisite to urinary incontinence. The fundamental clinical challenge at the bedside is to classify the disproportion between bladder pressure and sphincter competence (resistance).

Two Practical Classifications of Incontinence Mechanisms

While a bewildering array of terms has been proposed to classify urinary incontinence,

Table 24.1. Anatomic classification of incontinence mechanisms	
Bladder Malfunction	*Urethral Malfunction*
Bladder contracts when it should not contract	Urethral resistance is too high
Bladder does not contract when it should	Urethral resistance is too low

there are only five basic mechanisms that can occur singly or in combination to produce urinary incontinence.

The anatomic approach classifies the mechanism as either a bladder malfunction or a urethral problem: 1) the bladder contracts when it should not contract, or 2) it does not contract when it should; 3) the urethral resistance is too high, or 4) it is too low. Finally, 5) the incontinence issue may be due to a mechanism not in the urinary system.

Another way to think about this is to consider the basic functional mechanisms: *Problems of storing urine*, where the bladder contracts when it should not contract or the urethral resistance is weak, and *problems of bladder emptying*, where the bladder contractions are too weak to overcome the normal resistance to expel urine, or the urethral resistance is too high (outlet obstruction).

CLINICAL CLASSIFICATION OF INCONTINENCE

Given the five basic mechanisms, a simple taxonomy of urinary incontinence can be developed.

Detrusor instability refers to bladder contractions that overcome urethral resistance (a problem of storage).

Overflow incontinence means that urine only flows at large bladder volumes (a problem of bladder emptying).

Stress incontinence defines the situation where the outlet resistance is reduced (a problem of storage).

Functional incontinence refers to urologically normal people who cannot or will not void appropriately.

Iatrogenic incontinence is urinary incontinence caused by physician-related factors.

Clinical Features of Detrusor Instability

Detrusor instability refers to urinary incontinence caused by uninhibited bladder contractions of sufficient magnitude to overcome normal bladder resistance. It is the most common type of incontinence (up to 70%).

Detrusor instability can be caused by three potential mechanisms. Defects in CNS inhibition (Loop 1) cause the system to revert to the primary reflex arc. These CNS lesions need to be bilateral and involve the frontal parasaggital cortex, or thalamus.

A second mechanism producing detrusor instability is hyperactivity of the afferent pathways (Loop 2). Significant urinary tract infection, bladder stone, or bladder mass can

Table 24.2. Functional mechanisms producing urinary incontinence	
Problems of Holding Urine	*Problems of Bladder Emptying*
Bladder contracts when it should not contract	Bladder does not contract when it should
Urethral resistance is too low	Urethral resistance is too high

create such hyperactivity that the normal Loop 1 controls are overwhelmed.

The third mechanism is deconditioned voiding reflexes where people learn to be incontinent. While this sounds farfetched, elderly people can develop urinary incontinence through either of two common scenarios. Embarrassment over a single episode of incontinence may lead the person to void frequently in an attempt to keep the bladder empty to avoid another accident. Or the person may cut back on fluids to decrease urine output. Both strategies cause the bladder wall to contract and lose its capacity to stretch, thereby increasing irritability and reducing bladder capacity. The result is further episodes of incontinence. Loss of bladder reflexes caused by physicians can result when toileting becomes associated with uncomfortable equipment such as a cold bed pan or toilet seat, or when the increased physical or verbal attention brought on by the incontinence makes the incontinent person feel rewarded.

There are no characteristic features on history or physical examination except for "urge" symptoms. There is a characteristic urodynamic profile, but the specificity of these findings is unknown.

Clinical Features of Overflow Incontinence

Overflow incontinence occurs when the bladder cannot empty normally. This is generally the result of either very poor bladder contractions (detrusor inadequacy) or an elevated resistance to urine flow. The bladder that does not contract is sometimes called an atonic bladder or neurogenic bladder, and usually occurs in connection with severe diabetes mellitus or disease of the lower spinal cord. Resistance to urine flow implies bladder outlet obstruction (either anatomical or functional). A third mechanism producing overflow incontinence is impaired proprioception.

Generally, people with overflow incontinence have the feeling that their bladder has not emptied completely, experience difficulty starting to void, and note that their urinary stream is weak and dribbly.

Physical examination often reveals a palpable or percussible bladder (post-voiding), which is a highly specific finding. Urine flow rates are usually markedly reduced (below 15ml/second), and there is increased post-void residual urine (greater than 50 cc).

Clinical Features of Stress Incontinence

Stress incontinence is very common in older women and occurs when urethral resistance to flow is reduced. The most likely causes are changes in the lining in the urethra after the menopause related to the decline in circulating estrogens, combined with an earlier weakening in the pelvic muscles following childbirth. This weakness produces geometric alterations in the bladder, especially an increase in the posterior urethrovesical angle. In addition, urinary tract infections may precipitate stress incontinence. Stress incontinence in men usually occurs only with urinary tract infection, after surgery, or as the result of severe neurological disease.

The features of stress incontinence include the loss of urine following coughing, laughing, straining, sneezing, jogging, bending over, or any other condition that abruptly increases abdominal pressure. Pelvic examination may show atrophic vaginitis, bladder prolapse, or other abnormalities. Pushing on the abdomen and seeing urine flow confirms the diagnosis.

Clinical Features of Functional Incontinence

Functional incontinence occurs in people who have a normal urinary system but who cannot or will not reach the toilet in time. A history of accidents on the way to the bathroom suggests this problem. Musculoskeletal limitations are often present. Unfamiliar settings, lack of convenient toilet facilities, or other environmental factors can aggravate the disorder. People with dementia may not be able to recognize the need to void or to locate and use toilet facilities.

Sometimes incontinence is part of a psychiatric condition. Psychological difficulties can precipitate "spiteful" incontinence that occurs sporadically and usually not at night. There are often elements of depression, hostility, or anger in the presentation. Extreme humiliation can also precipitate urinary incontinence.

Clinical Features of Iatrogenic Incontinence

Iatrogenic factors can aggravate or unmask any other etiologies of urinary incontinence. Potent diuretics or physical restraints may create problems for normally continent older persons. Psychoactive medications may reduce attention to normal bladder cues. Medications may cause detrusor instability, overflow incontinence, and urinary retention, or may compromise sphincter competence.

THE CLINICAL EVALUATION OF INCONTINENCY

Overview

The evaluation of the patient with urinary incontinence has three objectives: 1) to identify and manage the factors that may be contributing to the incontinence, 2) to determine if further diagnostic testing is required, and 3) to develop a management plan.

The basic rationale is to document the incontinence, identify the patient who requires immediate urodynamic evaluation, and classify the disproportion between bladder

pressure and urethral pressure. All individuals who cannot be easily classified should be empirically treated for detrusor instability (since it is the most likely cause and does not produce consistent findings), reserving urodynamic studies for treatment failures.

Documentation

Have the patient or family member keep an incontinence chart to show the presence and pattern of urine loss. The pattern may have diagnostic and prognostic value, for example, loss associated with diuretics or incontinence that only happens at a specific time, such as nighttime.

Key Elements of the Medical History

Symptoms of an intense urge to void suggest detrusor instability.

Small volume loss associated only with increases in intra-abdominal pressure suggests stress incontinence.

Recent GU surgery suggests the need to obtain urodynamic studies and urologic consultation.

Medication use can produce incontinence through multiple mechanisms. The incontinence should resolve with appropriate modification.

Key Points on the Physical Examination

The physical examination is oriented toward the abdominal, genital and neurological examinations.

The abdominal examination (Chapter 16) focuses on percussing and palpating the bladder (after voiding) and searching for any areas of hypogastric tenderness. A palpable bladder suggests overflow incontinence.

The rectal examination (Chapter 16) can evaluate perianal sensation and sphincter tone,

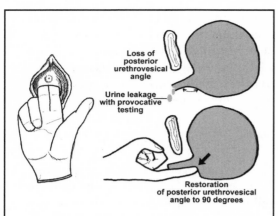

Loss of
posterior
urethrovesical
angle

Urine leakage
with provocative
testing

Restoration
of posterior urethrovesical
angle to 90 degrees

Figure 198. Bonney-Read-Marchetti Test.
This first part of the test is to gently push on
the abdomen during pelvic examination while
observing the urethral orifice. If urine leakage is
observed, then the patient has stress incontinence
by definition. The second part of the test is to
gently elevate the urethra approximately a centimeter with your forefinger and middle finger,
and push on the abdomen again. No urine flow
is a positive test and suggests loss of the posterior urethrovesical angle.

and can confirm prostate size and the presence
of a fecal impaction.

Pelvic examination (Chapter 19) can check
sensation, vaginal atrophy, bladder or rectal
prolapse, the presence of a mass, and the integrity of the posterior urethrovesicular angle
(with the Bonnie-Reed-Marchetti test). Urine
loss on provocative testing, such as pushing
gently on the abdomen, suggests stress incontinence.

Neurological examination (Chapter 21) can
determine mental function, balance and gait
abnormalities, focal neurological signs and
sacral reflexes. Sacral neurological signs suggest
overflow incontinence and the need for urgent
evaluation. Physical restraints or severe arthritis suggest functional incontinence.

Simple Laboratory Studies

Abnormal urinalysis suggests local diseases
and warrants further evaluation.

Abnormal serum glucose, calcium or elec-
trolytes suggest polyuric syndromes or metabolic complications of systemic illness, such
as diabetes mellitus or malignancy.

Abnormal vaginal smear suggests atrophic
vaginitis or malignancy.

Reduced urine flow rate or elevated post-
void residual suggests overflow incontinence.

Principles of Treating
Urinary Incontinence

An accurate pathophysiologic classification improves the likelihood of effective cure.
Most patients can expect significant improvement or total cure. Associated illnesses should
be optimally managed. Palliative treatments,
such as in-dwelling catheters or absorptive
pads, are appropriate for temporary control
or as last-resort options. Behavioral approaches
are useful additions to every treatment
plan.

A variety of products that are not excessively bulky under the clothing are available
to keep incontinent people dry and to control
odor. These items include rubber or plastic
pants with absorbent pads, intermittent catheterization, and external catheters and collecting systems. Generally, these are used only as
last resorts and only after careful evaluation
and treatment have failed to resolve the incontinence. Because the vast majority of people
with urinary incontinence can be successfully
managed or cured, these items should be used
sparingly.

Treating Detrusor Instability

For detrusor instability the goal of treatment is to decrease the bladder contractions
and to improve bladder capacity. Non-drug
treatments include bladder training programs,
pelvic floor exercises, and biofeedback. In general, anticholinergic medications are given to
reduce bladder contractions, and occasionally
medications are given to increase the resistance
of the urethral sphincter.

Treating Overflow Incontinence

The goal of treatment for overflow incontinence is to drain the bladder. Generally a non-drug strategy works best in this condition. Surgery is preferred in those cases where there is obstruction to outflow caused by a large prostate, cancer or stone. When the overflow is the result of detrusor inadequacy, it can be decompressed for about two weeks with an in-dwelling catheter. If bladder function is not restored, an in-dwelling catheter may be required for adequate drainage. Sometimes the obstruction can be overcome by the use of alpha-adrenergic blockers that relax the urethral sphincter.

Treating Stress Incontinence

The goal of treatment for stress incontinence is to increase the outlet resistance. For mild to moderate stress incontinence in women, using medication to reinforce urethral resistance (alpha-adrenergic agonists) is about as effective as doing exercises that strengthen the pelvic floor muscles. Estrogens offer beneficial effects on the tissues around the urethra and are sometimes part of a treatment regimen, but the extent of their helpfulness is unclear. In addition to strengthening the pelvic floor muscles through specific exercises, increased walking is helpful. Walking improves bladder proprioception. In cases that do not respond to these treatments, surgical procedures may be necessary. Injection of substances into the periurethral tissue is sometimes an option.

Treating Functional Incontinence

Functional incontinence is best managed by a simple approach. Physical and environmental impediments to effective voiding should be recognized and corrected. To avoid inadvertent conditioning toward incontinent behavior, the person should not be asked to use the toilet immediately after an episode of incontinence. A toileting program can be established based on an evaluation of the person's voiding pattern. To accomplish this, the person is checked every two hours over a two-day period and a record is kept of whether the person is wet or dry. The optimal toileting schedule can then be established to allow toilet use at a time when the bladder is most likely to be full. Successful toileting should be positively reinforced.

CHAPTER 25

Geriatric Skin Conditions

"Human subtlety will never devise an invention more beautiful, more simple nor more direct than does Nature, because in her inventions nothing is lacking and nothing is superfluous."

— **Leonardo da Vinci**

"The young man knows the rules, but the old man knows the exceptions."

— **Oliver Wendell Holmes**

"It is the mark of an educated mind to be able to entertain a thought without accepting it."

— **Aristotle**

This chapter is not a comprehensive review of geriatric dermatology. There are complete books that cover geriatric skin conditions in detail. It is a worthwhile investment to buy such a handbook or atlas and use it as a reference. Rather, this chapter is meant to be a practical guide to evaluating general skin disorders commonly encountered in geriatric patients.

INFORMATION TO BE GAINED

One of the first things we notice about another person (after their gender) is their skin. The skin is the largest organ of the body and a number of important clues and useful clinical signs appear on the skin. In the past, clinicians paid considerable attention to skin findings and appreciating the skin signs of internal disease. Moreover, the skin is immediately accessible for the clinician to examine.

The important point is that the skin examination is one of active intellectual inquiry. Do not wait for the patient to point out a skin lesion. Look for skin abnormalities and ask yourself why they are where they are. Assume that the presence of a skin lesion has meaning and is not simply a coincidence.

FUNDAMENTAL DERMATOLOGICAL QUESTIONS

Much of dermatology is pattern recognition, and there are some basic questions to consider in organizing your approach.

What Is the Distribution of the Process?

First consider the location and extent of skin involvement. Generalized lesions involve most of the body. Conditions along a dermatome suggest a limited differential related to sensory nerves, such as herpes zoster or malignancy. Other limited locations include the extremities (centrifugal) or the trunk (centripetal). Additional considerations are the areas *not* involved by the process and whether the process is symmetrical or not.

What Is the Color of the Skin?

The next set of questions involves changes in skin color. Look for sites of trauma and both sun-exposed (face and hands) and sun-protected areas (abdomen and pelvis). Generalized decreased pigmentation suggests albinism or pallor, while circumscribed loss of pigmentation suggests vitiligo.

Areas of increased pigmentation are generally most evident in skin folds, scars or areas of pressure from clothing. Generalized increased pigmentation suggests Addison's disease or hemachromatosis.

Limited increased pigmentation over sun-exposed areas, such as the dorsum of the hands, suggests pellagra. Pigmentation over the anterior shins suggests venous stasis change. If the hyperpigmentation has straight borders, consider thermal injury from a heating pad or old radiation injury.

What Is the Nature of the Border?

The next basic issue is to describe the border of any visible lesion. For example, is the border well-circumscribed, serpiginous, diffuse, etc.?

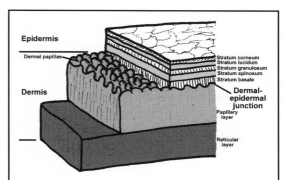

Figure 199. Cross Section of Normal Skin.
Normal skin is composed of five strata, comprising the epidermis, and two layers of the dermis. The most superficial layer, the stratum corneum, is affected in ichthyosis vulgaris. Lichen simplex and hyperkeratosis affect the stratum lucidum. The stratum granulosum contains the target for the staphylococcal scalded-skin syndrome toxin. Pemphigus vulgaris IgG against desmolein affects the stratum spinosum. Bullus pemphigoid has basement membrane-associated antibodies that cleave in this level. The abnormal keratinocytes of psoriasis are seen in all five epidermal strata. The papillary layer of the dermis is the cleavage plane for the Stevens-Johnson syndrome. Dermatitis herpetiformis, Sweet's syndrome, porphyria cutanea tarda, and systemic lupus erythematosis all affect the dermal epidermal junction. The reticular layer of the dermis is the site of involvement of erythema nodosum.

What Is the Type of Lesion?

The descriptive language of dermatology is important to learn because it allows precise communication of visually complex findings. This linguistic precision also sharpens our perceptive capabilities by forcing more complete analysis of what we observe and how we will describe the finding.

Macules are nonpalpable flat lesions up to a centimeter in size. (If you can feel it with

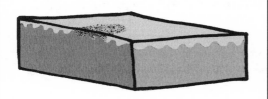

Figure 200. Macules and Patches.
Macules are nonpalpable flat lesions up to a centimeter in size. (If you can feel it with your eyes closed, it is not a macule.) A freckle is an example of a macule. Patches are macular lesions that are larger than a centimeter.

your eyes closed, it is not a macule.) A freckle is an example of a macule.

Patches are macular lesions that are larger than a centimeter.

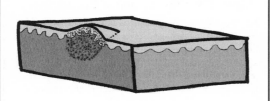

Figure 201. Papules and Plaques.
Papules are elevated, palpable, well-circumscribed, superficial, solid lesions up to a centimeter in size. A plaque is an elevated, well-circumscribed, solid lesion that is larger than a centimeter.

Papules are elevated (palpable), well-circumscribed, superficial, solid lesions up to a centimeter in size.

A *plaque* is an elevated, well-circumscribed, solid lesion that is larger than a centimeter.

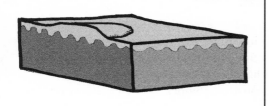

Figure 202. Wheal.
A wheal is a transient edematous papule. A mosquito bite produces a wheal.

A *wheal* is a transient edematous papule. A mosquito bite produces a wheal.

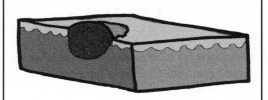

Figure 203. Nodules and Tumors.
A nodule is a solid lesion (a lump) up to a centimeter in size that may extend beneath the skin surface. Tumors are solid lesions greater than a centimeter in size (big lumps) that may extend below the skin surface.

A *nodule* is a solid lesion (a lump) up to a centimeter in size that may extend beneath the skin surface.

Tumors are solid lesions greater than a centimeter in size (big lumps) that may extend below the skin surface.

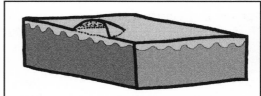

Figure 204. Fluid-filled Lesions.
Vesicles are serous fluid-filled lesions in the epidermis up to a centimeter in size. Bullae are serous fluid-filled lesions in the epidermis greater than a centimeter in size. Pustules are circumscribed fluid-filled lesions in the epidermis containing purulent material.

Pustules are circumscribed fluid-filled lesions in the epidermis containing purulent material.

Vesicles are serous fluid-filled lesions in the epidermis up to a centimeter in size.

Bulla are serous fluid-filled lesions in the epidermis greater than a centimeter in size.

Cysts are fluid-filled lesions that elevate the epidermis.

Petechiae are deposits of blood, generally a millimeter in size.

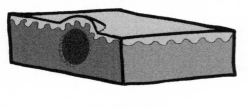

Figure 205. Cysts.
Cysts are fluid-filled lesions that elevate the epidermis.

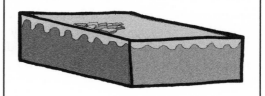

Figure 208. Scales.
Scales are a form of hyperkeratoses with heaps of epidermal cells that produce a raised mass.

Purpura is a deposit of blood greater than a centimeter in size.

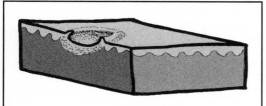

Figure 206. Ulcers.
Ulcers are irregularly shaped excavations in the skin.

Ulcers are irregularly shaped excavations in the skin.

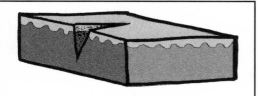

Figure 207. Fissures.
Fissures are clean cuts in the epidermis that produce a defect with sharp edges. Fissures tend to appear on thickened skin.

Fissures are clean cuts in the epidermis that produce a defect with sharp edges.

Fissures tend to appear on thickened skin.

Abrasions are superficial trauma to the skin.

Avulsions are deeper trauma to the skin.

Hyperkeratoses are heaps of epidermal cells that produce a raised mass such as scales and lichenification. A callus is a familiar example of a hyperkeratosis.

Additional Questions

These questions are useful to consider because the answers take us down different branches on the decision tree of pattern recognition.

Are the lesions single or grouped? Do the lesions itch? Is there any relationship to hair? Is there nail involvement? Are the mucous membranes involved?

PERFORMING THE EXAMINATION

General Points

Good lighting is absolutely essential. Direct sunlight is ideal. Examine the entire body if there is any question of a rash or other skin lesion. (There usually is.) Use a magnifying glass to inspect lesions for subtle findings. Sometimes examination under a Wood's light is helpful. Feel the lesions with your gloved hand to note consistency, nodularity, and extent. Be systematic, respectful, conscientious, and thorough.

General Inspection

Wrinkling of the skin suggests weight loss, recent fluid loss (fine lines over the previously edematous area), or vertebral compression fracture giving a transverse abdominal crease. Over-the-face wrinkling can suggest a former heavy smoker, while wrinkles over the back of the neck suggest excessive sun exposure (solar elastosis).

Shiny, tense skin suggests inflammation, edema, or underlying swelling.

Significant dryness raises the possibility of hypothyroidism, dehydration, Vitamin A or C deficiency, and scleroderma.

Significant skin moisture is an important sign in an elderly person. Cold, clammy periphery suggests shock. Moist feet suggest alcohol or benzodiazepine withdrawal. Moist palms suggest thyrotoxicosis. A moist brow and chest pain suggests significant physiological stress. Dermatomal moisture suggests metastatic disease.

A Limited Differential Diagnosis of Skin Lesions

◆ ERYTHEMATOUS LESIONS

Red macules suggest drug reaction, viral illness, and secondary syphilis.

Red papules suggest cherry angioma (scattered and bright cherry-red), dermatitis, scabies (often along the wrist, the belt line and between the fingers), insect bite, psoriasis, folliculitis (along a hair follicle), leukocytoclastic vasculitis, pyogenic granuloma, urticaria, and keratosis pilaris.

Red plaques suggest psoriasis, lichen planus, tinea versicolor, seborrheic dermatitis, T-cell lymphoma, Sweet's syndrome, secondary syphilis, dermatitis, and Paget's disease.

Well-circumscribed red patches in the groin or intertriginous locations suggest tinea cruris. If it involves the scrotum or labia, consider candida. If it spares the scrotum or labia, consider dermatophytes. If the patient is on steroids or has uncontrolled diabetes, consider erythrasma (Corynebacterium minutissimum) infection. Red patches and maceration on feet and between the toes suggests tinea pedis. Red

patch with central clearing suggests ringworm (tinea corporis).

Bright red rash on trunk that radiates centrifugally to the extremities suggests drug eruption.

◆ PURPLE LESIONS

Purple macules suggest senile purpura or an ecchymosis.

Purple papules suggest venous lake (often on the lip), lichen planus, angiokeratoma, mycosis fungoides, lymphoma, melanoma, Kaposi's sarcoma, and blue nevus.

◆ HYPOPIGMENTED LESIONS

Hypopigmented macules suggest radiation effect, tinea versicolor, vitiligo, post-inflammatory change, and tuberous sclerosis.

◆ PIGMENTED LESIONS

Brown macules suggest freckles, café-au-lait lesions, stasis dermatitis, lentigo, various nevi (Becker's nevus, junctional nevus), photosensitivity reaction, tinea nigra, erythrasma, and melasma.

Blue macules suggest lice (maculae ceruleae) or tattoo.

Brown papules suggest seborrheic keratoses (looking like mud stuck on a wall), warts, malignant melanoma, moles (nevi), and dermatofibroma (pinch it to see if it dimples).

◆ SKIN-COLORED PAPULES

Skin-colored papules suggest skin tags (achrodoron), sebaceous gland hyperplasia, lichen sclerosis et trophicus, adenoma sebaceum, basal cell epithelioma, molluscum contagiosum (umbilicated dome), and neurofibroma.

◆ VESICULAR LESIONS

Vesicular lesions suggest herpes zoster (along a dermatome), herpes simplex, dermatitis herpetiformis, erythema multiforme, lichen planus, porphyria cutania tarda, scabies (consider Norwegian scabies), acute eczema, and cat-scratch disease.

♦ BULLOUS LESIONS

Bullous lesions suggest bullous pemphigoid (Nikolsky sign negative), pemphigus vulgaris (Nikolsky sign positive), SLE, fixed drug eruption, and extreme immobility (often over a pressure point).

Pyotr V. Nikolsky (1858–1940) was a Russian dermatologist. The Nikolsky sign was first described by him as a characteristic sign of pemphigus foliaceus, in a thesis on that disease published in 1895. Pierre Louis Alphée Cazenave, founder of the first journal dedicated entirely to dermatology, actually documented the first description of pemphigus foliaceus in 1844. Nikolsky described lateral extension of the preexisting erosion due to lifting up the blister (and when applying lateral pressure to the clinically intact skin), whereas Asboe-Hansen described extension of the intact blister due to pressure applied to its roof.

In his textbook published in 1927, Nikolsky stated, "The skin in pemphigus foliaceus shows a weakened coherence among its layers (especially between the horny and granular layers), even in places between lesions on the seemingly unaffected skin. This characteristic behavior of the skin may be demonstrated by two methods: First, by pulling the ruptured wall of a blister one can detach the horny layer for a long distance, even on a seemingly healthy skin; and second, by slightly rubbing the epidermis between blisters one exposes the moist surface of the granular layer."

♦ PUSTULAR LESIONS

Pustular lesions suggest candidiasis, scabies, herpes virus, folliculitis, rosacea, keratosis pilaris, and pyoderma gangrenosum.

♦ ULCERATING LESIONS

Ulcerating lesions suggest pressure ulcer, stasis ulcer, vesiculobullous diseases, neoplasm, necrobiosis lipoidica diabetacorum, and factitious illness.

♦ NODULES, MASSES OR EXCRESCENCES

Nodules or masses suggest erythema nodosum, hemangioma, carbuncle, furuncle, lipoma (firms up with ice or cooling), sporotrichosis (rose gardener), wart, xanthoma, prurigo nodularis, and malignancies (basal cell carcinoma, squamous cell carcinoma, cutaneous T-cell lymphoma, melanoma, lymphoma, Kaposi's sarcoma, and metastatic cancer).

Moriz Kohn Kaposi (1837–1902), the Hungarian physician and dermatologist, concerned himself primarily with syphilitic lesions of the skin, and contributed many original articles to the dermatological literature of his day. During his training under the tutelage of then-famous Austrian dermatologist Ferdinand von Hebra, Kaposi courted and later married Hebra's daughter. Because she was Catholic and he Jewish, Moriz Kohn changed his name to Moriz Kohn Kaposi, with "Kaposi" being a play on the name of the village of his birth, Kaposvár, Hungary.

Kaposi is better known for "a particular form of malignant, multifocal vascular neoplasm characterized by multiple dark, bluish macular skin lesions, nodules and plaques, enlarging from 1 to 3cm in diameter that eventually may become sarcomatous." The malignancy tends to invade along superficial veins in a symmetric pattern along the distal appendages, but can occur anywhere, with men affected ten times more than women. Known as Kaposi's sarcoma, these lesions were once considered rare, occurring usually in elderly people, but now are more commonly associated with the immunosuppressed patient, especially those with AIDS.

♦ FINE SCALY LESIONS

Fine scaly lesions suggest dermatophytes, xerosis, seborrheic dermatitis (oily scales), psoriasis, and pityriasis rosea.

♦ DESQUAMATION

Desquamation suggests toxic shock, Kawasaki syndrome, staphylococcal scalded skin, or Stevens-Johnson syndrome.

SPECIAL CIRCUMSTANCES

These clinical situations are given with a limited differential diagnosis, as examples of presenting skin conditions. The list is far from comprehensive.

The Elderly Patient with Scaling or Crusting Scalp Lesions

Scaling lesions with thick scales suggest psoriasis. If there are fine scales that also appear in the eyebrows or around the ears and nose, consider seborrheic dermatitis. Fine scales in the setting of widespread dermatitis suggest atopic eczema. Also look for nits attached to the shaft of the hair, which indicate head lice. (The patient may also have posterior cervical lymphadenopathy.)

Crusting lesions suggest tinea capitis, acute inflammation or allergic contact eczema.

The Elderly Person with Hair Loss

An obvious decrease in the density of the hair, with fine hair, is a normal finding in advanced age.

Diffuse hair loss occurring over a few months with no discrete bald spots suggests anagen effluvium or telogen effluvium. If the person has been on cytotoxic drugs, such as chemotherapy, then anagen effluvium is most likely. Anagen hairs have the follicle on them, so look at a few strands of the patient's hair. If the patient has had major surgery or severe illness, then consider telogen effluvium (no follicle on the base of the hair). Telogen effluvium can cause hair to come out very easily and is usually fully reversible.

Other causes of diffuse hair loss in a well-appearing elderly patient are hypothyroidism, iron deficiency, anticoagulant therapy, or diffuse alopecia areata. (Look for hairs that resemble exclamation points and patterned pitting of the finger nails.) If the patient appears ill, then consider systemic lupus or secondary syphilis.

Focal areas of hair loss with a normal appearing scalp suggest alopecia areata (look for exclamation point hairs along the border, and white or blond hair regrowing), traction alopecia if the hair has been tensely braided, or trichotillomania in a psychiatric patient. If the scalp is abnormal, with scaling and itching, then consider psoriasis, pityriasis amantacea, lichen simplex or dermatophyte infection.

Focal bald areas, with scarring of the scalp, suggest previous scalp injury, such as herpes zoster, burn, trauma, radiation therapy, squamous cell carcinoma (especially if there is an advancing ulcer), or morphea. Seeing several lesions with red scaly plaques suggests discoid lupus or lichen planus. Pustular scalp lesions suggest bacterial infection.

The Elderly Person with an Erythematous Facial Rash

Acute transitory lesions predominantly around the mouth or tongue suggest urticaria or angioedema.

Acute persistent lesions, such as papules or plaques on the face without swelling, suggest eczema, seborrhea, or contact allergen. If there has been significant sun exposure, then consider drug-induced photosensitivity reaction (this should spare the upper eyelids behind the ears, and sometimes the upper neck) or polymorphic light eruption. Polymorphic light eruption is often pruritic. Small blisters on an erythematous base in a sun-exposed area can be acute sunburn.

A single blister on a red base that recurs at the same site suggests a fixed drug eruption.

Clustered blisters or vesicles forming crusts suggest herpes simplex or herpes zoster infection. Small blisters, especially around the eyelids with swelling, can indicate contact dermatitis. Large blisters in an ill-appearing elderly person with well demarcated erythema suggest erysipelas.

Chronic erythematous facial papules or plaques with telangiectasia over the cheeks, nose, or chin can be a manifestation of rosacea. Telangiectasias can be seen anywhere steroid creams have been used for long periods of time. Small papules around the mouth or eyelids suggest dermatitis. Papules with a central punctum suggest insect bites. A round, slowly enlarging lesion with a pearly border and rolled edge suggests a basal cell carcinoma.

If the surface is scaly, then feel it and scratch it with your fingernail. If the lesion feels rough like sandpaper, then consider solar keratosis. If there is abundant silver scaling on scratching, then psoriasis is most likely the condition. If the scale sticks to the lesion, then look at the color of the lesion. Atrophy with a pink discoloration suggests discoid lupus erythematosis, while orange or purple lesions suggest lupus vulgaris or lupus pernio. Biopsy may be necessary to confirm these conditions.

A large macule suggests a solar keratosis, while a dark purple lesion is a port wine stain. Linear lesions suggest dermatitis artefacta.

Soft, swollen lesions limited to a man's beard suggest tinea barbae. Staph aureus infection can produce small papules called sycosis barbae.

The Elderly Person with a Skin Lesion Involving the Ears

Involvement of the entire ear with vesicles or crusting suggests eczema.

A lesion on the helix of the ear can be a solar keratoses (feels like sandpaper), squamous cell carcinoma, keratoancanthoma (horny and appearing over a few months) or chilblain (a tender, violaceous nodule produced by the cold).

A lesion on the antihelix of the ear suggests gouty tophi (chalky white), rheumatoid nodule (check the extensor surface of the arm for others), granuloma annulare (look for other lesions), or chondrodermatitis nodularis helicis chronicus (tender papule when lying on the ear).

A lesion on the earlobe suggests contact dermatitis, epidermal inclusion cyst (skin-colored), chilblain (tender, purple nodule that appears in cold weather).

A scaly plaque along the external canal suggests seborrhea or psoriasis.

A lesion behind the ear can be due to basal cell carcinoma (round with heaped-up edge),

epidermoid cyst, or granuloma fissuratum (where eyeglasses produce trauma).

The Elderly Person with a Lesion on the Lips

An acute lesion with erosions and target lesions on the body suggests Stevens-Johnson syndrome.

A single painless ulcer or nodule suggests basal cell carcinoma (on upper lip), lichen planus (lower lip), squamous cell carcinoma (lower lip), or primary syphilis (less commonly in elderly people). Biopsy of a single ulcer is indicated.

A purple discoloration on the lip is a venous lake.

Multiple pigmented lip lesions suggest hereditary hemorrhagic telangiectasia (if they are red), Peutz-Jegher syndrome (if they are brown), and Fordyce spots (if they are pale yellow).

Redness and scaling at the fissures suggest angular chelitis.

A discrete rough rash on the lips, with similar lesions in other places, suggests lichen planus or discoid lupus.

The Elderly Person with Oral Lesions

A single painful oral ulcer suggests apthous ulcer (small and round with yellow center), Behcet's disease (look for genital ulcerations), lichen planus, squamous cell carcinoma, lymphoma, sarcoma, and leukemia. A painless ulcer that grows quickly suggests primary or tertiary syphilis.

Multiple ulcers in an ill patient suggests erythema multiforme (look for target lesions on the arms), herpes zoster (unilateral on the anterior two-thirds of the tongue), leukemia (multiple small ulcers), Behcet's disease (look for genital ulcers) or secondary syphilis (irregular, serpiginous ulcers with lymphadenopathy).

Multiple oral ulcers in a well appearing

person suggests pemphigus vulgaris, bullous pemphigoid (large tense bullae on body), lichen planus (look for Wickham's striae), or discoid lupus (often with scaly plaques on the face).

White plaques on the oral mucosa suggest candidiasis (painful red base), lichen planus (look for Wickham's straie), leukoplakia (thick, adherent plaque), or trauma from cheek biting (where teeth oppose).

The Elderly Person with an Erythematous Rash Over the Trunk and Extremities

An acute transitory erythematous rash suggests urticaria.

An acute, bright red rash that becomes confluent suggests drug reaction or enterovirus (Cocksackie or Echo) infection. If the patient is febrile, with a red or purple rash that becomes confluent, and develops red palms and soles, stomatitis and lymphadenopathy, then consider Kawasaki's disease. If the febrile patient with sore throat and abdominal pain develops desquamation of the skin over the hands and feet and anterior cervical lymphadenopathy, then consider scarlet fever.

A diffuse macular-papular rash over most of the body (75%–80%) suggests erythroderma. The patient may complain of feeling chilled and the skin feels warm to the touch. Look for medication effect or occult malignancy (lymphoma or carcinoma). If less than 75% of the skin is involved and the skin is painful and shears off, then consider toxic epidermal necrolysis or staphylococcal scalded-skin syndrome. If the skin is normal-appearing but red with distinct papules, then consider toxic erythema from medications.

An erythematous nodule that rapidly increases in size and bleeds easily, but is non-tender, suggests pyogenic granuloma. A painful, rapid-growing nodule suggests a carbuncle or infected epidermoid cyst.

Erythematous pustules suggest pustular psoriasis (patient looks unwell and the pustules are on scaly, red skin), folliculitis (should involve hair follicles and is often seen on the legs or buttocks, scattered between areas of completely normal appearing skin), or disseminated herpes zoster infection (pustules on the face and trunk that develop crusts).

Pruritic papules along the fingers, wrists or beltline suggest scabies.

Scattered papules with defined individual lesions can sometimes be determined by the color. One or a few scattered, chronic, cherry-red lesions suggests a cherry angioma (Campbell de Morgan spot). Red lesions with a central capillary and extending vessels that disappear when they are pressed suggest a spider angioma. Firm, purple, rounded lesions suggest sarcoidosis, lymphoma, Kaposi's sarcoma, or metastatic cancer. Flat, purple lesions with lacy, white strands (Wickham's striae) suggest lichen planus. Some pink-colored lesions can be due to insect bites.

A large (greater than a centimeter), round lesion with pale papules in a circle suggests granuloma annulare. Expanding, migrating lesions that change shape, with central clearing, suggests annular erythema. Circular lesions with multicolored rings (target lesions) suggest erythema multiforme. An expanding fixed lesion can also be due to Lyme disease (erythema migrans). Large lesions with scales or crusts and involvement of the skin between the lesions can be due to eczema. A large nodule or plaque also suggests basal cell carcinoma, lymphoma, leukemia, or metastatic cancer.

Chronic, large, scaly plaques can reflect eczema or lichen simplex if they are extremely pruritic. Non-pruritic plaques with a rolled border suggest a basal cell carcinoma. If the border is well-defined, consider psoriasis, Bowen's disease, solar keratoses (feels like sandpaper) or dermatophyte infection (tinea versicolor). If there is a larger herald patch, consider pityriasis rosea, but also think about secondary syphilis if the patient is ill or has lymphadenopathy.

Chronic blisters or bullae that are tense suggest bullous pemphigoid. If the oral mucosa is involved and the bullae are shallow, then think of pemphigus vulgaris (Nikolsky sign positive).

The Elderly Person with an Erythematous Rash Over Intertrigenous Areas

A bright red, non-scaling rash with satellite papules that involves the scrotum or labia suggests candida infection. A bright red, well-defined rash superimposed on opposing skin surfaces suggests intertrigo. If there is psoriasis in other locations, also consider psoriatic rash, especially along the gluteal crease.

A pink rash with scaling along the margin suggests tinea cruris. (This tends to spare the scrotum or labia.) Also look for maceration between the toes for tinea pedis. A pink rash with an indistinct margin suggests eczema.

A scaly, orange-tan rash in the axilla suggests erythrasma. (It will fluoresce pink under a Wood's light.)

Painful, red nodules suggest a boil. Multiple lesions with sinuses suggest hidradenitis suppurtiva.

The Elderly Person with an Erythematous Rash Over the Lower Extremities

Rapidly progressing erythema with swelling and pain suggests cellulitis. Erythema and large vesicles or bullae in a febrile patient suggest erysipelas.

Red, clustered lesions suggest insect bites, contact allergy, or leukocytoclastic vasculitis (palpable purpura).

Painful, red nodules lasting about a week may be erythema nodosum. Similar-appearing lesions that last for several months are more characteristic of vasculitis or panniculitis.

A well-defined plaque with a hyperpigmented border, telangiectasia and central yellow color suggests necrobiosis lipoidica diabeticorum. A pale pink, homogeneous plaque suggests granuloma annulare. A large red

plaque over the knee with lots of scaling suggests psoriasis. (There should be other psoriatic plaques.) A single plaque with scaling can be a sign of Bowen's disease (basal cell carcinoma).

Other conditions causing leg plaques include lichen planus (thick and purple with white lacy striae), lichen simplex (pruritic and usually on the lateral ankle), or eczema (associated with varicose veins or dry skin).

The Elderly Person with a Lower Extremity Ulcer

Lower extremity ulcers are often due to underlying vascular or neurological disease. If the pulses and basic sensation are intact, and if there are associated varicose veins and hyperpigmentation, then consider venous stasis ulceration. If there are absent pulses, with signs of vascular insufficiency, then an ulcer over the tibia is likely to be due to arterial insufficiency. If the patient has diabetes mellitus and a callus over a painless ulcer, then consider a neuropathic, diabetic ulcer.

Slow growing nodules or ulcers surrounded by normal skin can be signs of malignancy, including squamous cell carcinoma, malignant melanoma, basal cell carcinoma, or metastatic cancer. Other conditions to consider include pyoderma gangrenosum (undermined edge and purple border) and arteriovenous fistula. (Feel for a thrill and listen for a bruit.)

Ulcers within a rash suggest vasculitis, radiation damage (look for atrophy and telangiectasias), necrotizing fasciitis (ill patient with pain disproportionate to the lesion), or necrobiosis lipoidica diabeticorum (yellow center with telangiectasias).

The Elderly Person with Pigmented Lesions Over the Lower Extremities

Palpable purpura suggests leukocytoclastic vasculitis (a hypersensitivity vasculitis sometimes associated with drug reaction, Hepatitis C, and collagen vascular disease).

Purpura involving the lower extremity can also be a sign of thrombocytopenic purpura. (Check for purpura elsewhere, renal and neurological manifestations and schistocytes on the peripheral blood smear.)

Rust-colored pigmentation can be a post-inflammatory change or due to venous stasis with hemosiderin deposition.

Multiple, round, hypopigmented lesions suggest guttate hypomelanosis.

The Elderly Person with Pigmented Lesions Over the Trunk

Irregular, hyperpigmented, raised lesions that resemble mud stuck on a stucco wall are seborrheic keratoses. If the patient is fair skinned, and the lesions are on sun-exposed skin and feel like sandpaper, consider solar keratosis.

A large macular lesion that is stable in size may be a lentigo. If the macular lesion is growing and has an irregular border, consider lentigo maligna. If the lesion is palpable, then consider a superficial spreading melanoma.

Multiple, tan-colored, superficial lesions with a scale when scratched suggest tinea versicolor.

Dark, velvety, pruritic patches around the posterior neck, axillary fold, or groin suggest acanthosis nigricans. (Look for an internal malignancy in a non-obese patient.) Obese patients can develop acanthosis nigricans as part of an insulin-resistance syndrome.

Small papules with a black center suggest giant comedone.

A slowly growing pigmented lesion can be a malignant melanoma or a pigmented basal cell carcinoma. (All suspicious or uncertain lesions should be referred to a specialist for possible biopsy.)

A large volcano-like horn that appears over a few months could be a keratoacanthoma. A slower growing horn with an ulcer in a sun-exposed location suggests a squamous cell carcinoma.

The Elderly Person with Hypopigmented Lesions Over the Trunk

Normal-appearing skin with an irregular hypopigmented border suggests vitiligo. A hypopigmented area in the site of previous inflammation or injury can be post-inflammatory hypopigmentation.

Hypopigmented macules that produce a scale with scratching suggest tinea versicolor.

A hypopigmented area with shiny, wrinkled, atrophic skin and genital lesions suggests lichen sclerosus et atrophicus.

Pendunculated skin-colored lesions around the neck or axilla suggest skin tags (acrochordons).

The Elderly Person with a Rash on the Arms and Hands

A single nodule on the hand suggests a paronychia (if along a nail fold), a pyogenic granuloma (bright red and friable), orf (if a sheep farmer), or a staphylococcal abscess.

Target lesions suggest erythema multiforme.

Linear purple lesions along the fingers, with ivory plaques over the knuckles (Gottren's papules) suggest dermatomyositis.

Pruritic papules after sun exposure suggest polymorphic light eruption.

Small pruritic vesicles along the fingers suggest eczema.

A single papule producing a depression in the fingernail is most likely a mucous cyst.

Plaques over the hands suggest eczema, solar keratoses (feels like sandpaper), psoriasis (lots of scales) or scabies (check between the fingers)

An erythematous, scaly rash near a ring or piece of metal jewelry suggests contact eczema (possibly nickel sensitivity).

Table 25.1. Additional dermatological pearls

Sign	Manifestation
Asboc-Hansen	Purpura and petechiae on brown macules suggesting urticaria pigmentosa
Borsieri's	Presence of a white line that turns bright red when the fingernail is lightly stroked over the skin suggesting scarlet fever
Charcot-Vigouroux	Decreased electrical skin resistance in hyperthyroidism
Darier's	Producing urticaria and severe itching on rubbing the skin suggesting urticaria pigmentosa
Fitzpatrick's	Dimpling of a dermatofibroma on pinching
Grisolle's	Papule of smallpox can be felt through stretched skin
Hess's	Fragile capillary bleeding in scurvy
Leser-Trelat	Sudden appearance of seborrheic keratoses, telangiectases, or pigmented, warty lesions suggesting internal malignancy
Magnan's	Sensation of grit under the skin that changes location suggesting cocaine addiction
Meyer's	Sense of insects crawling on the skin when the hands are soaked in cold water suggesting scarlet fever
Nikolsky's	Rubbing the skin and producing a bulla suggesting pemphigus vulgaris
Osler's	Small, painful, red nodules on the palms and soles suggesting bacterial endocarditis
Peau d'Orange	Skin overlying a tumor resembles an orange peel when pinched
Sergent's	Lymphatic obstruction is suggested when the scratched skin does not redden
Verco's	Striae or punctate hemorrhages under the fingernails in erythema nodosum

A unilateral, red, scaly rash on the dorsum or palm of the hand suggests tinea manuum.

Palmar vesicles and target lesions suggest erythema multiforme.

Palmar hyperkeratosis suggests psoriasis, eczema, arsenic poisoning (look for Mee's lines on the fingernails) or tylosis (look for GI malignancy).

White, hard nodules with a salmon discoloration are likely to be gouty tophi or calcinosis cutis.

Rough nodules on the hands can be warts, solar keratoses (feels like sandpaper), callosities, squamous cell carcinoma (sun-exposed location and ulcerated base), or keratoacanthoma (growth over a few months, with a volcano shape).

The Elderly Person with a Rash on the Feet

A rash on the dorsum of the foot is usually due to eczema, tinea pedis, or bacterial superinfection.

A rash on the instep of one foot suggests tinea pedis (if bilateral, also consider tinea rubrum and eczema).

Hyperkeratosis of the soles suggests tylosis (look for GI malignancy), psoriasis, or eczema.

A rash between the toes can be due to tinea pedis, candida, eczema, psoriasis, or erythrasma.

Useful References

As mentioned in the preface, this book is not an evidence-based review of the literature on geriatric physical diagnosis. Rather it is a handbook of my general approach to the examination of an older person. Specific references have not been given because my intention was to give the learner a feel for the examination. However, no originality is claimed for any of the material. Many of the signs were transmitted to me orally during my medical education as part of a culture of bedside-teaching rounds. Nonetheless, a number of useful references have strongly informed my bedside skills. Some are true classics and all are worthy of the student's attention.

Sapira, Joseph D. *The Art and Science of Bedside Diagnosis*. Baltimore: Urban & Schwarzenberg, 1990. An extraordinary textbook that has an educational density unmatched by other works. It is sometimes challenging to get a clear image from the text how a particular technique is performed. For older clinicians it has the nostalgia of bedside-teaching rounds back in the days when physical diagnosis was considered a cornerstone of medical teaching. A modern classic and deliberately placed at the head of this otherwise alphabetical list.

Adams, F. Dennette. *Physical Diagnosis*, 14th edition. Baltimore: Williams and Wilkins, 1961. An updated version of Cabot's classic, with enough new information to warrant a careful examination.

Bailey, Hamilton. *Demonstrations of Physical Signs in Clinical Surgery*, 13th edition. Baltimore: Williams & Wilkins, 1960. A classic. Any edition is worth reading but this one is probably the best.

Beaven, D.W., and **S.E. Brooks.** *A Colour Atlas of the Nail in Clinical Diagnosis*. London: Wolfe Medical Books, 1984. A useful reference on nail changes in various medical diseases.

Berg, Dale. *Advanced Clinical Skills*, 2nd edition. Malden, MA: Blackwell-Science, 2004. An excellent modern handbook, especially strong on the musculoskeletal examination.

Bickley, Lynn S., and **Peter G. Szilagyi.** *Bates' Guide to the Physical Examination and History Taking*, 8th edition. Philadelphia: Lippincott, Williams and Wilkins, 2003. The most recent edition of a comprehensive text loaded with illustrations of common findings on physical examination.

Cabot, Richard C. *Physical Diagnosis*, 11th edition. Baltimore: William Wood, 1934. Another classic that systematically presents physical diagnosis with numerous pearls relevant to the diseases of the day, including tuberculosis, syphilis and advanced infectious disease complications.

Cope, Zachary, and **William Silen.** *Cope's Early Diagnosis of the Acute Abdomen*, 15th edition. New York: Oxford University Press, 1979. Another classic with essential information on the abdominal examination.

De Berker, David, R. Baran, and **R.P.R. Dawber.** *Handbook of Diseases of the Nails and Their Management.* Cambridge, MA: Blackwell Science, 1995. An excellent atlas of nail changes in systemic and local disease.

DeGowin, Elmer Louis, and **Richard L. DeGowin.** *Bedside Diagnostic Examination*, 2nd edition. London: Macmillan, 1969. A comprehensive handbook with hundreds of useful illustrations by the senior author. His skill and clarity inspired me to add line drawings to this book.

Fitzgerald, Faith T., and **Lawrence M. Tierney Jr.** "The bedside Sherlock Holmes." *Western Journal of Medicine* 137 No. 2 (August 1982) 169–175. Not a book but an amazing article that inspired my clinical observations and formed the basis of Chapter 3.

Hadler, Nortin M. *Medical Management of the Regional Musculoskeletal Diseases.* Orlando: Grune & Stratten, 1984. A comprehensive review of musculoskeletal illness with careful original thinking and critique of the clinical literature. Excellent clinical advice.

Lindsay, Kenneth W., Ian Bone, and **Robin Callander.** *Neurology and Neurosurgery Illustrated*, 2nd edition. Edinburgh: Churchill Livingstone, 1991. A useful book with a wealth of illustrations that clarify many neurological conditions and examination techniques.

Major, Ralph Hermon, Mahlon H. Delp, and **Robert T. Manning.** *Major's Physical Diagnosis*, 8th edition. Philadelphia: Saunders, 1975. An easily readable classic in the style of Cabot and Adams. Excellent initial chapter on the history of the physical examination.

Patten, John. *Neurological Differential Diagnosis*, 2nd edition. New York: Springer, 1995. Another gem with inspiring, unique illustrations by the author. Several of the illustrations served as inspirations for my figures. The text uses a case-based approach that is helpful and interesting. A very useful neurological text for the non-neurologist.

Reilly, Brendan M. *Practical Strategies in Outpatient Medicine.* Philadelphia: Saunders, 1984. An extraordinary book that uses a case-based approach to teach how an expert clinician uses physical diagnosis and skillful reasoning. Very useful chapters on a number of common conditions such as shoulder pain, low back pain, knee pain, office gynecology and dizziness. Several of the illustrations inspired my figures.

Stevenson, Ian. *Medical history-taking.* New York: Hoeber, 1960. A rare book that provides a holistic approach to taking the history. The author shares a wealth of practical advice that includes observations to make during the interview.

Index

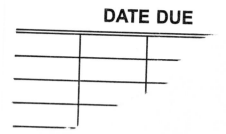

DATE DUE